# Essentials in Total Knee Arthroplasty

# Essentials in Total Knee Arthroplasty

*Edited by*

*Javad Parvizi, MD*
*Rothman Institute*
*Department of Orthopedic Surgery*
*Thomas Jefferson University*
*Philadelphia, Pennsylvania*

*Brian A. Klatt, MD*
*Assistant Professor*
*Department of Orthopedic Surgery*
*University of Pittsburgh Physicians*
*Pittsburgh, Pennsylvania*

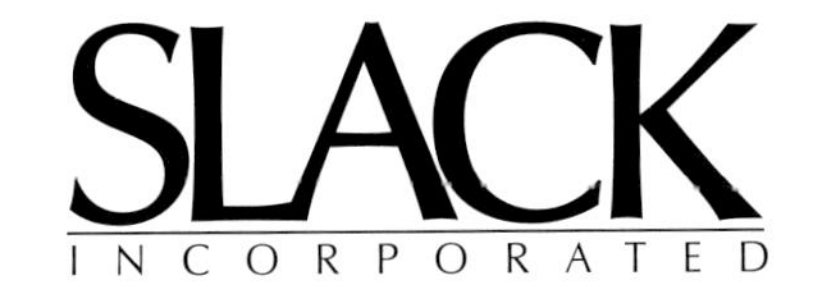

**www.slackbooks.com**

ISBN: 978-1-55642-851-7



The procedures and practices described in this book should be implemented in a manner consistent with the professional standards set for the circumstances that apply in each specific situation. Every effort has been made to confirm the accuracy of the information presented and to correctly relate generally accepted practices. The authors, editor, and publisher cannot accept responsibility for errors or exclusions or for the outcome of the material presented herein. There is no expressed or implied warranty of this book or information imparted by it. Care has been taken to ensure that drug selection and dosages are in accordance with currently accepted/recommended practice. Due to continuing research, changes in government policy and regulations, and various effects of drug reactions and interactions, it is recommended that the reader carefully review all materials and literature provided for each drug, especially those that are new or not frequently used. Any review or mention of specific companies or products is not intended as an endorsement by the author or publisher.

SLACK Incorporated uses a review process to evaluate submitted material. Prior to publication, educators or clinicians provide important feedback on the content that we publish. We welcome feedback on this work.

Published by: SLACK Incorporated
6900 Grove Road
Thorofare, NJ 08086 USA
Telephone: 856-848-1000
Fax: 856-853-5991
www.slackbooks.com



Contact SLACK Incorporated for more information about other books in this field or about the availability of our books from distributors outside the United States.

Library of Congress Cataloging-in-Publication Data

Essentials in total knee arthroplasty / edited by Javad Parvizi, Brian A. Klatt.
p. ; cm.
Includes bibliographical references and index.
ISBN 978-1-55642-851-7 (alk. paper)
1. Total knee replacement. I. Parvizi, Javad. II. Klatt, Brian A.
[DNLM: 1. Arthroplasty, Replacement, Knee--methods. 2. Arthroplasty, Replacement, Knee--adverse effects. 3. Knee--surgery. WE 870 E78 2011]
RD561.E87 2011
617.5'820592--dc22

2010023417



Last digit is print number: 10 9 8 7 6 5 4 3 2 1

# Dedication

To my students, residents, and fellows who enlighten and inspire me. — *JP*

# Contents

*Dedication* ... v
*Acknowledgments* ... ix
*About the Editors* ... ix
*Contributing Authors* ... xi
*Preface* ... xv
*Foreword* by Richard H. Rothman, MD, PhD ... xvii

Chapter 1 Applied Anatomy of Total Knee Arthroplasty ... 1
*Arjun Saxena, MD; Sarah Lombardo, MD; and Javad Parvizi, MD*

Chapter 2 Knee Biomechanics and Biomaterials ... 9
*Nitin Goyal, MD and William Hozack, MD*

Chapter 3 Arthritides ... 19
*Bruce Hopper, MD*

Chapter 4 Nonsurgical Alternatives/Conservative Management ... 23
*Peter C. Vitanzo Jr, MD and Barry E. Kenneally, MD*

Chapter 5 Surgical Alternatives to Total Knee Arthroplasty ... 33
*Hany Bedair, MD and David Backstein, MD, MEd, FRCSC*

Chapter 6 The History of Modern Total Knee Arthroplasty ... 43
*Jennifer K. Bow, MD, FRCSC and Javad Parvizi, MD*

Chapter 7 Indications for Total Knee Arthroplasty ... 55
*Harvey E. Smith, MD and Craig J. Della Valle, MD*

Chapter 8 Preoperative Patient Evaluation for Total Knee Arthroplasty ... 61
*Benjamin Bender, MD; Ashok L. Gowda, BS; and Javad Parvizi, MD*

Chapter 9 Surgical Approaches to Total Knee Arthroplasty ... 65
*Gregg R. Klein, MD and Mark A. Hartzband, MD*

Chapter 10 Operating Room Set-Up ... 73
*Manny Porat, MD and William Hozack, MD*

Chapter 11 Surgical Principles of Total Knee Arthroplasty ... 79
*Gregory K. Deirmengian, MD and Carl A. Deirmengian, MD*

Chapter 12 Avoiding and Overcoming Your Nightmares ... 91
*Michael R. Pagnotto, MD and Brian A. Klatt, MD*

Chapter 13 Postoperative Analgesia Options for the Total Knee Arthroplasty Patient ........ 101
*Eric Schwenk, MD; Kishor Gandhi, MD MPH; and Eugene R. Viscusi, MD*

Chapter 14 Controversies in Total Knee Arthroplasty ........ 109
*James J. Purtill, MD and Khalid A. Azzam, MD*

Chapter 15 Early Failure in Primary Total Knee Arthroplasty ........ 121
*William V. Arnold, MD, PhD*

Chapter 16 Mechanisms of Failure in Total Knee Arthroplasty ........ 129
*Peter F. Sharkey, MD and Omar Abdul-Hadi, MD*

Chapter 17 Patella Fracture Following Total Knee Arthroplasty ........ 141
*Alvin Ong, MD*

Chapter 18 Periprosthetic Fractures in Total Knee Arthroplasty ........ 151
*Garen Daxton Steele, MD and Brian A. Klatt, MD*

Chapter 19 Total Knee Infection ........ 161
*Michael Williamson, MD and Javad Parvizi, MD*

Chapter 20 Aseptic Loosening ........ 167
*Zachary Post, MD*

Chapter 21 Complex Primary Total Knee Arthroplasty ........ 175
*Benjamin Bender, MD; Luis Pulido, MD; and Javad Parvizi, MD*

Chapter 22 Total Knee Arthroplasty Revision ........ 187
*Matthew S. Austin, MD and Eric L. Grossman, MD*

Chapter 23 Total Knee Arthroplasty Rehabilitation ........ 201
*Catherine J. Fedorka, MD; Katie O'Shea, PT, DPT, MBA; Kristen Vogl, PT, DPT; and Kristen Huber, PT, MSPT*

*Financial Disclosures ........ 209*

*Index ........ 211*

## About the Editors

*Javad Parvizi, MD* completed his medical training in the United Kingdom, graduating from University of Sheffield in 1991. He then completed his surgical training at the Mayo Clinic in Rochester, MN, where he also attained a master's degree from the Mayo Foundation in Molecular Biology involving evaluating bone healing and cartilage repair, which sparked his interest in both basic science and clinical research in the field of orthopedics. His fellowship training was completed under the direction of Professor Reinhold Ganz at Inselspital, Bern, Switzerland. Dr. Parvizi is currently a Professor of Orthopedic Surgery at Rothman Institute and Thomas Jefferson University in Philadelphia, PA. He also is the director of clinical research and a member of the education committee. His dedication to education encompasses a number of activities including publication of numerous books and book chapters, and over 240 peer-reviewed publications.

Dr. Parvizi's desire to provide succinct, accurate, and relevant information was the impetus behind this book.

*Brian A. Klatt, MD* graduated from the University of Pittsburgh School of Medicine in 1997. After completing his orthopedic surgery residency at the University of Pittsburgh, he served 4 years on active duty with the United States Air Force. The final 2 years in the military were spent working with the residency program at Wilford Hall Medical Center, and it was there that his commitment to education was solidified. After an honorable discharge from the military, Dr. Klatt completed a fellowship in adult reconstruction at the Rothman Institute, Thomas Jefferson University in Philadelphia. His decision to attend a fellowship at the Rothman Institute was a direct result of meeting Dr. Rothman at a lecture in San Antonio. Dr. Klatt has been lucky to be mentored by many of the great names in orthopedic surgery today. He is currently an Assistant Professor of Orthopedic Surgery at the University of Pittsburgh. Dr. Klatt returned to the University of Pittsburgh, where he continues to dedicate himself to the education of medical students and residents. His research interests are varied and encompass both clinical and basic science topics. He was honored to work with Dr. Parvizi in producing this text. Dr. Klatt hopes that this book will provide a quick and easy source for residents who seek to understand the essential information required to master total knee arthroplasty.

# Contributing Authors

*Omar Abdul-Hadi, MD (Chapter 16)*
Southern Oregon Orthopedics
Medford, Oregon

*William V. Arnold, MD, PhD (Chapter 15)*
Department of Orthopedic Surgery
Rothman Institute at Thomas Jefferson University Hospital
Philadelphia, Pennsylvania

*Matthew S. Austin, MD (Chapter 22)*
Assistant Professor
Department of Orthopedic Surgery
Rothman Institute at Thomas Jefferson University Hospital
Philadelphia, Pennsylvania

*Khalid A. Azzam, MD (Chapter 14)*
Joint Reconstructive Research
Rothman Institute at Thomas Jefferson University Hospital
Philadelphia, Pennsylvania

*David Backstein, MD, MEd, FRCSC (Chapter 5)*
Associate Professor of Surgery
Hip and Knee Reconstruction
Mt. Sinai Hospital Toronto
Director, Undergraduate Surgical Education
University of Toronto
Toronto, Ontario, Canada

*Hany Bedair, MD (Chapter 5)*
Instructor
Department of Orthopedic Surgery
Massachusetts General Hospital
Harvard Medical School
Boston, Massachusetts

*Benjamin Bender, MD (Chapters 8, 21)*
Hip and Knee Specialist
Joint Replacement Specialist
Assuta Hospital
Tel-Aviv, Israel

*Jennifer K. Bow, MD, FRCSC (Chapter 6)*
Adult Reconstruction Fellow
Department of Orthopedic Surgery
Rothman Institute at Thomas Jefferson University Hospital
Philadelphia, Pennsylvania

*Carl A. Deirmengian, MD (Chapter 11)*
Clinical Assistant Professor of Orthopedic Surgery
University of Pennsylvania School of Medicine
Philadelphia, Pennsylvania
Director of Comprehensive Arthritis and Joint Replacement Research
Lankenau Institute for Medical Research
Wynnewood, Pennsylvania

*Gregory K. Deirmengian, MD (Chapter 11)*
Assistant Professor
Department of Orthopedic Surgery
Rothman Institute at Thomas Jefferson University Hospital
Philadelphia, Pennsylvania

*Craig J. Della Valle, MD (Chapter 7)*
Associate Professor of Orthopedic Surgery
Director, Adult Reconstructive Fellowship
Rush University Medical Center
Chicago, Illinois

*Catherine J. Fedorka, MD (Chapter 23)*
Orthopedic Surgery Resident
Drexel University College of Medicine
Hahnemann University Hospital
Department of Orthopedic Surgery
Philadelphia, Pennsylvania

*Kishor Gandhi, MD/MPH (Chapter 13)*
Department of Anesthesiology and Acute Pain Management
Thomas Jefferson University Hospital
Philadelphia, Pennsylvania

*Ashok L. Gowda, BS (Chapter 8)*
Valhalla, NY

*Nitin Goyal, MD (Chapter 2)*
Adult Reconstruction Fellow
Rothman Institute at Thomas Jefferson University Hospital
Philadelphia, Pennsylvania

*Eric L. Grossman, MD (Chapter 22)*
Chief Resident
Department of Orthopedic Surgery
Rothman Institute at Thomas Jefferson University Hospital
Philadelphia, Pennsylvania

*Mark A. Hartzband, MD (Chapter 9)*
Hartzband Center for Hip and Knee Replacement
Paramus, New Jersey
Hackensack University Medical Center
Hackensack, New Jersey

*William Hozack, MD (Chapters 2, 10)*
Professor of Orthopedic Surgery
Rothman Institute at Thomas Jefferson University Hospital
Philadelphia, Pennsylvania

*Bruce Hopper, MD (Chapter 3)*
Rothman Institute at Thomas Jefferson University Hospital
Philadelphia, Pennsylvania

*Kristen Huber, PT, MSPT (Chapter 23)*
Department of Rehabilitation Medicine
Thomas Jefferson University Hospital
Philadelphia, Pennsylvania

*Barry E. Kenneally, MD (Chapter 4)*
Sports Medicine Specialist
Rothman Institute
Philadelphia, Pennsylvania

*Gregg R. Klein, MD (Chapter 9)*
Hartzband Center for Hip and Knee Replacement
Paramus, New Jersey
Hackensack University Medical Center
Hackensack, New Jersey

*Sarah Lombardo, MD (Chapter 1)*
Thomas Jefferson University Medical School
Philadelphia, Pennsylvania

*Alvin Ong, MD (Chapter 17)*
Clinical Instructor
Department of Orthopedic Surgery
Thomas Jefferson University Hospital
Philadelphia, Pennsylvania

*Katie O'Shea PT, DPT, MBA (Chapter 23)*
Thomas Jefferson University Hospital
Department of Rehabilitation Medicine
Philadelphia, Pennsylvania

*Michael R. Pagnotto, MD (Chapter 12)*
Fellow, Adult Reconstruction
Mayo Clinic
Rochester, Minnesota

*Manny Porat, MD (Chapter 10)*
Resident
Department of Orthopedic Surgery
Thomas Jefferson University
Philadelphia, Pennsylvania

*Zachary Post, MD (Chapter 20)*
Utah Orthopedics
Ogden, Utah

*Luis Pulido, MD (Chapter 21)*
Rothman Institute at Thomas Jefferson University Hospital
Philadelphia, Pennsylvania

*James J. Purtill, MD (Chapter 14)*
Associate Professor of Orthopedic Surgery
Rothman Institute at Thomas Jefferson University Hospital
Philadelphia, Pennsylvania

*Arjun Saxena, MD (Chapter 1)*
Department of Orthopedic Surgery
Thomas Jefferson University Hospital
Philadelphia, Pennsylvania

*Eric Schwenk, MD (Chapter 13)*
Resident
Department of Anesthesiology and Acute Pain Management
Thomas Jefferson University Hospital
Philadelphia, Pennsylvania

*Peter F. Sharkey, MD (Chapter 16)*
Professor of Orthopedic Surgery
Rothman Institute at Thomas Jefferson University Hospital
Philadelphia, Pennsylvania

*Harvey E. Smith, MD (Chapter 7)*
Methodist Center for Orthopedic Surgery
Houston, Texas

*Garen Daxton Steele, MD (Chapter 18)*
Wilmington Orthopedic Group
Wilmington, North Carolina

*Eugene R. Viscusi, MD (Chapter 13)*
Department of Anesthesiology and Acute Pain Management
Thomas Jefferson University Hospital
Philadelphia, Pennsylvania

*Peter C. Vitanzo Jr, MD (Chapter 4)*
Sports Medicine Specialist
Director, Division of Non-Operative Sports Medicine
Rothman Orthopedic Institute
Philadelphia, Pennsylvania

*Kristen Vogl, PT, DPT (Chapter 23)*
Thomas Jefferson University Hospital
Department of Rehabilitation Medicine
Philadelphia, Pennsylvania

*Michael Williamson, MD (Chapter 19)*
Rothman Institute at Thomas Jefferson University Hospital
Philadelphia, Pennsylvania

# Preface

In today's world of orthopedic surgery, the adult knee is the area operated most frequently. Total knee replacement is the second most commonly performed procedure, directly behind knee arthroscopy. *Essentials in Total Knee Arthroplasty* is a concise text with the information needed to grasp the core principles of this common surgery. The editors created a colorful text that contains a unique look into the world of total knee arthroplasty, including an in-depth history of the procedure and strategies to treat as well as to prevent complications.

The editors have recruited a resident and an attending for each chapter. By capturing the perspective of both resident and staff, the book provides a unique perspective into the facts and issues in total knee replacement. The descriptive text is written in a user-friendly, "easy to read" style and supplemented by full-color visuals.

We believe this will be the "go-to" book for residents and fellows training in orthopedics or related surgical disciplines. We hope you will find the material in this book as valuable as it is intended to be.

# FOREWORD

The concept of reconstruction of the arthritic or damaged knee using total knee arthroplasty has been widely utilized for decades. It has helped to revolutionize not only the specialty of orthopedic surgery, but has also changed the quality of life for elderly patients struck down by incapacity due to knee disease. It has been studied extensively by the orthopedic community and a vast amount of material has been published in peer-reviewed journals to bring the latest knowledge to interested and concerned surgeons. This textbook will serve as a compendium of the latest knowledge, judgment, and information in this area available to scholars.

The authors are notable for their deep fund of knowledge in reconstruction and their interest in clinical research. Without a broad view and judgment, new knowledge is a mixed blessing. In arthroplasty, the failure rate approximates 1% to 2% at the end of 10 years on a mechanical basis. Therefore, innovation brings both potential advantages and potential worsening of outcomes. A broad contextual view and judgment are needed before radical changes are incorporated into clinical practice.

The focus on minimal incisions is a good example of an idea that seems to be an obvious step forward in clinical practice and yet has led to mixed outcomes in a variety of reconstructive centers. This again highlights the need for perspective in terms of time, comparison of studies from many centers, and controlled data. Without this, new information is of little value.

In this monograph, readers are provided with the history and depth of knowledge to place new developments in their proper role. The text is eloquent and well illustrated to help appreciate new technical advances.

The reader is offered a wide scope of knowledge in regard to the various surgical approaches for total knee arthroplasty, as well as enlightened discussion of the indications and contraindications for surgery. Postoperative failures are placed in their proper context to allow better understanding and prevention of these catastrophes. Their treatment is well outlined.

I believe this text will assume its proper position as a classic guide for orthopedic surgeons concerned with reconstruction of the knee.

*Richard H. Rothman, MD, PhD*
*James Edwards Professor*
*Thomas Jefferson University*
*Rothman Institute*
*Philadelphia, Pennsylvania*

1

# Applied Anatomy of Total Knee Arthroplasty

*Arjun Saxena, MD; Sarah Lombardo, MD; and Javad Parvizi, MD*

The knee is a complex hinged joint that allows for movement in multiple directions. The knee is involved in functions such as running, jumping, and changing direction. Movements at the knee joint include flexion and extension, internal and external rotation, translation, and abduction and adduction. This large variety and range of motion is assured by the shallow articular surface shared by the tibia and femur, as well as the mobility of the medial and lateral menisci on the tibial plateau. Conversely, stability is provided in the form of many large, powerful muscles crossing the joint and a strong, fibrous joint capsule coupled with thick band-like ligaments. A great deal of research has been dedicated to the neurovascular, muscular, cartilaginous, and bony anatomy. The various surgical approaches and techniques have been developed through the application of this research. This chapter focuses on the role of anatomy during total knee arthroplasty (TKA).

## Examination

The first aspect of applying anatomy for any surgical procedure comes from the physical exam. During the physical exam of the knee, one has the opportunity to observe the deformities that may cause or be caused by a patient's pathology. Recognizing these deformities preoperatively will allow for proper surgical planning.

In the sagittal plane, a flexion contracture or a hyperextension deformity may exist. A flexion contracture about the knee can be observed by visualization and/or a patient's inability to completely extend the knee. Treating a knee with a flexion contracture may require modification of surgical technique. For a contracture less than 10 degrees, removal of osteophytes and a posterior capsular release may be adequate. A contracture greater than 10 degrees may require a slightly larger distal femoral resection. Conversely, if the knee hyperextends on the preoperative exam, the surgeon needs to be careful to not take more than the minimal distal femur resection. The posterior capsule may need to be left intact so as not to make the knee too loose in extension. A knee that lacks flexion may need a smaller femoral component to help improve motion.

In addition, the nature of the coronal plane deformity about the knee should be noted. The most common deformity is the varus (bow-legged) deformity. A standard approach requires a medial release, but a varus deformity of greater than 10 degrees may necessitate a larger medial release. This involves releasing the deep medial collateral ligament (MCL) off of the proximal tibia and elevating the superficial MCL. A more extensive elevation of the MCL can be done as needed. The pes anserinus expansion can be released on the medial tibia. The 3 muscles that insert at the pes anserinus are the sartorius, semitendinosus, and the gracilis. Also, the posteromedial tibia requires full release in a knee with a large varus deformity; the insertion of the semimembranosus is included in this release. All osteophytes should be removed, and the medial bone can be trimmed to allow better medial balance.

A large valgus (knock-knee) deformity may indicate a need to perform a lateral release. The first structure released



Parvizi J, Klatt B.
*Essentials in Total Knee Arthroplasty* (pp 1-8).

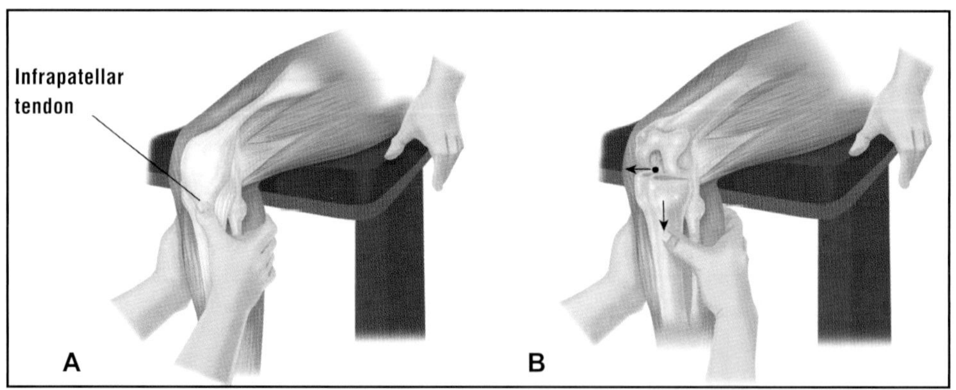


**Figure 1-1.** (A) Palpation of the infrapatellar tendon. (B) Palpation of the infrapatellar tendon and tibial tubercle.

is the iliotibial (IT) band at the knee. For a partial release, the tendon can be pie crusted with a blade. The popliteal tendon is usually released second. It is elevated off of the periosteum on the lateral femoral condyle. A partial release may be all that is needed. The IT band has a greater impact in extension, and the popliteal tendon is more important in flexion. In addition, if the deformity is severe, the lateral collateral ligament may need release off the femoral condyle. As with the medial side, all osteophytes should be resected. Some surgeons accomplish the lateral release by performing a lateral parapatellar approach in the severe valgus knee.

## Bony Architecture/Landmarks

Prior to surgery, palpation of major landmarks about the knee joint is imperative for orientation. The patella is the easiest, most superficial structure to palpate; the patellar ligament may also be felt as it arises from the inferior pole of the patella and inserts on the tibial tuberosity (Figure 1-1). For the medial parapatellar approach, the skin incision should lie just medial to the tibial tubercle. The pes anserinus inserts and infrapatellar bursa lies just inferior to the tubercle (Figure 1-2).

The medial and lateral femoral condyles are of importance because the line connecting them marks the epicondylar axis of the knee (Figure 1-3). These distal aspects of the femur are best palpated with the knee in 90 degrees of flexion or greater.[1] Accurate assessment of the epicondyles is important for surgeons who choose to use the epicondylar axis for aligning femoral rotation.

## Nerves

A longitudinal incision made on the medial aspect of the knee will reveal the infrapatellar branch of the saphenous nerve running transversely across the operative field (Figure 1-4). This small nerve is sacrificed to gain access to the joint capsule and, consequently, patients can expect some degree of numbness on the lateral aspect of the knee postoperatively.[2] The blunt end of the severed nerve should be buried in fat to prevent formation of a painful neuroma. However, due to contributions from branches of the obturator nerve, much of the sensory innervation to the skin at the knee joint is preserved.

The saphenous nerve, which appears in this plane from between the gracilis and sartorius muscles, joins with the saphenous vein to continue its descent along the inferior border of the sartorius. Care should be taken not to injure either structure, as the saphenous nerve provides sensory innervation to medial aspects of the lower leg, while the saphenous vein can be used as a graft in future coronary artery bypass surgeries.

The tibial nerve is the larger of the 2 divisions of the sciatic nerve. It courses through the popliteal fossa, in the posterolateral aspect of the knee just medial to the popliteal artery. It gives off muscular branches to the deep and superficial compartment muscles of the leg before terminating distal to the ankle as the medial and lateral plantar nerves. In addition, the sural nerve, responsible for sensory innervation of the lateral aspect of the foot, arises from the tibial nerve and the common peroneal nerve proximal to the knee joint.

The common peroneal nerve, the smaller of the 2 divisions of the sciatic nerve, courses through the popliteal fossa laterally to the tibial nerve. The nerve runs between the biceps femoris tendon and the lateral head of the gastrocnemius and posterior to the fibular head where it wraps around the lateral aspect of the fibular neck before dividing into a superficial and deep peroneal nerve. The deep peroneal nerve innervates the muscles of the anterior compartment of the leg while the superficial innervates the lateral compartment muscles. Both also function in sensory innervation of the foot. The common peroneal nerve can be affected during TKA when a significant valgus deformity with a flexion

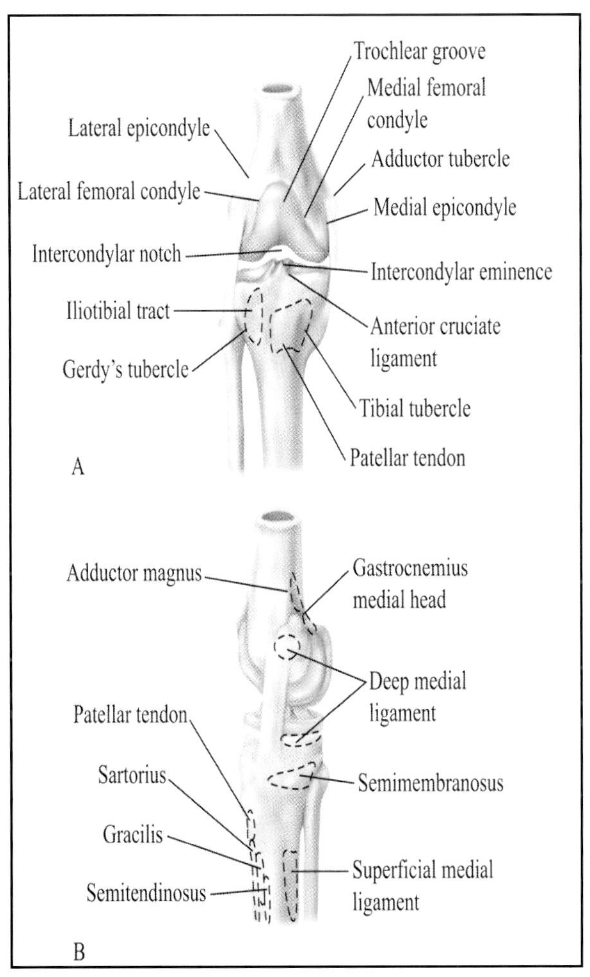


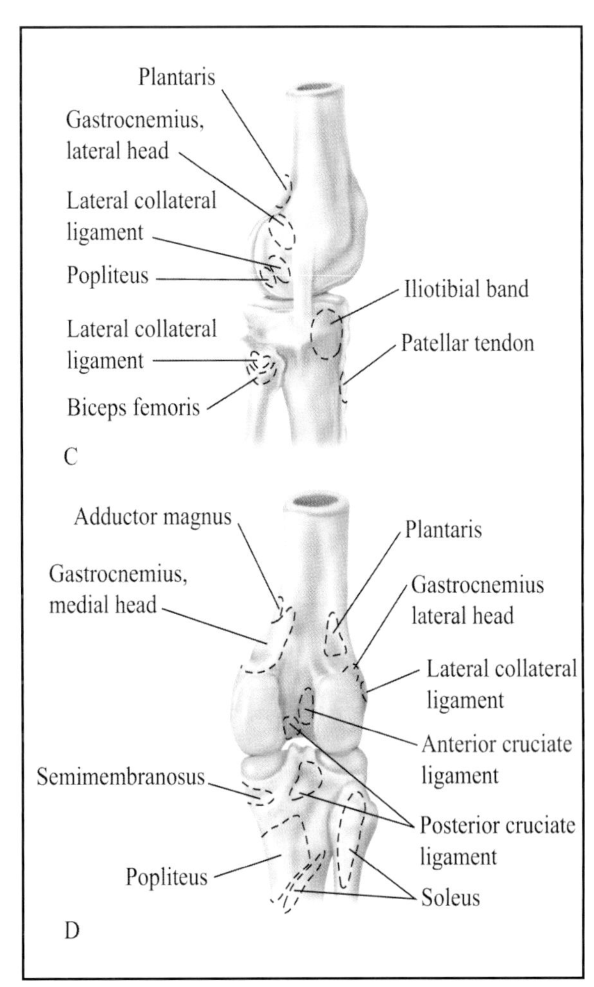


**Figure 1-2.** Bony landmarks with ligament and tendon attachment sites. (A) Anterior aspect, (B) medial aspect, (C) lateral aspect, and (D) posterior aspect.

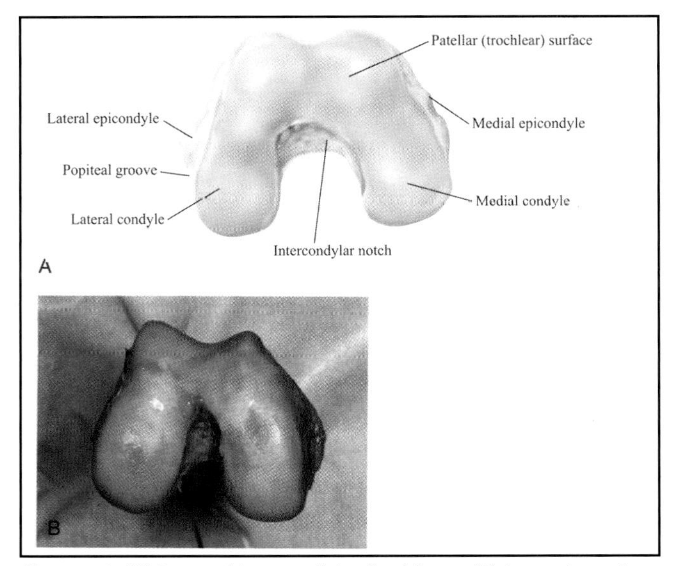


**Figure 1-3.** (A) Bony architecture of the distal femur. (B) Anatomic specimen of the distal femur.

contracture is corrected; this can place the nerve on stretch and lead to a peroneal nerve palsy.[3]

## Blood Supply

Blood supply to the knee is provided by the periarticular genicular anastomoses of approximately 10 small vessels originating from the femoral, popliteal, anterior tibial recurrent, and circumflex fibular arteries (see Figure 1-4). In the anterior knee, these vessels run in the superficial layers and most can be preserved by making a single clean incision to the level of the deep fascia before retracting to enlarge the surgical field.[4] A longitudinal, medially placed incision will likely sacrifice the superior and inferior medial genicular arteries, both of which arise from the popliteal artery to course around the medial femoral epicondyle and medial tibial condyle, respectively. The middle genicular branch of

**Figure 1-4.** Superficial neurovascular structures of the anterior aspect of the knee.

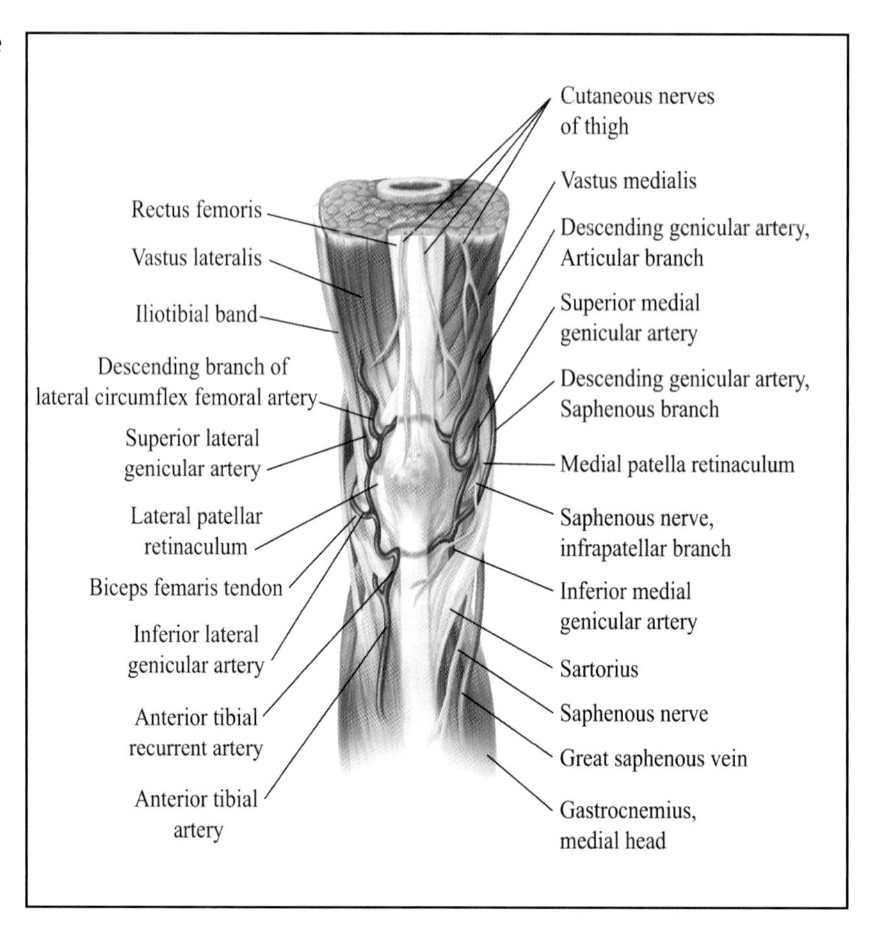


the popliteal artery pierces the joint capsule posteriorly to supply the cruciate ligaments, the synovial membrane, and the menisci.[5] When excising the cruciates, the notch should be inspected and the middle genicular branch should be cauterized. Along the lateral meniscus, a lateral genicular branch is often found that should also be cauterized.

The popliteal artery is located posterolaterally in the knee. The popliteal artery is the sole blood supply to the lower leg. This is especially important when using a retractor to expose the tibial plateau and when dislocating the knee. A section of Chapter 12, Avoiding and Overcoming Your Nightmares is devoted to a description of how to protect the neurovascular structures in the posterior aspect of the knee.

## The Knee Capsule and Surrounding Soft Tissue

The important stabilizing elements of the knee joint lie deep to the superficial layers. Stability depends on the strength and action of the surrounding muscles, as well as contributions from various ligaments connecting the femur and tibia. At this level, the anatomy becomes increasingly complex, because many of the ligamentous stabilizing structures are not easily defined from the underlying joint capsule.

The deep fascia gives rise to the lateral and medial parapatellar retinaculum anteriorly, which blend with the underlying structures to insert along the lateral and medial borders of the patella and on the proximal aspect of the tibial plateau. Investing fascia of the sartorius, gracilis, and semitendinosus also continues posteriorly to contribute to the fascial roof of the popliteal fossa. Traversing the posteromedial aspect of the knee joint, in anterior to posterior order, the sartorius, semitendinosus, and gracilis descend to attach at the pes anserine on the medial surface of the tibia, 4 to 6 cm distal to the tibial plateau. Deep to the retinaculum, the patellofemoral ligaments descend from the medial and lateral femoral epicondyles to insert on the superomedial and superolateral poles of the patella, respectively.

Deep to the distal patella and the patellar tendon is the infrapatellar fat pad. The fat pad may play a role in shock absorption, but the role of the fat pad is controversial. Some consider the fat pad to be a nonessential component of the knee joint that can be excised, and others feel that it should be maintained. Removal of the fat pad improves visibility, but may be accompanied by increased pain postoperatively.[6]

## Musculature About the Knee

During TKA, a portion of the extensor mechanism (ie, quadriceps femoris, quadriceps tendon, and patellar tendon) is sacrificed to gain access to the joint. In addition to knee extension, the quadriceps muscle group is the most important contributor to knee stabilization, so care should be taken to minimize injury to this muscle group. The quadriceps becomes aponeurotic distally to yield the quadriceps tendon, which attaches to the superior pole of the patella. The patellar tendon then descends from the inferior pole to attach at the tibial tuberosity.

The quadriceps muscle group is composed of the rectus femoris, vastus medialis and vastus medialis oblique (VMO), vastus lateralis, and vastus intermedius. These muscles are innervated by the femoral nerve, L2-4. The rectus femoris has a dual origin; the straight head arises from the anterior inferior iliac spine and the reflected head from a groove just above the acetabulum. It forms the superficial, central part of the quadriceps tendon. The main origin of the vastus medialis is the medial lip of the linea aspera of the femur; this muscle forms the lateral wall of the adductor (Hunter's) canal. The vastus lateralis is the largest of the quadriceps muscles; its main origin is the lateral aspect of the linea aspera of the femur. Lastly, the vastus intermedius originates in the anterior and lateral surfaces of the proximal femur and its fibers make up the deep part of the quadriceps tendon.

On the medial aspect, the VMO blends with the superior border of the medial patellofemoral ligament to insert on the superomedial border of the patella.[7] Together these structures limit lateral tracking and lateral subluxation of the patella. Medial tracking and subluxation is kept in check by the actions of the vastus lateralis and lateral patellofemoral ligament. Dislocation of the patella, as necessitated for TKA, requires the disruption of both the parapatellar retinaculum and the patellofemoral ligaments of one side. Depending on the approach and the degree of exposure required, a portion of the VMO attachment may be retained.

The posterior muscles of the knee are often referred to as the hamstrings. This group of muscles consists of the semitendinosus, semimembranosus, and the biceps femoris. These muscles function collectively to flex the knee joint. The semitendinosus, semimembranosus, and biceps femoris long head are innervated by the tibial division of the sciatic nerve, L5, S1-2. The biceps femoris short head is innervated by the common fibular division of the sciatic nerve, L5, S1-2. The semitendinosus is in the posteromedial thigh and arises from the ischial tuberosity. The muscle inserts on the anteromedial aspect of the proximal tibia between the sartorius and the gracilis to complete the pes anserinus. The semimembranosus is also located posteromedially in the thigh and also arises from the ischial tuberosity. Distally, at the level of the knee, the tendon divides into 5 components that all have attachments in the medial aspect of the knee; the main attachment is on the posterior aspect of the medial tibial condyle. The biceps femoris lies in the posterolateral aspect of the thigh. The long head originates from the ischial tuberosity whereas the short head originates from the lateral aspect of the linea aspera of the femur. The tendon inserts on the head of the fibula.

The gastrocnemius is the most superficial muscle in the posterior aspect of the lower leg; it has 2 heads that arise from the medial and lateral condyles of the distal femur. Distally, it forms the calcaneal tendon, which inserts on the calcaneal tuberosity. This muscle's main function is plantar flexion of the foot and it is innervated by the tibial nerve, S1-2.

The popliteus is one of the few muscles in the body that has its insertion proximal to its origin. It originates on the medial tibia posteriorly and inserts on the lateral surface of the lateral femoral epicondyle. The popliteal tendon ascends laterally over the joint capsule, passing between the lateral meniscus and lateral collateral ligament (LCL). Action of the popliteus laterally rotates the femur during full extension, unlocking the knee to permit flexion.

## Collateral Ligaments

Intimately related to the joint capsule, the collateral ligaments contribute to joint stability during full extension by limiting medial and lateral rotation of the tibia. A primary valgus stabilizer, the MCL (tibial collateral) originates at the medial femoral epicondyle and inserts on the medial tibial shaft, just proximal to the pes anserine. It is composed of a deep ligament and a superficial ligament. The deep fibers are a capsular thickening that adheres to the medial meniscus. This intimate connection likely contributes to the frequent concomitant injury of both structures.[5] When performing a medial meniscectomy during TKA, care must be taken to avoid iatrogenic damage to the MCL. As stated in the section on inspection, a varus deformity may require a medial release, which most commonly entails removing osteophytes and releasing the deep MCL.

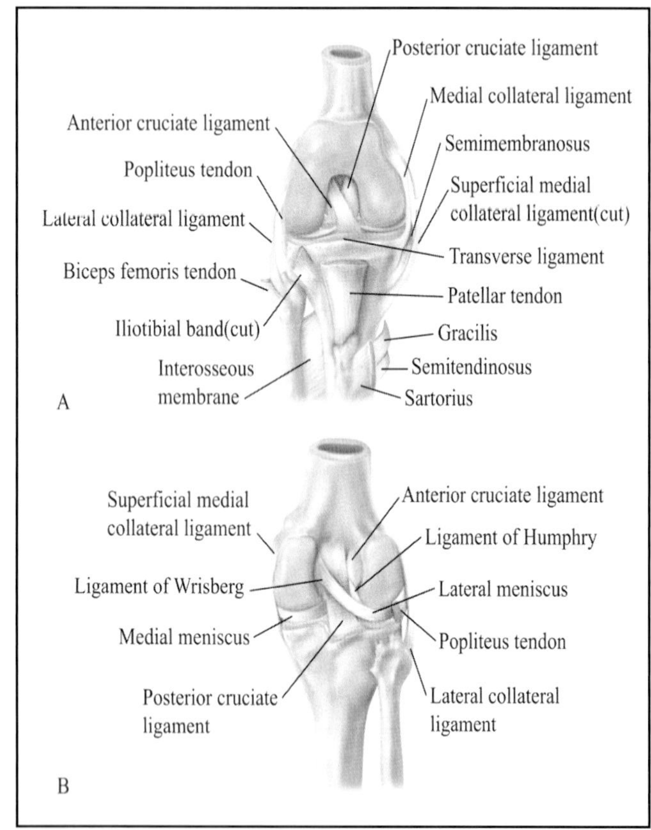


**Figure 1-5.** The ligaments and tendons of the knee from the (A) anterior aspect and (B) posterior aspect.

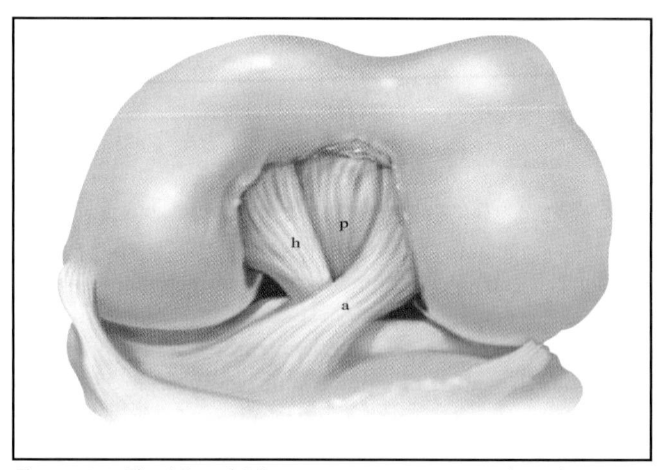


**Figure 1-6.** The ACL and PCL in an anatomic specimen from the anterior aspect.

The LCL is a strong, cord-like band running from the lateral epicondyle of the femur to the blend with the biceps femoris in its attachment to the fibular head. Unlike the MCL, the deep fibers of the LCL do not adhere to the lateral meniscus, instead allowing passage of the popliteal tendon. The LCL is a major varus stabilizer of the knee; in cases with a severe valgus deformity, it may be released as a last resort to correct coronal plane imbalance.

Preservation of both the MCL and the LCL during TKA is possible given their more posterior location along the medial and lateral surfaces of the joint capsule, respectively. The integrity of these ligaments ensures greater joint stability for the mobile patient postoperatively. Injury to either ligament may require a switch to a more constrained prosthesis.

## Cruciate Ligaments

Within the joint capsule, yet excluded from the synovial capsule, lie the anterior and posterior cruciate ligaments (Figures 1-5 and 1-6). Together, these ligaments convert most anterior and posterior rolling motions to spinning motions, with the intercondylar space as the central axis.

The anterior cruciate ligament (ACL) descends from the posteromedial aspect of the lateral femoral notch to attach at the anteromedial intercondylar area of the tibia. The weaker of the 2 intra-articular ligaments, the ACL limits posterior migration of the femur on the tibial plateau during flexion and prevents joint hyperextension and anterior displacement of the tibia. The ACL must be sacrificed in TKA to dislocate the knee and expose the tibial plateau.

Originating on the lateral surface of the anteromedial femoral notch and descending to a posterolateral tibial insertion, the posterior cruciate ligament (PCL) crosses the ACL in the intercondylar space. Individually, the PCL limits anterior rolling of the femoral condyles on the tibial plateau and prevents anterior displacement of the femur and joint hyperflexion. The PCL may be sacrificed or retained during TKA depending on the type of implant that is employed.

## Menisci

The menisci are intra-articular, fibrocartilaginous structures that serve the dual function of deepening the accepting surface of the tibial plateau and acting as shock absorbers (Figures 1-7 and 1-8). The medial meniscus is C shaped, with a broader posterior region tapering to a thin attachment at the anterior tibial border. Its thicker exterior edge is adherent to the joint capsule (specifically deep fibers of the MCL), whereas the interior region is thin and unattached. The lateral meniscus is nearly circular, smaller than the medial meniscus, and more mobile, because it is not fused with the LCL. The exterior edges of both menisci are

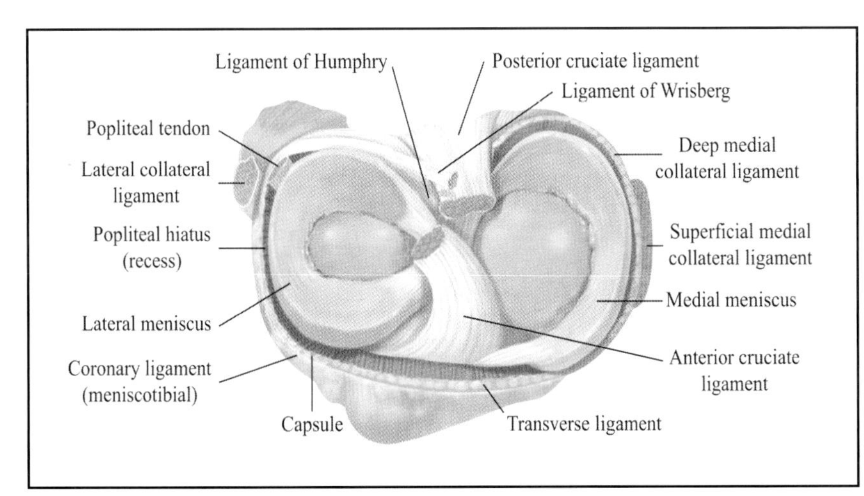


**Figure 1-7.** Drawing of the superior aspect of the tibial plateau.

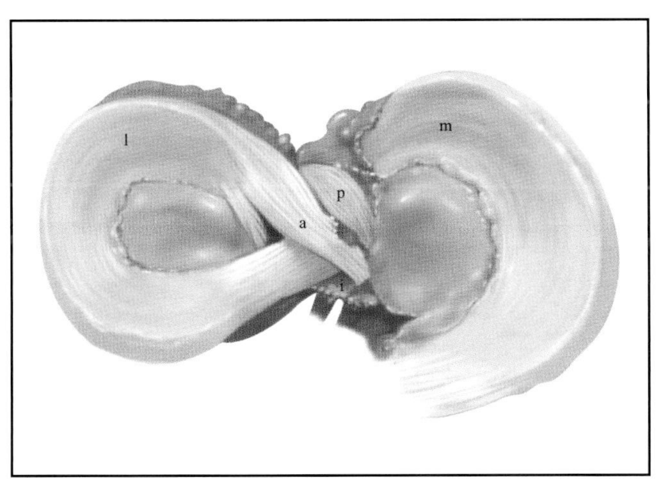


**Figure 1-8.** The superior aspect of the tibial plateau in an anatomic specimen.

attached to the tibial condyles by the coronary ligaments, extensions of the joint capsule. Removal of the menisci and coronary ligaments is necessary before the tibial plateau can be reshaped and fitted for the appropriate TKA prosthesis. Given the intimate relationships of the medial meniscus with the MCL and of the lateral meniscus with the popliteus tendon, care must be taken not to damage these important structures.

## Posterior Aspect

The posterior aspect of the knee joint consists of the posterior joint capsule, the popliteus muscle, and a superficial depressed region containing the neurovascular structures supplying the lower leg. Nestled between the medial and lateral heads of the gastrocnemius inferiorly and the semimembranosus and semitendinosus superiorly, the popliteal fossa houses the popliteal artery and vein, the tibial nerve, the common peroneal nerve, lymph tissue, and varying amounts of fat. As stated previously, the neurovascular structures lie posterior to the medial aspect of the lateral tibial plateau.

In a posterior approach, the popliteal fossa is encountered first, followed by the popliteus. Deeper still, the posterior joint capsule is incomplete to allow passage of a portion of the popliteus to its proximal attachment on the lateral surface of the lateral femoral epicondyle.

## References

1. Hoppenfeld S. *Physical Examination of the Spine and Extremities.* Norwalk, CT: Appleton-Century-Crofts; 1976.
2. Chambers GH. The prepatellar nerve: a cause of suboptimal results in knee arthrotomy. *Clin Orthop Related Res.* 1972;82:157-159.
3. Nercessian OA, Obinwanne, FC, Sangdo P. Peroneal nerve palsy after total knee arthroplasty. *J Arthroplasty.* 2005;20:1068-1073.
4. Haertsch PA. The blood supply to the skin of the leg; a post mortem investigation. *Br J Plast Surg.* 1981;34:470-477.
5. Moore KL, Dalley AF. *Clinically Oriented Anatomy.* 5th ed. New York, NY: Lippincott Williams & Wilkins; 2005.
6. Meneghini RM, Pierson JL, Bagsby D, Berend ME, Ritter MA, Meding JB. The effect of retropatellar fat pad excision on patellar tendon contracture and functional outcomes after total knee arthroplasty. *J Arthroplasty.* 2007;22:47-50.
7. Hoppenfeld S, deBoer P. *Surgical Approaches in Orthopaedics: The Anatomic Approach.* 3rd ed. New York, NY: Lippincott Williams & Wilkins; 2003.

# 2

# Knee Biomechanics and Biomaterials

*Nitin Goyal, MD and William Hozack, MD*

## Biomechanics

An in-depth understanding of normal native knee joint geometric anatomy and biomechanics is vital to the understanding of success in total knee arthroplasty (TKA). The geometry and biomechanics of the knee joint have been extensively researched. In this section, we will discuss the normal geometric anatomy of the knee, the resulting functional and structural properties, and the biomechanics and kinematics of the tibiofemoral and patellofemoral joints. Finally, we will discuss the various biomechanical aspects that shape a successful TKA.

### Geometric Anatomy

The knee joint involves articulation between the femur, proximal tibia, and the patellar portion of the extensor mechanism. The distal femur enlarges approximately 3 times the normal width of the shaft into the medial and lateral condyles. The condyles are rounded articular structures that are joined at the center by the arch of the intercondylar notch.[1,2] The condyles are joined together anteriorly to form the patellofemoral articulation (the patellofemoral groove), while the inferior and posterior rounded aspects of the condyles articulate with the tibial plateau. The intercondylar fossa separates the condyles inferiorly and provides area for the cruciate ligaments. Both medial and lateral condyles have a posterior offset in relation to the femoral shaft, which allows for the tibial rotation that is necessary in deep flexion (> 160 degrees).[2,3] The medial condylar surface is more flat anteriorly and more curved posteriorly than the lateral, whereas the lateral condyle has greater posterior excursion. The femoral portion of the patellofemoral articulation is formed predominantly from the lateral condyle. The articulating surface of the tibia-tibial plateau is formed as the tibia flares out into the medial and lateral condyles. There is a femoral-tibial offset present in the native knee that results in the center of the tibia being lateral and posterior to the center of the femur. The rim of each plateau is lined by the medial and lateral menisci. An intercondylar eminence with 2 tubercles is formed between the 2 articular surfaces of the tibia. These tubercles interlock with the intercondylar notch of the distal femur, imparting stability to medial and lateral shear stresses while preventing hyperextension without limiting flexion. The tibial plateaus and the menisci in combination provide conduits for the femoral condyles that provide stability in flexion and rotation without the problem of joint overconstraint.

### Knee Joint Stabilizers

Functional biomechanics of the knee joint can be evaluated in terms of static and dynamic elements. Static elements that contribute to native knee joint stability are imparted by intrinsic and extrinsic anatomic biomechanical structures. This intrinsic form of stability in the knee joint is created by the bony structures with the described geometry of the articulating surfaces, the capsule, the menisci, and the 4 principal ligaments. The principal bony anatomy described above functions as an innate stabilizer of the joint. Knee motion is further constrained by the cruciate and collateral



Parvizi J, Klatt B.
*Essentials in Total Knee Arthroplasty* (pp 9-18).

ligaments, which act as tensile checkreins, which permit a limited range of motion. The medial and lateral collateral ligaments impart resistance to varus/valgus angulation forces while the anterior and posterior cruciate ligaments bestow stability in the sagittal plane. Extrinsic stability of the knee is provided by the muscular structures of the lower extremity. The muscles of the thigh and calf produce the force to articulate and provide motion of the knee joint, but they also prove invaluable as increased stability to resist abnormal stresses to the extremity. Anterior motion control is through the quadriceps extensor mechanism, posterior control through the hamstrings, and anterior-lateral control by way of the iliotibial complex. In combination, the 3 groups allow for the rotational glide of the tibia over the femoral articulating surfaces. The dynamic elements in stability are the coordinated activity of the muscles that cross the knee joint, which use proprioceptive feedback to optimize the biomechanical function of the joint.

In the native knee joint, the 4 primary ligaments impart significant stability by acting as restraints to translation and rotation. The anterior cruciate ligament (ACL) is the most tensile in full extension, and decreases as the knee flexion decreases to approximately 40 degrees. The ACL is composed of 2 major ligamentous tissue bands, the anteromedial and posterolateral bundles. From 0 to 45 degrees of knee flexion, the posterolateral bundle is the primary restraint to anterior translation of the knee joint. At 45 degrees flexion, the contribution of the posterolateral and the anteromedial bundle as restraints to translation are equivalent. Beyond 45 degrees flexion, the anteromedial bundle is the primary restraint. The posterior cruciate ligament (PCL) primarily resists posterior translation of the tibia on the femur. The PCL is also composed of 2 bundles, the anterolateral and posteromedial, which share the force evenly from extension to 30 degrees flexion. After approximately 30 degrees of knee flexion, the primary force is carried through the anterolateral bundle. ACL force is maximized with anterior translation along with a varus moment and internal rotation, whereas PCL force is maximized with posterior translation with a valgus moment and internal rotation. In essence, the cruciate ligaments ensure anterior/posterior stability while allowing hinge movements of the tibiofemoral joint. The ACL is stretched by extension and helps to limit hyperextension; conversely, the PCL is stretched by flexion.

The medial collateral ligament (MCL) is the dominant restraint to medial opening of the joint, with smaller, variable contributions from the capsule, ACL, and PCL. This is paralleled at the lateral joint, with the lateral collateral ligament (LCL) as the primary restraint to lateral joint space opening, with similar contributions from the ACL/PCL and capsule.

# Functional Mechanics/Kinematics

## Knee Joint Forces

Normal joint loading can be divided into 2 distinct components: the normal compressive force that is applied primarily along the axis of the tibia (and perpendicular to the knee joint) and a shearing force that is applied tangential to the knee joint surface.[4] When walking on level terrain, the principal force is along the axis of the tibia, and the knee can experience a compressive force that is up to 6 times the body weight and shear forces up to twice the body weight.[5] At the toe-off segment of gait, the knee extensors contract to extend the knee and propel the body forward. Those extension forces are applied through the knee joint. Joint forces have been evaluated in the past by several researchers[5-12] through use of experimental methods, modeling, and utilization of the laws of mechanics/kinetics to approximate joint forces. These experimental results are especially vital in the development and implantation of knee prostheses in that implants are subjected through numerous diverse loads and must remain well fixed over time considering the average individual takes over 1,900,000 steps per year.[13] The total joint force for the knee joint equals the vector sum of the forces applied by the quadriceps, hamstrings, and gastrocnemius muscles in addition to the force applied from contact with the ground.

## Tibiofemoral Kinematics

The principal motion of the knee joint is flexion and extension in the sagittal plane. In 1836, Weber described knee motion as a combination of rolling, sliding, and axial rotation at the tibiofemoral joint.[2] With a pure rolling motion alone, the femoral condyle would roll off of the tibial plateau as the knee was flexed more than 100 degrees (as the circumference of the femoral condyle is almost twice the length of the tibial plateau), and with gliding alone, there would be impingement between the tibia and the femoral shaft. During the early phases of flexion, the femur and tibia predominantly undergo a rolling motion, whereas as further flexion occurs, the sliding motion predominates. A combined rolling/sliding motion accommodates for the full range of flexion of the knee joint. Femoral-tibial roll/slide is dependent on a multitude of factors. The ACL and the PCL significantly impact this rolling/sliding motion of the knee in a comparatively passive manner; during flexion while the femur rolls in a posterior direction, the ACL pulls the femur and causes it to slide anteriorly. In parallel, the PCL causes the femoral condyle to slide posteriorly while it rolls in an anterior direction during extension. Additionally, the knee extensors actively produce sliding during knee extension when they pull the tibia anteriorly under the femur, while the knee flexors cause the tibia to glide posteriorly during flexion.

Traditionally, it has been said that both medial and lateral femoral condyles roll/slide back; however, recent magnetic resonance imaging studies have implied that the medial femoral condyle is only able to rotate like a ball in a socket and produce flexion/longitudinal rotation as the medial femoral-tibial articular surfaces have congruency that obstructs any sliding. Conversely, the lateral surface is comparatively flat, which permits the lateral condyle to roll and slide.

Within the arc of active flexion (0 to 120 degrees), the lateral femoral condyle has much more significant posterior translation (15 mm) than the medial condyle (2 mm). The end result of this varied translation is external rotation of the femur of approximately 30 degrees around a medial axis. Axial rotation of the tibia relative to the femur results from numerous force couples. The screwhome mechanism, which is caused by the distinct shapes of the medial and lateral tibial plateaus, and the disparate radii of curvature/lengths of the 2 femoral condyles results in external rotation of the tibia on the femur as the knee is extended from 20 degrees flexion. Additional axial rotation results from the application of the force applied by the musculature and the ground reactive force. The ligaments and capsular structures oppose these rotational forces.

### Patellofemoral Mechanics

The patella lies within the tendinous expansion of the quadriceps femoris muscle and acts as a pulley mechanism, increasing the lever arm of the quadriceps mechanism by increasing the moment arm of the quadriceps muscle force from the center of rotation of the knee joint. Therefore, the patella increases the extension moment that the quadriceps muscle can apply. It is generally recognized that the principal function of the patella is to augment the quadriceps efficiency by increasing the lever arm of the knee extensor mechanism. The Q angle is the angle between the longitudinal axis of the femur, the patella, and the tibial tubercle, and it forms the valgus load at the patellofemoral joint when the quadriceps mechanism contracts. The Q angle has a direct impact on the amount of compressive force at the patellofemoral joint, as does the degree of knee flexion.[14]

Patellofemoral joint reactive forces are consequences of the tension that develops in the quadriceps and patellar tendons during quadriceps contraction. These forces can be more than 0.5 times the body weight for level walking at 9 degrees of knee flexion, more than 3 times the body weight for stair climbing/descending with 60 degrees of knee flexion, and almost 8 times the body weight with deep knee bends.

## Biomechanics of Total Knee Arthroplasty

The principal goals of TKA are to alleviate pain and restore full function at the knee joint. In TKA, the geometry of the implants and the materials from which they are made are crucial. These factors determine the alignment, kinematics, load transmission, wear, and overall performance of the knee joint.

### Stability

The stability of the modern TKA is dependent on many factors: the shape and size of the implant, the location and orientation of the bone cuts, and the tension in the ligaments and muscles around the knee.

At present, most prostheses in primary total knee replacement are semi-constrained. The majority of the native ligaments and muscles are used to provide stability to the TKA. Complex revisions may require fully constrained implants. This is required in situations where the native medial and lateral stabilizers are gone.

The ACL and sometimes PCL are removed during the surgery. These implants must add kinematic features that replace the function of these ligaments to provide joint function. For example, if a semiconstrained implant is used and the PCL is sacrificed, the implant must have a restraint to impede posterior sliding of the tibia on the femur and to provide femoral rollback. This is done with a post mechanism on the tibial polyethylene. This prevents posterior instability and provides femoral rollback as the knee is flexed. As a result of this restraint, however, shearing forces will be transmitted through the implant to the bone-implant interface, which may subsequently result in loosening. Therefore, the shape of the implant itself can impart stability. However, the more constrained the prosthesis, the more significant the amount of force transmitted to the bone-prosthesis interface.

### Kinematics

Most recent TKA implants control knee flexion and extension motion by the design geometry of the implant femoral condyles. Most of the newer implants emulate the anatomical shape of the femoral condyles using 2 radii of curvature: a larger anterior radius for extension and a smaller posterior radius for knee flexion. Attempts to maximize the kinematics of knee flexion have also been affected by one of the larger controversies in total knee replacement—PCL-sparing versus PCL-sacrificing implants. It is argued that PCL-retaining implants have more natural knee kinematics and that the proprioceptive nature of the ligament is preserved; however, studies have shown that appropriately balancing the PCL can be difficult, it often does not stay functional,[15] and proprioceptive capabilities are equal in PCL-sparing versus PCL-sacrificing replacements.[16,17] In PCL-sparing prostheses, it is of utmost importance that the surgeon maintain the anatomic joint line, otherwise the kinematics of the knee joint will be altered secondary to the PCL laxity/rigidity, resulting in larger contact stresses or mechanical wear.

PCL-sacrificing implants exploit a post-and-cam mechanism and a posteriorly positioned equilibrium point to attain posterior translation with knee flexion. The post-and-cam mechanism essentially functions as a substitute for the PCL. The post-and-cam mechanism is specifically designed to reproduce the dynamic progressive rollback function of a native PCL. Downfalls to the PCL-sacrificing implants include a larger bone resection from the intercondylar notch to accommodate the post-and-cam mechanism, as well as the potential wear from impingement of the tibial post with the femoral component.[18,19] Advantages of PCL-sacrificing knees include the surgical technique is easier to perform, minimal tibial resection is possible because the surgeon is not limited to a depth of bone that balances the PCL, and results that have shown through fluoroscopic studies that PCL substitution results in more normal knee kinematics.[20,21]

## Contact Stress Distribution

Contact stress is an important factor that directly affects the long-term success of total joint arthroplasty. Optimal outcomes are obtained when bone at the prosthesis–bone interface is not subjected to loads high enough to cause local mechanical failure at the interface or to diminished stress that can produce stress shielding and bone resorption. When loads become concentrated and the contact area between femoral and tibial components is reduced, there is a substantial increase in the polyethylene wear. The effects of polyethylene wear have been shown to be substantial, causing mechanical or aseptic loosening secondary to wear debris that activates an inflammatory response.

A primary mechanism of wear and loosening is fixation of a prosthesis with a low contact area resulting in large compressive forces through a comparatively smaller portion of the polyethylene to the prosthesis–bone interface. The goal of component fixation therefore is to uniformly distribute the stress at the prosthesis–bone interface by maximizing the contact area. Long-term success after TKA is reliant on optimal distribution of stress at the bone–prosthesis interface.

Generally, a tibial component that is smaller than 6 mm is not used because it is too flexible and is likely to mechanically deform. Additionally, a thicker tibial component will provide for increased distribution of stress at the bone–prosthesis interface. However, as a thicker tibial component is used, there is an increase in the effective lever arm to the shearing forces at the surface, increasing the risk of loosening.

The primary mechanism of failure of a TKA is loosening. There are 2 other chief mechanisms that are responsible for aseptic loosening in addition to the one mentioned above: micromotion at the bone-prosthesis interface and excessive stress. Stress that surpasses the failure limit of the components or the interface will result in micromotion of the components. In 1986, Miegel et al demonstrated that cemented tibial components increased the uniformity of the contact stress distribution as compared to noncemented tibial components.[22] This is likely secondary to biologic factors as bone ingrowth is not uniform, resulting in areas of stress shielding in addition to areas of disproportionately increased stress. Several studies with finite element models[23-25] have argued against the theory that noncemented tibial components have disproportionate distribution of stress. It must be noted, however, that the finite element models assume that there is a precisely level tibial resection, which is not always the case.

The addition of a metal tibial tray beneath the polyethylene provides a stiffer foundation for the polyethylene, therefore resulting in more uniform distribution of stress at the bone-prosthesis interface as shown by Bartel et al.[26] The metal tray reduces the overall compressive stresses and distortion in the underlying cancellous bone. It has been demonstrated by Walker et al that the tibial cortex should be included in the fixation and maximal coverage of the resected surface is optimal for stress distribution.[27] Generally, the stress distribution is proportional, so an increase in the coverage area by 10% will lower the overall stress by 10%.

In addition to the aforementioned factors affecting loosening and motion, it is of utmost importance that precise bone resection, component sizing, and alignment be obtained to anatomically restore the joint line and recreate the anatomical mechanical load vectors. Joint line malposition can potentially change the kinematics around the knee joint, affecting loosening. Additionally, if anatomical alignment is not obtained, the joint reactive forces and load vectors may be shifted and subsequently result in increased stress at the bone–prosthesis interface on the respective side. Finally, proper ligamentous tension is crucial so as to avoid subjecting the components to eccentric loading (if the ligaments are too lax) and increase contact stresses (if the ligaments are too tight).

### Fixation

The mode of fixation in TKA can considerably affect the biomechanics of the knee and eventual success of the prosthesis. The method of fixation must transmit stress to the bone at a degree that is favorable for bone formation. Undue stress will fatigue bone and cause loosening, while stress shielding will result in resorption of bone. The total knee prosthesis can be implanted using either cement or cementless techniques that use screws and/or pegs. Considerable controversy exists over the best method, but it is clear that precise surgical technique in implantation is required regardless of the type of fixation.

## Biomaterials

Ideally, the materials chosen as bearing surfaces for TKA should demonstrate similar friction and wear characteristics to normal knee cartilage. This poses a challenge because biologic tissues remodel in response to stress. Because there is clearly no remodeling potential, the ideal TKA materials must endure the rigorous daily demands of the knee joint with minimal degeneration. TKA materials must demonstrate biocompatibility, a low coefficient of friction, as well as a high resistance to wear. Current knee arthroplasty materials used as bearing surfaces are either metallic or polymeric. The 2 metals most commonly used in TKA are cobalt-chromium and titanium alloy. The polymer that is used is ultra-high molecular weight polyethylene (UHMWPE). Most current prostheses have a metal femoral component articulating with a polyethylene component (tibial and patellar components).

### *Metals*

Metallic alloys have a long track record of use in a variety of orthopedic applications, particularly in joint replacement. Orthopedic prosthesis implants are classically made of cobalt-chromium–based alloys and titanium alloys. These metals are fitting due to their biocompatibility and their innate metallic properties, including their ductility, strength, hardness, and corrosion resistance. These intrinsic properties of the metals allow for surgical use in a variety of situations, including fracture care and on load-bearing surfaces. The properties for each alloy are distinct because each is composed of individual elements, and the subsequent metallic bonds and crystalline microstructure that develops (as the liquid form of the metal cools) forms the properties of each alloy.

There are multiple processes by which the metal implants can be manufactured. Most common orthopedic total joint implants are either cast (ie, metal is melted and poured into a mold) or forged (ie, metal is pressed, under pressure, into a given shape). Forging generally yields components with greater strength than casting because heat working of a material during the forging process refines the grain flow orientation, which imparts predictable strength and reliability at stress points in the material. This type of refinement is not possible in the casting process. Additionally, forgings are dense and free from porosity that may be present in the casting process.

Metal alloys may corrode in vivo by means of galvanic, crevice, stress, and fretting corrosion. Corrosion is a significant molecular/chemical entity when evaluating metals for orthopedic implantation. The high corrosion resistance of cobalt and titanium-based alloys have made them the principal alloys used in implant manufacturing. If corrosion becomes more critical, it can affect the mechanical strength of the implant, and corrosion by-products can be extremely toxic. The high corrosion resistance of the cobalt/titanium alloys is in part due to the protective barriers that form on the surface of the alloys once implanted. These adherent oxide coatings that are formed (self-passivation) are composed of metal oxides that prevent transport of ions across the metal. The characteristics of this film are strictly based on the electrolytic solution in which the metal is placed and the film is composed. This is the reason surface treatments are used to strengthen the film barrier.

#### Cobalt-Chromium

Cobalt-chromium–based alloys are composed of approximately 65% cobalt and approximately 35% chromium. In addition, molybdenum (Mo) is added to improve the mechanical properties. These alloys have a high corrosion resistance that is predominantly due to the chromium content within the metal, which also forms a protective layer on the surface. The Co-Cr-Mo knee arthroplasty implants are generally cast into their final shape; however, forging is becoming more popular to compromise between strength and hardness.

#### Titanium

Titanium-based alloys used in total joint arthroplasty are usually stabilized by small percentages of vanadium and aluminum, and the mechanical properties of these alloys are very dependent on the processing. The main drawback of titanium when used in total joint arthroplasty is the significantly reduced wear resistance and high notch sensitivity as compared to Co-Cr-Mo–based implants. Due to this, titanium alloys are infrequently used as a bearing surface in TKA. They are still frequently used as a material for the base plate in fixed-bearing knees.

### Zirconium

Zirconium (Zr) is a strong transition metal that resembles titanium. It is highly biocompatible due to the spontaneous formation of a passive zirconium oxide film, which protects the metal from further oxidation. Zirconium alloy implants, which contain low levels of nickel, are marketed as an alternative for patients with metal allergies. Metal allergy in knee replacement is a controversial topic, and some claim that the allergy is a result of the nickel in alloys such as cobalt-chromium. Currently, the use of zirconium in knee replacement is limited to the femoral components of one company. The prosthetic femoral components made of zirconium are heated and infused with oxygen to create a ceramic surface on the metal. Oxidized zirconium may be well suited for bearing surface applications because of high levels of wear resistance and hardness (ceramic like). Oxidized zirconium has the advantage of the ceramics in terms of resistance to abrasive scratching, immunity to corrosive roughening, and low friction with less brittleness than the pure ceramic materials. However, ceramics such as zirconium do have lower fracture toughness than metals like cobalt-chromium, making them more brittle. It remains to be shown with long-term data that a ceramic surface is more durable than normal metals. The oxidized layer is microns thick, and long-term durability needs to be studied.

### Tantalum-Based Alloys

Tantalum (Ta) is being used in knee replacement by one company as a material for ingrowth implants. Tantalum implants are fabricated using elemental tantalum metal and vapor deposition techniques onto a carbon frame that create a metallic strut configuration similar to trabecular bone. Porous tantalum has high volumetric porosity (70% to 80%), a low modulus of elasticity, and high frictional characteristics that make it an optimal material for biologic fixation. The low modulus of elasticity may result in more physiologic transfer of loads and a relative increase in preservation of bone stock. Additionally, porous tantalum has been shown to have superior biocompatibility and ingrowth properties. Long-term studies on tantalum implants in knees are needed to determine the value of this technology.

## Polyethylene

UHMWPE is the primary tibial surface for articulation against the femoral component in TKA. Polyethylene is composed of a chain of linked carbon molecules each bonding to 2 hydrogen atoms. The molecular weight, crystalline organization, and thermal history as well as the sterilization methods are critical to forming the mechanical properties of UHMWPE that make it possible for use in total joint arthroplasty. Ultra-high molecular weight polyethylene is defined as having an average molecular weight of more than 3 million g per mol,[28] but the UHMWPE used in total joint implants generally has a molecular weight of 3 to 6 million g per mol.

Sterilization methods for implant use of UHMWPE have been shown to radically affect the mechanical properties of UHMWPE that is implanted. The current methods of sterilization include gamma irradiation, gas plasma, and ethylene oxide. Gamma irradiation in air results in free radicals that form from broken bonds in the polyethylene, which when combined with oxygen can cause chemical reactions that result in fragmentation of long polymer chains. It is well understood that gamma irradiation in air causes this chain scission, cross-linking, and long-term oxidative degradation of the polyethylene material. This can result in significantly reduced mechanical properties, including a reduction in fatigue/fracture strength.[29-32] This can be avoided by gamma irradiation in a vacuum.

In contrast to the negative effect of oxidation, gamma irradiation can prove favorable in respect to some wear properties when it results in cross-linking. Cross-linking is the formation of bonds between adjacent polyethylene molecules. Cross-linking has been shown to make the UHMWPE more resistant to deformation and wear in the plane perpendicular to the molecular axis. However, the mechanical concern with cross-linking in UHMWPE is that it causes a reduction in ultimate tensile strength, a decrease in fracture toughness, and a reduction in fatigue crack propagation resistance.[33,34] Because these properties are especially important mechanical properties of UHMWPE for the application as a bearing surface in TKA (as opposed to total hip arthroplasty), it is not yet clear if the benefits of the cross-linking outweigh the disadvantages. Most of the wear studies done with cross-linked UHMWPE have been in total hip arthroplasty, and the variable stresses of TKA may impact the wear and mechanical failure in a distinct manner. Other methods of sterilization including gas plasma and ethylene oxide do not result in cross-linking.

UHMWPE wear in TKA can be a result of multiple factors. As discussed previously in this chapter, the polyethylene wear increases with contact pressure and the wear is inversely proportional to the contact area. Wear in TKA may result from both abrasive wear and fatigue wear. Fatigue wear occurs in TKA as a result of cyclic contact stress, while abrasive wear is critically influenced by the roughness of the counterface. The counterface surface (the metal bearing) can be significantly increased by oxidative wear and scratching. A single scratch on the counterface can increase the UHMWPE wear rate by a factor of 10. Additionally, care must be taken to clear all bone fragments and polymethylmethacrylate (PMMA) fragments that can damage the articular surface of the UHMWPE. Abrasive materials such as particles of bone or PMMA have been shown to be a cause of scratching of the metal bearing surfaces, resulting in increased surface roughness and subsequent increased UHMWPE wear.[35,36] A scratch on the metal bearing surface results in a trough with a raised area of metal on both sides. This raised area above the rough causes the increase in wear by cutting into the opposite bearing surface. Wear is further influenced by the direction of scratches on the countersurface. A scratch that is transverse to the axis of motion results in significantly more wear than scratches that are longitudinal to the axis of motion.

One cause of loosening of the implant is directly related to the wear particles from the UHMWPE, resulting in a macrophage response. Although any particle in the joint space (UHMWPE, metal debris, ceramic debris, PMMA, bone debris) may cause osteolysis, the debris that is well known to result in an enhanced histiocytic response is UHMWPE, PMMA, cobalt-chromium, and titanium. Due to the fact that the UHMWPE is significantly softer than the other materials and due to the volume of UHMWPE debris generated, it is generally considered as the major source of the osteolysis process. Additionally, the size of the particles involved in osteolysis is very small (0.2 to 7 μm), further implicating the UHMWPE particles. These submicron particles must be ingested by the macrophages, which results in activation of several factors, including TNF-α, interleukin-6, and interleukin-1β that activate the osteoclast system and in combination cause the resorption of bone around the prosthesis. "Backside wear" (ie, unintentional micromotion between the UHMWPE tibial insert and the metal tibial tray) may also be a principal source of wear debris. Manufacturers have attempted to minimize this through better fixation between the 2 modular components; however, it is likely impossible to completely eliminate wear from this interface. Polyethylene thickness is critical in the process of catastrophic wear. The UHMWPE thickness must be at least 8 mm to keep joint contact stresses below the yield strength. In cases in which exceedingly thin UHMWPE inserts are used, the yield strength may be exceeded, leading to rapid failure of the prosthesis.

### Polymethylmethacrylate Bone Cement

The PMMA used in modern orthopedic surgery is a polymer that is usually stored in 2 separate states: separately as a liquid and in powder form. The liquid solution usually contains a methylmethacrylate (MMA) monomer, hydroquinone and dimethyl para-toluidine. The powder solution of PMMA typically contains polymerized PMMA mixed with comonomers of styrene, methyl acrylate, or butyl methacrylate, which adds to the strength of the final product. The powder and liquid solutions are mixed together at the appropriate time in the operation to form the final PMMA product.

Older generation techniques of mixing of the cement in open-air bowls by hand has more recently been supplanted by vacuum mixing and centrifugation, which has helped to reduce the porosity of the PMMA. Additionally, cement pressurization has been found to aid in improving the interface between the PMMA and bone. After pressurization, the cement mantle has increased interdigitation with the surrounding bone, thereby improving the shear strength.

PMMA is an extremely brittle material and the modulus of elasticity is approximately 10 times lower than that of the surrounding cortical bone and more than 100 times lower than that of the metal implant, which allows it to act as an elastic layer between the stiffer layers around it. It has poor tensile and shear strength and is strongest in compression. However, PMMA is still 50% weaker in compression and shear than cortical bone and, when used in load bearing, must be supported by bone to avoid fracture of the cement.

Debris from PMMA may elicit a macrophage response that results in osteolysis. Particle debris from PMMA up to 300 μm in size has been demonstrated to stimulate macrophages in vitro.[37] This macrophage stimulation activates the inflammatory cascade and has been implicated in local bone resorption through the osteoclastic response.

## Summary

A general knowledge of biomechanics and materials in total knee replacement is crucial. The choice of implants must be made by the surgeon. Understanding the geometry, function, and materials in various implants is crucial to determining what is best for the patient.

## REFERENCES


1. Elias SG, Freeman MA, Gokcay EI. A correlative study of the geometry and anatomy of the distal femur. *Clin Orthop.* 1990;260:98-103.
2. Muller W. *Kinematics*. New York, NY: Springer-Verlag; 1938:8-28.
3. Hefzy MS, Kelly BP, Cooke TD. Kinematics of the knee joint in deep flexion: a radiographic assessment. *Med Eng Phys.* 1998;20(4):302-307.
4. Nisell R. Mechanics of the knee: a study of joint and muscle load with clinical applications. *Acta Orthop Scand Suppl.* 1985;216(Suppl. 216):1-42.
5. Seireg A, Arvikar. The prediction of muscular lad sharing and joint forces in the lower extremities during walking. *J Biomech.* 1975;8(2):89-102.
6. Kettelkamp DB, Chao EY. A method for quantitative analysis of medial and lateral compression forces at the knee during standing. *Clin Orthop.* 1972;83:202-213.
7. Mena D, Mansour JM, Simon SR. Analysis and synthesis of human swing leg motion during gait and its clinical applications. *J Biomech.* 1981;14(12):823-832.
8. Mikosz RP, Andriacchi TP, Andersson GB. Model analysis of factors influencing the prediction of muscle forces at the knee. *J Orthop Res.* 1988;6(2):205-214.
9. Minns RJ. Forces at the knee joint: anatomical considerations. *J Biomech.* 1981;14(9):633-643.
10. Simon SR, Paul IL, Mansour J, Munro M, Abernethy PJ, Radin EL. Peak dynamic force in human gait. *J Biomech.* 1981;14(12):817-822.
11. Whittle MW. Dynamic assessment of knee joint function. *Eng Med.* 1986;15(2):71-75.
12. Harrington IJ. A bioengineering analysis of force actions at the knee in normal and pathological gait. *Biomed Eng.* 1976;11(5):167-172.
13. Walker P. Friction and wear in artificial joints. In: *Human Joints and Their Artificial Replacements.* Springfield, IL: Thomas; 1977:368-422.
14. Hungerford DS, Barry M. Biomechanics of the patellofemoral joint. *Clin Orthop.* 1979;144:9-15.
15. Incavo SJ, Johnson CC, Beynnon BD, Howe JG. Posterior cruciate ligament strain biomechanics in total knee arthroplasty. *Clin Orthop.* 1994;309:88-93.
16. Simmons S, Lephart S, Rubash H, Borsa P, Barrack RL. Proprioception following total knee arthroplasty with and without the posterior cruciate ligament. *J Arthroplasty.* 1996;11(7):763-768.
17. Cash RM, Gonzalez MH, Garst J, Barmada R, Stern SH. Proprioception after arthroplasty: role of the posterior cruciate ligament. *Clin Orthop.* 1996;331:172-178.
18. Puloski SK, McCalden RW, MacDonald SJ, Rorabeck CH, Bourne RB. Tibial post wear in posterior stabilized total knee arthroplasty: an unrecognized source of polyethylene debris. *J Bone Joint Surg Am.* 2001;83-A(3):390-397.
19. Mestha P, Shenava Y, D'Arcy JC. Fracture of the polyethylene tibial post in posterior stabilized (Insall Burstein II) total knee arthroplasty. *J Arthroplasty.* 2000;15(6):814-815.
20. Dennis DA, Komistek RD, Hoff WA, Gabriel SM. In vivo knee kinematics derived using an inverse perspective technique. *Clin Orthop.* 1996;331:107-117.
21. Stiehl JB, Komistek RD, Dennis DA, Paxson RD, Hoff WA. Fluoroscopic analysis of kinematics after posterior-cruciate-retaining knee arthroplasty. *J Bone Joint Surg Br.* 1995;77(6):884-889.
22. Miegel RE, Walker PS, Nelson PC, Inadomi J, Needelman L, Maxine M. A compliant interface for total knee arthroplasty. *J Orthop Res.* 1986;4(4):486-493.
23. Cheal EJ, Hayes WC, Lee CH, Snyder BD, Miller J. Stress analysis of a condylar knee tibial component: influence of metaphyseal shell properties and cement injection depth. *J Orthop Res.* 1985;3(4):424-434.
24. Vasu R, Carter DR, Schurman DJ, Beaupre GS. Epiphyseal-based designs for tibial plateau components--I. Stress analysis in the frontal plane. *J Biomech.* 1986;19(8):647-662.
25. Garg A, Walker PS. The effect of the interface on the bone stresses beneath tibial components. *J Biomech.* 1986;19(12):957-967.
26. Bartel DL, Burstein AH, Santavicca EA, Insall JN. Performance of the tibial component in total knee replacement. *J Bone Joint Surg Am.* 1982;64(7):1026-1033.
27. Walker PS, Greene D, Reilly D, Thatcher J, Ben-Dov M, Ewald FC. Fixation of tibial components of knee prostheses. *J Bone Joint Surg Am.* 1981;63(2):258-267.
28. Kurtz SM, Muratoglu OK, Evans M, Edidin AA. Advances in the processing, sterilization, and crosslinking of ultra-high molecular weight polyethylene for total joint arthroplasty. *Biomaterials.* 1999;20(18):1659-1688.
29. Collier JP, Sperling DK, Currier JH, Sutula LC, Saum KA, Mayor MB. Impact of gamma sterilization on clinical performance of polyethylene in the knee. *J Arthroplasty.* 1996;11(4):377-389.
30. Sutula LC, Collier JP, Saum KA, et al. The Otto Aufranc Award. Impact of gamma sterilization on clinical performance of polyethylene in the hip. *Clin Orthop.* 1995;319:28-40.
31. Rose RM, Crugnola A, Ries M, Cimino WR, Paul I, Radin EL. On the origins of high in vivo wear rates in polyethylene components of total joint prostheses. *Clin Orthop.* 1979;145:277-286.
32. McKellop HA, Shen FW, Campbell P, Ota T. Effect of molecular weight, calcium stearate, and sterilization methods on the wear of ultra high molecular weight polyethylene acetabular cups in a hip joint simulator. *J Orthop Res.* 1999;17(3):329-339.
33. Baker DA, Bellare A, Pruitt L. The effects of degree of crosslinking on the fatigue crack initiation and propagation resistance of orthopedic-grade polyethylene. *J Biomed Mater Res A.* 2003;66(1):146-154.
34. Baker DA, Hastings RS, Pruitt L. Study of fatigue resistance of chemical and radiation crosslinked medical grade ultrahigh molecular weight polyethylene. *J Biomed Mater Res.* 1999;46(4):573-581.

35. Davidson JA. Characteristics of metal and ceramic total hip bearing surfaces and their effect on long-term ultra high molecular weight polyethylene wear. *Clin Orthop.* 1993;294:361-378.
36. Jasty M, Bragdon CR, Lee K, Hanson A, Harris WH. Surface damage to cobalt-chrome femoral head prostheses. *J Bone Joint Surg Br.* 1994;76(1):73-77.
37. Holt G, Murnaghan C, Reilly J, Meek RM. The biology of aseptic osteolysis. *Clin Orthop.* 2007;460:240-252.

# 3

# ARTHRITIDES

*Bruce Hopper, MD*

The definition of arthritis is joint inflammation. The knee joint contains several specific tissues: articular cartilage, meniscus cartilage, synovium, synovial fluid, capsule, ligaments, periarticular muscles, and subchondral bone.[1] Arthritis has 2 general categories: inflammatory and noninflammatory. The most common form of noninflammatory arthritis is osteoarthritis, or degenerative joint disease, which is the mechanical "wear and tear" of joints associated with aging. The knee joint is one of the most commonly affected joints in humans from both inflammatory and noninflammatory perspectives. The inflammatory arthritides about the knee include several etiologies: rheumatoid, lupus-mediated, crystalline, infectious, viral, septic, and psoriatic. Furthermore, inflammatory arthritis is associated with more than 100 other rheumatic diseases. There are currently 46 million Americans living with some type of arthritis. It is the most common cause of adult disability in the United States, affecting 19 million Americans.[2]

## OSTEOARTHRITIS/OSTEOARTHROSIS

Osteoarthritis is the most common form of arthritis, but the term is somewhat of a misnomer. A more accurate term is *osteoarthrosis*, which implies chronic, degenerative changes. To be academically precise, I will use the term osteoarthrosis (OA) hereafter. Primary OA is the mechanical "wear and tear" that naturally occurs to the articular cartilage with aging. As the OA progresses, more joint tissues become involved. These changes are seen in the synovium, synovial fluid, joint capsule, ligaments, and subchondral bone. Secondary OA is defined as the destruction of articular tissues due to another condition. Common causes of secondary OA include avascular necrosis (AVN), sickle cell disease, and post-traumatic OA.

The intra-articular space within the medial and lateral tibiofemoral compartments is exposed to several types of mechanical stresses, including rotatory, torsional, axial, and compressive forces. At first, the smooth, articular hyaline surface is intact without discontinuity. With exposure to athletics, trauma, or awkward knee movements, the hyaline surface develops small irregularities called fibrillations. Fibrillations may advance into small tears, which advance to larger tears, which may then peel off the subchondral plate.

Subchondral bone continuously maintains a dynamic remodeling homeostasis under normal conditions, but when it is damaged, it will remodel inappropriately into dense, sclerotic, weaker bone. This degenerative phenomenon is not completely understood. There are complex biochemical signaling pathways that break down at the intracellular level. There is a genetic component, poorly understood at this time, due to the observation that it runs in families. About 20% to 35% of knee OA may have a genetic component.[3,4]

When compressive forces axially load the advanced OA joint, bone will grind against bone, causing intense pain. This process can progress quickly or at a very slow rate. In fact, the time between a patient's first visit with a physician and the time when a patient needs arthroplasty may span more than 30 years. Typically, patients first seek a physician's advice around age 40, and the age when they undergo surgery is around age 60.



Parvizi J, Klatt B.
*Essentials in Total Knee Arthroplasty* (pp 19-22).

## Rheumatoid Arthritis

Rheumatoid arthritis (RA) is the most common inflammatory arthritis. Incidence among Americans is 25 per 100,000 for men and 54 per 100,000 for women.[5] The economic burden associated with RA is immense. Nine million outpatient visits and 250,000 hospitalizations are due to RA.[6] Up to 30% of untreated RA patients will become disabled within 3 years of diagnosis.[7]

There is no definitive etiology to RA. The working hypothesis is that an environmental trigger, or antigen, initiates an autoimmune phenomenon in genetically susceptible individuals. The unknown antigen stimulates T-cells that, in turn, make cytokines that activate β-cells to make antibodies. These antibodies, or rheumatoid factors (RF), then bind to immunoglobulins to form immune complexes, which embed themselves into synovium and articular cartilage. A cascade of chronic inflammation ensues.

RF is a laboratory test collected in the diagnostic work-up for RA. It has 80% sensitivity, and thus, a high false negative rate; if the result is negative, then the patient may still have RA. If there is any clinical suspicion for RA, even in the presence of a negative test, referral to a rheumatologist is appropriate for further diagnostic testing. Although often the end result of RA is knee replacement, RA can be a multiorgan system disease. There are effective medical treatments available now that either stabilize or slow down the disease process. There is a role for synovectomy to treat a knee with inflammation that will not respond to medications.

## Systemic Lupus Erythematosus Arthritis

Systemic lupus erythematosus (SLE) is a chronic, relapse-remitting, inflammatory autoimmune disorder that affects connective tissue, skin, joints, heart, lungs, blood vessels, liver, and the nervous system. Between 270,000 and 1.5 million Americans have SLE. Women are 9 times more likely to be diagnosed than men. It is a relatively common cause of polyarthritis (ie, arthritis of more than 4 joints).

Arthritis is one of the most common symptoms SLE patients develop over time.[8] SLE-mediated arthritis is rarely erosive and rarely leads to knee arthroplasty. Treatments are designed to slow progression and alleviate symptoms. It is important to identify this disorder as a cause of knee pain because there are effective interventions that need to be monitored and treated by a rheumatologist. There is no surgical intervention available to treat or delay the progression of symptoms in the knee.

## Crystalline Arthritis

There are a variety of microcrystals that can precipitate in joint tissues and cause arthritic changes. Before electron microscopy and X-ray diffraction techniques, there was no way to classify these crystals, and physicians assumed that the lucent lesions on X-ray were all the same. With these more accurate techniques, physicians now understand there are several different types of crystal deposition. These are normal chemical structures that are present in abnormal amounts in those who suffer from metabolic disorders. The more common crystals are monosodium urate (MSU) and calcium pyrophosphate dihydrate (CPPD), and the lesser common crystals are calcium apatite (CaA) and calcium oxalate (CaOx).

Gout can occur without hyperuricemia; however, hyperuricemia is a common feature of gout, so its presence supports a diagnosis of gout. Dietary intake has been implicated in causing gouty exacerbations. There is a strong association with the consumption of alcohol, sugar, meat, and seafood. High-protein foods such as sardines, seafood, and hotdogs have high levels of purines (the amino acids alanine and guanine), which are metabolized to urate. The urate merges with calcium in the blood and precipitates as MSU in synovial tissues. This process is very painful and causes erythematous joint effusions. Diagnosis is confirmed by microscopic analysis of joint aspirate, revealing negatively birefringent needle-shaped crystals. The most common site for gouty effusions is the first metatarsophalangeal joint. The second most common site is the knee.

Treatment can be accomplished with medical measures or by aspiration with glucocorticoid injection. Patients with infrequent attacks are treated with colchicine, nonsteroidal anti-inflammatory drugs (NSAIDs) such as Indocin, or intra-articular aspiration and glucocorticoid injection. Colchicine is incredibly effective for resolving an acute attack. Colchicine inhibits the deposition of urate crystals. The usual dose to abort an attack is 1 mg. This dose is followed by 0.5 mg every hour until pain is relieved or until diarrhea ensues. Articular pain and swelling typically improve by 12 hours. Any NSAID can be used for the treatment of inflammation and should be dosed appropriately for acute inflammation. If attacks are frequent, then prophylactic allopurinol is prescribed.

CPPD is another crystal type that builds up deposits in the joint tissues. This phenomenon is called pseudogout. CPPD crystals appear positively birefringent and rhomboid, rectangular, and rod shaped under a microscope. Patients are pain free most of the time. Most frequently, CPPD crystals are seen incidentally on X-rays for evaluation of osteoarthritis. Ten percent to 15% of people aged 65 to 75 and 30% to 50% people over 85 years have pseudogout.

CaA crystals are associated with hypercalcemic states. Examples include hyperparathyroidism, chronic renal failure, and metastatic disease. Very rarely do these cases present with arthralgias as the first complaint. CaOx crystals are also quite rare. Primary oxalosis is a rare genetic metabolic disorder. Dysfunctional enzymes in the biochemical pathway lead to increased production of CaOx and deposition into joint tissues. CaOx crystals have variable birefringence, but they can commonly appear as bipyramidal shapes and have strong birefringence.

## Lyme Arthritis

The deer tick *Ixodes scapularis* transmits the bacterium *Borrelia burgdorferi* when it infects humans. The "bulls' eye" rash, erythema migrans, is diagnostic. There is no confirmed erythema migrans most of the time. Patients usually present with a subacute onset of knee pain and swelling without any significant medical history or precipitating event.

About 60% of untreated patients develop arthritis in large joints, especially the knee, several months after infection. *B. burgdorferi* attacks the synovium, leading to synovial hypertrophy, vascular proliferation, and infiltration of mononuclear cells. Lyme disease can be cured in most patients with a few weeks of antibiotics. Doxycycline, amoxicillin, and cefuroxime are commonly used for oral treatment. Even if patients are treated appropriately with antibiotics, there is still the possibility of persistent bouts of knee pain with effusion. Some doctors believe there is an autoimmune response for persistent, chronic episodes of joint pain and swelling. If one suspects infection without a confirmed history of tick bite or erythema migrans, then one should order the serum Lyme antibody "two-test": ELISA and Western blot.[9]

It is best to address Lyme disease early. Chronic Lyme disease can affect the skin, brain, nervous system, muscles, bones, and cartilage. Symptoms can include chronic arthritis, fatigue, headaches, joint inflammation in the knees and other large joints, memory loss, mood changes, and sleep disorders.

## Viral

Another cause of joint pain is from a virus. Usually, there is a chronological history of a viral prodrome followed shortly thereafter with joint pain. The joint pain is self-limiting most of the time and resolves after the concomitant infection. Common viruses include Adenovirus, Coxsackie, Rubella, Parvovirus, and Epstein-Barr. These infections are self-limiting and rarely lead to chronic synovitis. It is not uncommon for one to get arthritis after an immunization. Other viruses are associated with more serious organ involvement. These include hepatitis A, hepatitis B, hepatitis C, and human immunodeficiency virus (HIV). These chronic infections are usually associated with relapsing and remitting bouts of arthralgias. None of the viral arthritides leads to joint destruction requiring knee arthroplasty.[10]

## Septic Arthritis

Septic arthritis is a nongonococcal bacterial infection of a joint, usually the hip or knee. Transient bacteremia seeds into the joint space. Causative organisms are more frequently staphylococcus, *Streptococcus pneumoniae*, or group B streptococcus; less common infections are from *Mycobacterium tuberculosis* and *Candida albicans*.

Physical signs reveal a swollen, erythematous knee and symptoms demonstrate exquisite knee pain with both active and passive range of motion. A low-grade fever and subjective intermittent fever, chills, and sweating should lower the threshold for making a clinical diagnosis of septic arthritis. The joint must be aspirated. A diagnostic aspiration may draw pus or murky synovial fluid, which must be sent for gram stain with sensitivities and cell analysis with differential. It is typical to find synovial fluid leukocyte count above 50,000/mm$^3$ in an infection. A proportion of leukocytes in synovial fluid of 90% polymorphonuclear leukocytes (PMNs) also indicates infection. Certainly these numbers are not absolutes, and the judgment of the surgeon is needed to put the entire clinical picture together to form the diagnosis. A count of 30,000/mm$^3$ with 95% PMNs may indicate infection. One must also send peripheral blood for erythrocyte sedimentation rate, C-reactive protein, complete blood cell count with differential, and blood cultures with gram stain and sensitivities. If infection is diagnosed, a surgeon needs to imminently perform an open or an arthroscopic I&D to prevent damage to the cartilage of the knee.

## Psoriatic Arthritis

Psoriasis is a chronic epidermal immune-mediated skin condition. Approximately 2% of the American population has some form, in varying degrees, of psoriasis. It is responsible for approximately 1 million office visits per year.[11] The characteristic lesion is a well-demarcated erythematous plaque with silvery scale. Common lesion sites are symmetric on the elbows, ears, knees, umbilicus, gluteal cleft, and genitalia. Psoriasis can also involve the scalp and fingernails.[12] Skin changes over the joints typically occur on the extensor surfaces.

Joints are rarely affected prior to dermatologic manifestations, but it has been reported. Mild forms of psoriatic arthritis involve relapsing, self-limiting episodes of arthralgias. Aggressive forms lead to complete destruction of the joint, requiring total knee arthroplasty. An accurate diagnosis is essential because there are effective biologic treatments such as methotrexate and disease-modifying anti-rheumatic drugs (DMARDs) that have been proven to slow progression and disability.[13]

## Avascular Necrosis

AVN is the destruction of subchondral bone due to compromised blood flow to a segment of bone. Although not technically an arthritic process, it does lead to arthritis when the supporting bone collapses and disruption occurs to the overlying cartilage. About 10% of AVN occurs in the knee. The most common site is the hip, and other sites include the scaphoid, lunate, talus, femur, metatarsal, mandible, and the humerus. There are 2 subclasses of AVN: spontaneous osteonecrosis of the knee (SONK) and secondary causes.

SONK is commonly associated with osteoporosis. One plausible mechanism is fluid accumulates in the marrow space because of minor trauma to weak bone. As a result, high pressures build within the marrow space, leading to necrosis. Another mechanism is vascular in origin, rather than marrow. The vessels of the osseous microcirculation become corrupted and cut off blood flow to segmental bone, resulting in necrosis.

There are several secondary causes of AVN. Associations include alcohol, steroids, trauma, sickle cell disease, hypertension, vasculitis, medications, inflammatory forms of arthritis, and decompression sickness.

SONK can usually be treated nonoperatively, but secondary osteonecrosis usually leads to surgical treatment. If there is no joint collapse from SONK, then partial weightbearing or an unloader brace can afford recovery. Progression to joint collapse usually occurs quickly in secondary osteonecrosis. If secondary osteonecrosis is identified quickly before joint collapse, then core decompression may delay knee arthroplasty.[14] If joint collapse is already identified, however, then usually knee arthroplasty is necessary.

## Summary

The etiology of knee pain is diverse. There are several arthritides that can cause severe knee pain. Accurate diagnosis is essential so that patients can receive appropriate care. Oftentimes, clues to proper diagnosis require assessment of physical signs and symptoms away from the knee joint itself.

## References

1. Bernstein J, ed. *Musculoskeletal Medicine.* Rosemont, IL: American Academy of Orthopaedic Surgeons; 2003.
2. Summary Health Statistics for U.S. Adults: United States, 2005, Tables 7, 8, Appendix III Table VII
3. Felson DT, Zhang Y. An update on the epidemiology of knee and hip osteoarthritis with a view to prevention. *Arthritis Rheum.* 1998;41(8):1343–1355.
4. Felson DT. Risk factors for osteoarthritis. *Clin Orthoped Rel Res.* 2004;427S:S16–S21.
5. Firestein GS. Etiology and pathogenesis of rheumatoid arthritis. In: Ruddy S, Harris ED, Sledge CB, Kelley WN, eds. *Kelley's Textbook of Rheumatology.* 7th ed. Philadelphia, PA: WB Saunders; 2005:996-1042.
6. American College of Rheumatology Subcommittee on Rheumatoid Arthritis Guidelines. Guidelines for the management of rheumatoid arthritis: 2002 update. *Arthritis Rheum.* 2002;46:328-346.
7. Sokka T. Work disability in early rheumatoid arthritis. *Clin Exp Rheum.* 2003;21(5 suppl 31):S71-S74.
8. Cervera R, Khamashta MA, Font J, et al. Systemic lupus erythematosus: clinical and immunologic patterns of disease expression in a cohort of 1,000 patients—The European Working Party on Systemic Lupus Erythematosus. *Medicine (Baltimore).* 1993;72:113.
9. Steere AC. Lyme disease. *N Engl J Med.* 2001;345:115.
10. Siegel LB, Gall EP. Viral infection as a cause of arthritis. *Am Fam Physician.* 1996;54(6):2009-2015.
11. Fleischer AB Jr, Feldman SR, Bradham DD. Office-based physician services provided by dermatologists in the United States in 1990. *J Invest Dermatol.* 1994;102:93-97.
12. *Am Fam Physician.* 2000;61:725-733,736.
13. Khan MA. Psoriatic Arthritis: An Update From EULAR 2007 CME.
14. Mont MA, Tomek IM, Hungerford DS. Core decompression for avascular necrosis of the distal femur: long term followup. *Clin Orthop.* 1997;334:124-130.

# 4

# Nonsurgical Alternatives/ Conservative Management

*Peter C. Vitanzo Jr, MD and Barry E. Kenneally, MD*

The ultimate treatment for end-stage knee osteoarthritis (OA) is knee replacement. However, when patients first present to a clinic with knee OA, it is often too early for surgery. At this point, either the disease process is not that advanced, the pain intensity is not that severe, or the patient's functional disability is not that limiting. Furthermore, and quite frequently, the patient is just not "mentally prepared" for surgery. Nonsurgical modalities can effectively serve as a bridge to knee replacement. Since artificial joints have a finite lifespan, delaying surgery can minimize the need for multiple revision surgeries in younger patients. In addition, nonsurgical therapies may be the only option for patients of extreme age or with significant medical co-morbidities prohibiting them from getting such replacement surgeries. It is possible that these patients can be managed effectively with conservative options so that they will never require a joint arthroplasty procedure.

What is a clinician to do when a patient is not ready for surgery or not a good surgical candidate, but the pain is too severe to ignore? There is a vast array of nonsurgical treatment options that can be effectively incorporated into one's practice. These treatments are both pharmacological and nonpharmacological and include weight loss, physical therapy (PT), low-impact exercise, braces, complementary medicine, topical medicine, systemic medicine, and joint injection (Figures 4-1 and 4-2). Physicians should be familiar with all of these approaches in order to provide comprehensive and effective care to patients presenting with knee OA, regardless of their age.

The primary goals of therapy are to relieve pain and improve function of the knee. These 2 goals are inseparable. Knee pain, swelling, and inflammation stimulate neurons, which inhibit the firing of quadriceps motor units. The chronic knee pain of OA can lead to atrophy and weakness of the quadriceps muscle. By focusing on pain-free knee function, physicians can greatly enhance the OA patient's quality of life.

There are several factors to consider when developing a treatment plan and these include, but are not limited to, the following: demographics (including age and work requirements), risk factors (obesity, prior injury/surgery, polypharmacy, medical comorbidities), knee characteristics (malalignment, structural damage, trauma), level of inflammation (effusion), level of pain and disability, and the patient's desired level of activity. There are no evidence-based algorithms to help choose which therapies will work in different subgroups of patients. Therefore, this treatment protocol must be "individualized" for every patient with this condition. Essentially, it is collaboration between the patient and physician. Incorporating patient preference and lifestyle can have a large impact on compliance and effectiveness of treatment.

## Weight Loss

Obesity is probably one of the most significant risk factors for the development and progressive worsening of knee OA, and this risk is especially strong among women.[1] The extent



Parvizi J, Klatt B.
*Essentials in Total Knee Arthroplasty* (pp 23-32).

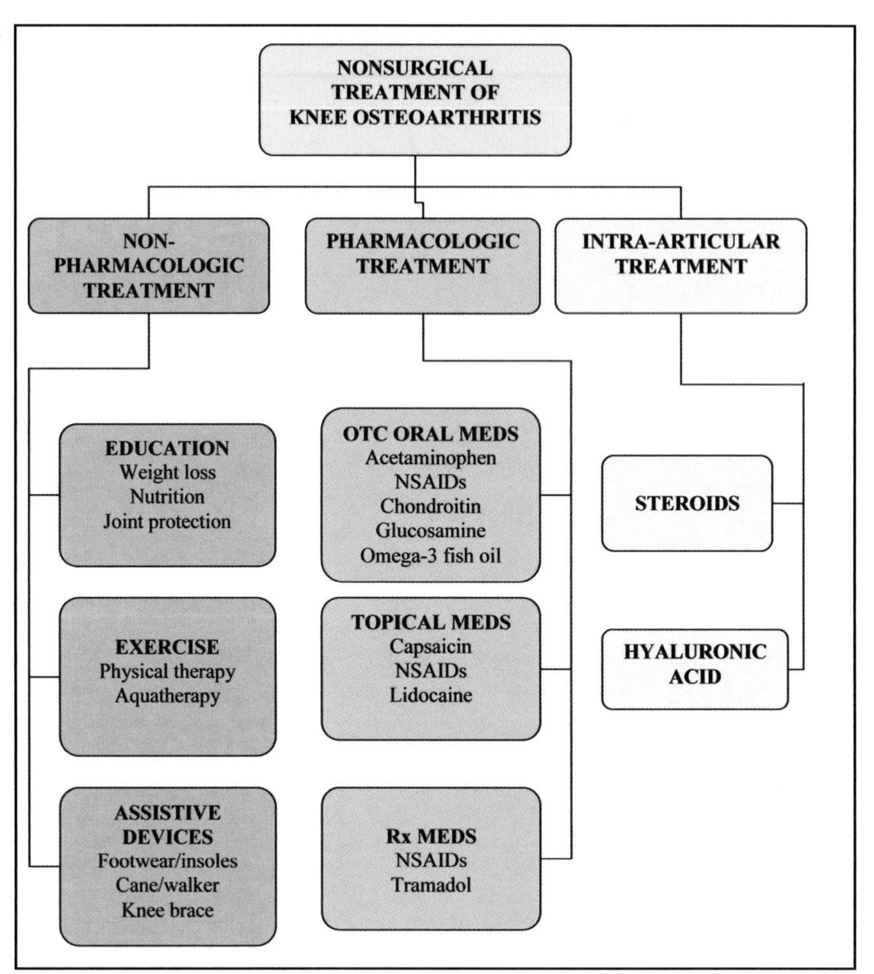


**Figure 4-1.** Nonsurgical treatment options for knee osteoarthritis.

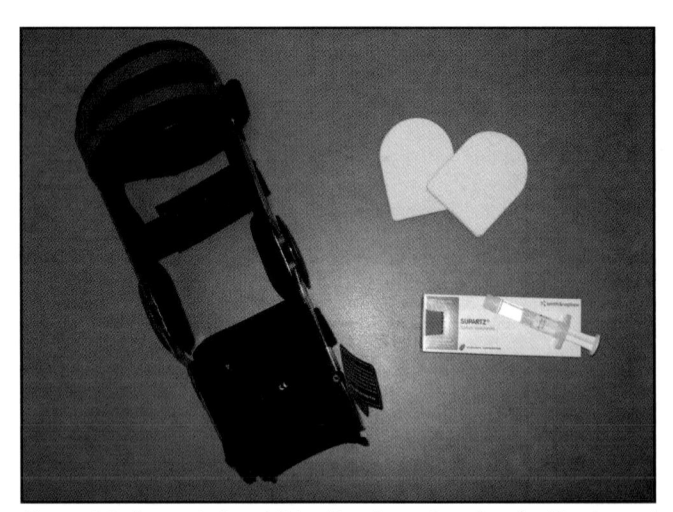

**Figure 4-2.** Nonsurgical modalities: Knee brace, lateral wedged insoles, and hyaluronic acid.

to which weight loss can affect the long-term progression of OA is somewhat less clear, but can certainly impact conservative and, ultimately, surgical outcomes. Body mass index (BMI) is commonly used in assessing knee OA patients and is associated with OA progression.[2] The traditional theory explaining the link between OA and obesity was that the extra weight caused increased "wear and tear" on joints. However, many patients with OA notice symptoms first in their nonweight-bearing joints such as their fingers. The traditional "wear and tear" hypothesis of OA may not fully explain this phenomenon. There is some recent evidence that the increased level of OA in the obese patient may be related to the proinflammatory effects of adipose tissue.[3-5] This information may yield new insights and treatments.

Whatever the mechanism linking obesity and knee OA, it stands to reason that weight loss would be helpful for knee OA patients. Indeed, weight loss has been shown to reduce pain and improve function in patients with knee OA.[6,7] The effects were even more dramatic when combined with exercise.[8] As with any patient fighting obesity, a combined program of aerobic exercise and appropriate nutrition will have the most substantial impact. Involving trained nutritionists/dieticians can greatly facilitate this treatment process. Furthermore, if patients are finding weight loss difficult despite their best efforts, it is not unreasonable to consider consultation for alternatives such as medications or even bariatric surgery.

## Exercise and Activity Modification

Low-impact exercise is an important component of treating knee OA. Exercise can help to improve strength, proprioception, and flexibility, as well as assist with weight loss. The effect of exercise interventions on pain and function in knee OA patients have been found to be equivalent to nonsteroidal anti-inflammatory drugs (NSAIDs).[9] However, high-impact physical activity may actually worsen knee OA, especially among obese individuals.[10] These high-impact activities tend to be occupational, involving kneeling, squatting, stair climbing, running, and heavy lifting.[11] Typically, knee OA progression does not occur with regular recreational activities such as light jogging.[12] It is possible that the data on vocational heavy activities are tainted with worker's compensation issues.

Knee OA patients should engage in exercise that is low impact and takes place in a controlled environment. Such activities include walking, aquatic exercise, cycling, yoga, Pilates, and Tai Chi. Patients should also be educated on proper shoe wear and sticking to "softer" surfaces such as padded tracks, grass, and boardwalks, which can minimize the impact on the joints. There are also various exercise machines with designs that minimize the impact on the knee, including elliptical machines, rowing machines, and stationary bicycles.

When prescribing an exercise program for a patient, it is important to combine aerobic and strengthening exercises. Although strengthening programs are more effective than aerobic in the short term, aerobic exercise has important advantages in the long term.[13] Aerobic activity also has a positive effect on mood not seen with strengthening exercises alone. No single exercise program has been found more effective than others.[14] Patients should be encouraged to pursue programs to their liking. Because knee OA is a chronic disease, any formal rehabilitation should be structured with progression to a home program.

## Topical Therapy

Patients will frequently use ice, heat, or even a combination for pain relief. Many patients even look toward massage therapy as an alternative approach for treating the pain of knee OA. In addition to these traditional topical therapeutic options, patients will also incorporate a variety of topical creams/ointments that are readily available over the counter.

Topical NSAIDs are effective alternatives to their systemic counterparts but with less systemic toxicity. There are a plethora of choices for these topical agents for patients. In some studies, topical NSAIDs have been found to be as effective as oral NSAIDs in treating knee OA.[15] Available formulations include diclofenac, salicylates, and ibuprofen. Although systemic levels are much lower than when taking oral NSAIDs, topical NSAIDs can be absorbed systemically.

Topical capsaicin is a safe and effective option for patients. It has been shown to be more effective than placebo at controlling pain in knee OA.[16] The chemical in this product is the active ingredient in hot peppers. Capsaicin therapy works by down regulating substance P in local tissues. No systemic side effects have been reported and capsaicin will not interact with any medications. Patients should be warned to use a glove when applying capsaicin and that there is an initial period of hypersensitivity before the substance P is down regulated.

Any topical agent can cause a local skin reaction. This is a fairly common occurrence and should resolve with discontinuation of the topical agent.

## Supplements

Although there are numerous nutraceutical products on the market, the potential benefits of glucosamine and chondroitin have been studied the most extensively. Chondroitin and glucosamine are derivatives of articular glycosaminoglycans. They are thought to promote chondrocyte glycosaminoglycan production and perhaps reduce inflammation in OA while at the same time reduce pain. There have been conflicting results on studies of these supplements in OA.[17-20] Initial studies had shown some promise, especially for chondroitin. Conversely, recent larger trials have shown little or no advantage over placebo. However, some of these trials showed that treatment may have some benefit in patients with moderate to severe disease.[19]

Although the compounds may have little or no effect on the progression of knee OA, it is apparent that many patients are convinced that they work at least for facilitating pain control. Whether this level of pain control is related to a placebo effect is debatable. There have been few side effects reported with either compound. The supplements may allow some patients to reduce the dose of more toxic medications. The recommended dose of chondroitin is 1200 mg per day

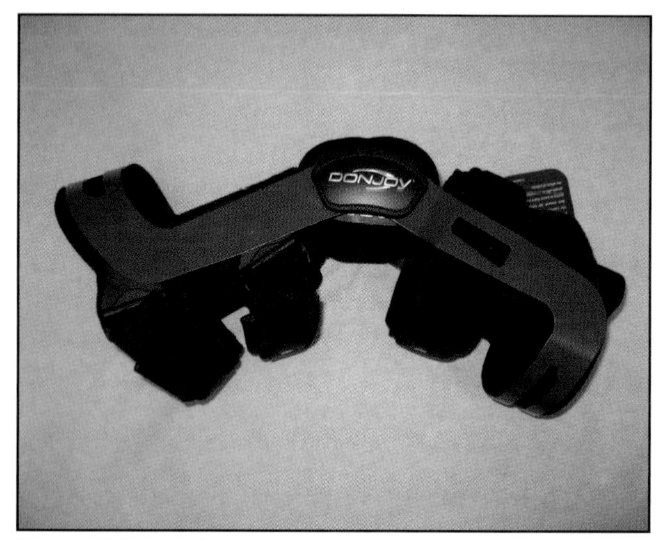


**Figure 4-3.** Unloader knee brace.

and for glucosamine 1500 mg per day. Glucosamine should not be used in patients with seafood allergy and should be used with caution in diabetics because it may elevate blood glucose levels, although studies have not consistently found this to be the case. The side effects of chondroitin tend to be mild gastrointestinal symptoms.

Fish oil is another supplement used to treat OA. The recommended fish oils are those high in omega-3 fatty acids. These fatty acids are typically found in cold water fish such as wild salmon, herring, mackerel, sardines, and anchovies. Although there are limited data on the use of fish oil in OA, it has been shown to improve the lipid profile of bone marrow and joint fluid, theoretically strengthening joints.[21] Fish oil supplements have also been shown to reduce production of proinflammatory cytokines.[22] Unfortunately, the clinical relevance of these findings is unclear. Nevertheless, many OA patients report a favorable response. Some clinicians express concerns over concentrated heavy metals and other pollutants in fish oil extracts. Simply increasing the amount of dietary omega-3 fatty acids may be safer.

## Assistive Devices

Various assistive devices can help to relieve the pain of knee OA. Unloading knee braces are a useful modality for patients with either isolated medial or lateral compartment knee OA that should be considered in your treatment regimen (Figure 4-3). In knee OA, the medial compartment is affected 10 times more often than the lateral compartment.[23] As the medial compartment degenerates, the knee shifts into a varus alignment. This can transfer up to 80% of the knee's load to the medial compartment.[24] To correct this malalignment, a valgus brace can be used to "unload" the medial compartment, transferring more weight to the lateral side. This does not seem to overload the lateral compartment but rather restores a more physiologic alignment.[26] Several studies have shown that valgus bracing reduces pain and improves activity levels in patients with isolated medial compartment OA.[25-30]

Lateral-wedged insoles are another device that addresses the varus knee deformity in medial compartment OA. Kinetic studies have shown that insoles of 5 to 10 degrees partially correct varus knee deformities.[31,32] Several clinical studies have also shown that the insoles improve pain and function.[25,31,33-36] Although lateral-wedged insoles have not been compared directly to knee braces, insoles have the advantage of being less cumbersome.

Crutches and contralateral canes may also be helpful, but these are more commonly used in OA of the hip. Many believe that the use of these assistive devices represents end-stage OA, making them candidates for total knee arthroplasty.

## Acupuncture

Acupuncture has been used to treat knee OA in Eastern countries for thousands of years. In recent years, acupuncture has seen growing popularity in the West. Although acupuncture studies are very complex given the difficulties of blinding and choosing a placebo, the most accepted design is to compare traditional acupuncture to sham acupuncture. Some studies show no effect[37,38] but others have shown marked improvement in pain scores.[39-42] A recent meta-analysis of 13 randomly controlled trials concluded that acupuncture was significantly superior to sham acupuncture for patients with chronic knee pain.[43] The major adverse event associated with acupuncture is infection. However, practitioners now have access to sterilized acupuncture needles and are subject to Food and Drug Administration (FDA) standards. Given the safety of acupuncture, it seems a reasonable complementary treatment for knee OA.

## Magnets

Static magnets are widely used to relieve pain of many types. Although there is some evidence that magnets reduce knee pain in OA patients,[44] much of the evidence is contradictory. There are inherent problems with interpreting studies using magnets. It is difficult to blind such studies when magnetism is so easy to detect. Also, a wide variety of magnets and diseases have been studied, making direct application difficult. A recent meta-analysis failed to provide sufficient evidence to recommend the use of magnets for pain relief.[45] Nevertheless, magnets are safe and warrant further study.

## Systemic Medications

The American College of Rheumatology and the European League Against Rheumatism recommend acetaminophen (or paracetamol, a European analog of acetaminophen) as the systemic medication of choice for knee OA patients who do not respond to nonpharmacological means.[46,47] Acetaminophen lacks the substantial side effects of NSAIDs and is almost as effective a pain reliever. Doses of up to 4 g per day are generally safe, but patients should be encouraged to use the lowest effective dose. However, hepatic toxicity can occur in chronic alcoholics. Once patients find their appropriate dose, they should take acetaminophen on a regular basis rather than sporadically. Many patients do well on a dose of 1 g twice daily.

NSAIDs are considered second-line analgesics for knee OA patients. The risk of gastrointestinal bleeding or perforation from NSAIDs has long been known.[48] In 2000, the American College of Rheumatology recommended hyaluronic acid (HA) for knee OA patients who have not responded to pharmacological therapy or patients who have a contraindication to NSAIDs. Since then, there has been new data on the cardiovascular side effects of both selective and nonselective NSAIDs.[49-53] Some selective cyclooxygenase (COX)-2 inhibitors have even been withdrawn from the market. Because of these substantial side effects, most experts recommend against using NSAIDs on a long-term basis in knee OA. Instead, they can be used for brief periods (~1 week) for patients with breakthrough pain or flares.

## Joint Injection

The major injection therapies for knee OA are steroids and HA. Although these are very different compounds, the technique for injection is the same. There are several sites that can be used, including the following: anterolateral, anteromedial, medial midpatellar, and lateral midpatellar. There is conflicting evidence as to the most accurate site for knee injection.[54,55] The authors prefer the anterolateral site for injection. If arthrocentesis is being performed, most physicians prefer the lateral midpatellar site.

## Intra-Articular Steroids

Intra-articular (IA) steroid injections are often used to treat knee OA. Acute inflammatory flares with effusions seem to respond particularly well to steroids. A combination of long-acting and/or short-acting anesthetic is traditionally injected with the steroid, often after arthrocentesis. IA steroids seem particularly effective in joints with effusions, especially when combined with arthrocentesis.[12] Some believe that large effusions represent a more inflammatory form of knee OA. Thus, such patients might be expected to respond better to the anti-inflammatory effects of steroids. The benefits of IA steroids tend to be short lived, but some patients do experience long-term relief of up to 24 weeks or longer.

IA steroids are safe and cost effective, but there are few studies supporting their efficacy. Repeated injections over short intervals can cause cartilage degradation so injections should be limited to 3 per year in any given joint. Although IA steroids work locally, systemic absorption does occur. Diabetics should be warned that they may experience poor glucose control in the days following IA steroid injections and should monitor their glucose levels closely. Rarely, a crystalline synovitis can be seen after IA corticosteroid injections. Also, there is a low risk of joint infection with any knee injection. Injecting a knee shortly before replacement is believed to increase the risk of TKA infection, but there are not true guidelines for how long to avoid injecting knees before replacement surgery.

## Viscosupplementation

Viscosupplementation, or now more commonly referred to as "joint fluid therapy," is one of the newer treatments for OA. It is the IA administration of HA, which is one of the major components of synovial fluid. The major tasks of synovial fluid are protecting the joint from trauma and acting as a transport medium for nutrients and waste products. HA seems to help with the former. Having both viscous and elastic properties, HA acts as both a lubricant (protection during slow movements) and a shock absorber (protection during rapid movements).

The properties of synovial fluid and HA are altered in OA, leading to dysfunction within the joint. In the osteoarthritic knee, HA may be reduced by as much as three-fold. Along with this reduction, the molecular weight falls and charge of HA changes in OA. As early as the 1960s, Balasz and Denlinger proposed that supplementation with HA would restore proper synovial function and reduce pain.[56]

Table 4-1

**VISCOSUPPLEMENTATION PRODUCTS AVAILABLE IN THE UNITED STATES**

| TRADE NAME | COMPONENT | NUMBER OF WEEKLY INJECTIONS | MOLECULAR WEIGHT (IN MILLIONS OF DALTONS) |
|---|---|---|---|
| Hyalgan | Sodium hyaluronate | 3 to 5 | 0.50 to 0.73 |
| Supartz | Sodium hyaluronate | 3 to 5 | 0.62 to 1.17 |
| Orthovisc | High-molecular weight hyaluran | 3 to 4 | 1.0 to 2.9 |
| Euflexxa | Sodium hyaluronate | 3 | 2.4 to 3.6 |
| Synvisc | Hyalan G-F 20 | 3 | 6.0 |

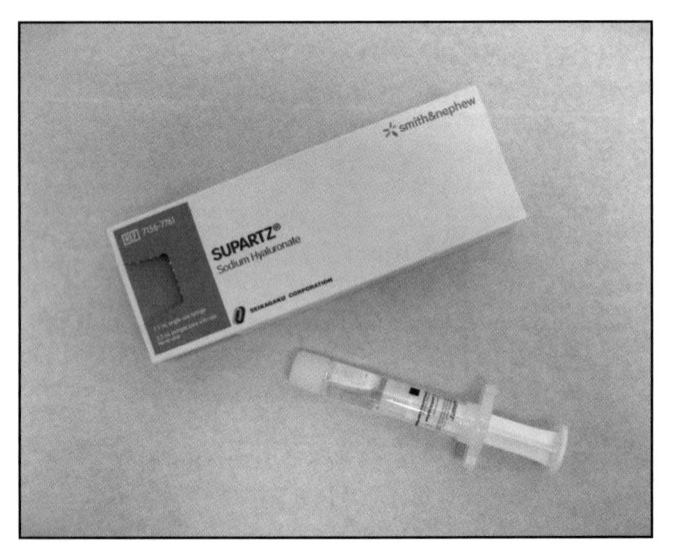


**Figure 4-4.** Hyaluronic acid single-dose kit.

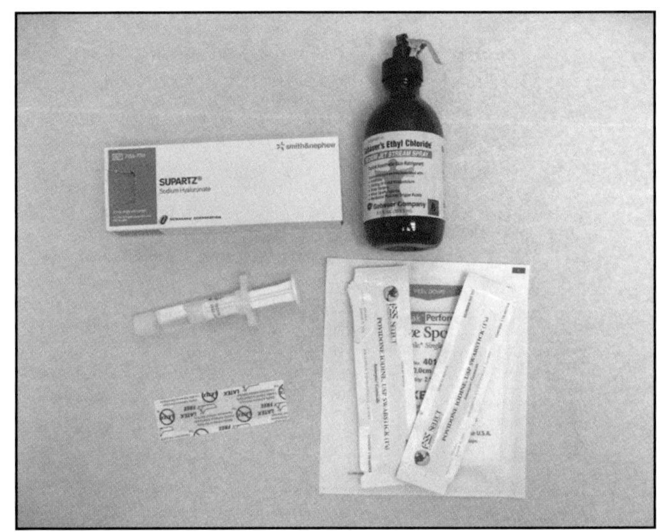


**Figure 4-5.** Injection supplies.

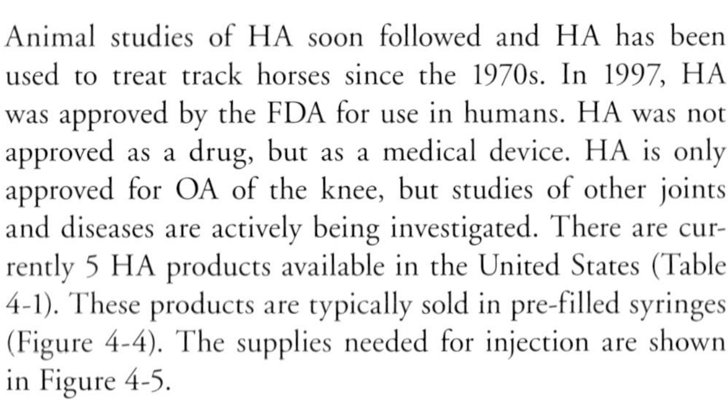

Animal studies of HA soon followed and HA has been used to treat track horses since the 1970s. In 1997, HA was approved by the FDA for use in humans. HA was not approved as a drug, but as a medical device. HA is only approved for OA of the knee, but studies of other joints and diseases are actively being investigated. There are currently 5 HA products available in the United States (Table 4-1). These products are typically sold in pre-filled syringes (Figure 4-4). The supplies needed for injection are shown in Figure 4-5.

HA's mechanism of action is unclear. There are 5 popular theories: 1) restoration of the viscoelastic properties of synovial fluid; 2) nociceptor analgesia; 3) stimulating HA production by synoviocytes; 4) suppressing inflammation; and 5) stimulating chondrocyte growth and collagen synthesis and decreasing chondrocyte apoptosis.[57]

There are numerous studies that lend credence to these theories. HA has been shown to reduce the levels of inflammatory mediators (prostaglandin, cytokines, cyclic adenosine monophosphate) in the synovial fluid of OA patients.[58-61] HA also directly effects leukocyte activity, reducing proliferation, migration, adherence, and phagocytosis.[62] In vitro studies have also shown that HA administration stimulates endogenous production of HA and other glycosaminoglycans.[62]

Studies of the clinical efficacy of viscosupplementation have been mixed (Table 4-2). Some believe that this is due to the fact that patients with more severe OA do not benefit as much as those with milder disease. Also, HA has been compared to many of the different modalities discussed above: NSAIDs, IA steroids, exercise, and PT. The varying design of the studies makes interpretation difficult. In most studies, HA was found to be at least equivalent to

Table 4-2

**STUDIES ON VISCO SUPPLEMENTATION**

| *STUDY, YEAR* | *N* | *HA TX REGIMEN* | *OTHER TX ARMS* | *PAIN SCALE* | *FOLLOW-UP* | *MEAN AGE* | *RESULTS* |
|---|---|---|---|---|---|---|---|
| Altman & Moskowitz 1998[69] | 495 | Hyalgan 5 weekly | placebo or naproxen | VAS, WOMAC | 26 weeks | 62 | HA naproxen |
| Carborn et al 1995[58] | 100 | Synvisc 3 weekly | IA triamcino-lone | VAS, WOMAC | 26 weeks | 63 | HA with longer duration |
| Huskisson & Donnelly 1999[70] | 100 | Hyalgan 5 weekly | IA saline | VAS | 6 months | 66 | HA superior |
| Jubb et al 2003[71] | 408 | Hyalgan 3 weekly Q 4 mos x 3 | IA saline | VAS, LFI | 1 year | 64 | HA with less joint space narrowing |
| Karlsson et al 2002[72] | 210 | Artzal 3 weekly, Synvisc 3 weekly | IA saline | WOMAC, LFI | 1 year | 71 | HA with longer duration benefit |
| Leopold et al 2003[73] | 100 | Synvisc 3 weekly | IA betametha-sone | VAS, WOMAC | 6 months | 66 | Tx arms equal |
| Wobig et al 1998[74] | 110 | Synvisc 3 weekly | LMW HA[b] 3 weekly | VAS, WOMAC | 12 weeks | 60 | Synvisc more effective |

LFI = Luquesne Functional Index; VAS = Visual Analog Scale; WOMAC = Western Ontario and McMaster University Osteoarthritis Index; IA = intra-articular; HA = hyaluronic acid; Tx = therapy; LMW = low molecular weight

continuous NSAIDs. IA steroids were found to be more effective than HA in the short-term. However, HA had longer-lasting effects, providing up to 6 months of relief. IA HA seems to be particularly effective at reducing pain on weight bearing between 5 and 13 weeks postinjection.

A recent Cochrane meta-analysis of 76 trials concluded that IA HA was an effective treatment for knee OA.[63] IA HA is also part of the American College of Rheumatology's protocol for the treatment of OA.[64] There is also some evidence attesting to the cost effectiveness of IA HA.[65,66] Some of the cost savings are related to the lack of toxicity from systemic medications.

Adverse effects from HA are few and tend to be local. These include needle breakage or separation, infection, hypersensitivity to local anesthetic or preservative, local discomfort, swelling, and pain. Local symptom flares may occur in 1% to 3% of patients. This pain and swelling typically subsides in 1 to 3 days. Some flares can be severe, however, resembling joint infection. These flares are called severe acute inflammatory reactions (SAIRs) or pseudoseptic reactions and seem to be more common with higher molecular weight HA preparations.[67] Some theorize that the reaction is a cell-mediated allergic reaction to cross-linked HA or to products used in manufacturing.

Some critics have cited the inconvenience of taking 3 to 5 weekly injections every 6 months. These multiple visits can lead to missed work and other inconveniences. However, the author's (Vitanzo) own extensive clinical experience with viscosupplementation has shown this to be quite the contrary. Patients are very willing to schedule the appropriate number of visits to receive this treatment option. In addition, one viscosupplementation product is now available as a single-shot dose.

IA HA can be used along with other OA treatments, such as IA steroid injections. The synergistic effect of the two IA regimens can provide earlier pain relief than treatment with HA alone.[68] This combination therapy seems especially effective when combined with arthrocentesis of knee effusions. Many feel that OA with effusion represents a more inflammatory form of OA.

## Summary

Osteoarthritis of the knee is a disease of multifactorial etiology. As such, it responds best to a treatment plan using multiple modalities. Treatment should be tailored to the individual patient and the patient should be directly involved. Important factors to consider include the patient's biomechanics, comorbidities, physical demands, as well as personal preferences. Such a task may seem daunting, but we can rely upon a large team of health care providers. This team includes physical therapists, pharmacists, nutritionists, fitness trainers, prosthetic specialists, and alternative practitioners. This team approach can maximize treatment effectiveness, minimize toxicity, and empower patients to manage their disease.

## References


1. Felson DT, Zhang Y, Hannan MT, et al. Risk factors for incident radiographic knee osteoarthritis in the elderly: the Framingham Study. *Arthritis Rheum.* 1997;40:728-733.
2. Felson DT, Goggins J, Niu J, Zhang Y, Hunter DJ. The effect of body weight on progression of knee osteoarthritis is dependent on alignment. *Arthritis Rheum.* 2004;50:3904-3909.
3. Toussirot E, Streit G, Wendling D. The contribution of adipose tissue and adipokines to inflammation in joint diseases. *Curr Med Chem.* 2007;14:1095-1100.
4. Rojas-Rodriguez J, Escobar-Linares LE, Garcia-Carrasco M, Escarcega RO, Fuentes-Alexandro S, Zamora-Ustaran A. The relationship between the metabolic syndrome and energy-utilization deficit in the pathogenesis of obesity-induced osteoarthritis. *Med Hypotheses.* 2007;69:860-868.
5. Dayer JM, Chicheportiche R, Juge-Aubry C, Meier C. Adipose tissue has anti-inflammatory properties: focus on IL-1 receptor antagonist (IL-1Ra). *Ann N Y Acad Sci.* 2006;1069:444-453.
6. Toda Y. The effect of energy restriction, walking, and exercise on lower extremity lean body mass in obese women with osteoarthritis of the knee. *J Orthop Sci.* 2001;6:148-154.
7. Huang MH, Chen CH, Chen TW, Weng MC, Wang WT, Wang YL. The effects of weight reduction on the rehabilitation of patients with knee osteoarthritis and obesity. *Arthritis Care Res.* 2000;13:398-405.
8. Messier SP, Loeser RF, Miller GD, et al. Exercise and dietary weight loss in overweight and obese older adults with knee osteoarthritis: the arthritis, diet, and activity promotion trial. *Arthritis Rheum.* 2004;50:1501-1510.
9. Bischoff HA, Roos EM. Effectiveness and safety of strengthening, aerobic, and coordination exercises for patients with osteoarthritis. *Curr Opin Rheumatol.* 2003;15:141-144.
10. McAlindon TE, Wilson PW, Aliabadi P, Weissman B, Felson DT. Level of physical activity and the risk of radiographic and symptomatic knee osteoarthritis in the elderly: the Framingham Study. *Am J Med.* 1999;106:151-157.
11. Cooper C, Coggon D. Physical activity and knee osteoarthritis. *Lancet.* 1999;353:2177-2178.
12. Felson DT, Niu J, Clancy M, Sack B, Aliabadi P, Zhang Y. Effect of recreational physical activities on the development of knee osteoarthritis in older adults of different weights: the Framingham Study. *Arthritis Rheum.* 2007;57:6-12.
13. Bennell K, Hinman R. Exercise as a treatment for osteoarthritis. *Curr Opin Rheumatol.* 2005;17:634-640.
14. Roddy E, Zhang W, Doherty M, et al. Evidence-based recommendations for the role of exercise in the management of osteoarthritis of the hip or knee: the MOVE consensus. *Rheumatology (Oxford).* 2005;44:67-73.
15. Biswal S, Medhi B, Pandhi P. Longterm efficacy of topical nonsteroidal antiinflammatory drugs in knee osteoarthritis: meta-analysis of randomized placebo controlled clinical trials. *J Rheumatol.* 2006;33:1841-1844.
16. Zhang WY, Li Wan Po A. The effectiveness of topically applied capsaicin: a meta-analysis. *Eur J Clin Pharmacol.* 1994;46:517-522.
17. Monfort J, Pelletier JP, Garcia-Giralt N, Martel-Pelletier J. Biochemical basis of the effect of chondroitin sulfate on osteoarthritis articular tissues. *Ann Rheum Dis.* 2007;67(6):735-740.
18. Reichenbach S, Sterchi R, Scherer M, et al. Meta-analysis: chondroitin for osteoarthritis of the knee or hip. *Ann Intern Med.* 2007;146:580-590.
19. Clegg DO, Reda DJ, Harris CL, et al. Glucosamine, chondroitin sulfate, and the two in combination for painful knee osteoarthritis. *N Engl J Med.* 2006;354:795-808.
20. Mazieres B, Hucher M, Zaim M, Garnero P. Effect of chondroitin sulphate in symptomatic knee osteoarthritis: a multicentre, randomised, double-blind, placebo-controlled study. *Ann Rheum Dis.* 2007;66:639-645.
21. Pritchett JW. Statins and dietary fish oils improve lipid composition in bone marrow and joints. *Clin Orthop Relat Res.* 2007;456:233-237.
22. Curtis CL, Rees SG, Cramp J, et al. Effects of n-3 fatty acids on cartilage metabolism. *Proc Nutr Soc.* 2002;61:381-389.
23. Ahlback S. Osteoarthrosis of the knee: a radiographic investigation. *Acta Radiol Diagn (Stockh).* 1968;Suppl 277:7-72.
24. Prodromos CC, Andriacchi TP, Galante JO. A relationship between gait and clinical changes following high tibial osteotomy. *J Bone Joint Surg Am.* 1985;67:1188-1194.
25. Pollo FE, Otis JC, Backus SI, Warren RF, Wickiewicz TL. Reduction of medial compartment loads with valgus bracing of the osteoarthritic knee. *Am J Sports Med.* 2002;30:414-421.
26. Hewett TE, Noyes FR, Barber-Westin SD, Heckmann TP. Decrease in knee joint pain and increase in function in patients with medial compartment arthrosis: a prospective analysis of valgus bracing. *Orthopedics.* 1998;21:131-138.
27. Matsuno H, Kadowaki KM, Tsuji H. Generation II knee bracing for severe medial compartment osteoarthritis of the knee. *Arch Phys Med Rehabil.* 1997;78:745-749.
28. Gaasbeek RD, Groen BE, Hampsink B, van Heerwaarden RJ, Duysens J. Valgus bracing in patients with medial compartment osteoarthritis of the knee: a gait analysis study of a new brace. *Gait Posture.* 2007;26:3-10.

29. Finger S, Paulos LE. Clinical and biomechanical evaluation of the unloading brace. *J Knee Surg.* 2002;15:155-158; discussion 159.
30. Lindenfeld TN, Hewett TE, Andriacchi TP. Joint loading with valgus bracing in patients with varus gonarthrosis. *Clin Orthop Relat Res.* 1997;344:290-297.
31. Kerrigan DC, Lelas JL, Goggins J, Merriman GJ, Kaplan RJ, Felson DT. Effectiveness of a lateral-wedge insole on knee varus torque in patients with knee osteoarthritis. *Arch Phys Med Rehabil.* 2002;83:889-893.
32. Crenshaw SJ, Pollo FE, Calton EF. Effects of lateral-wedged insoles on kinetics at the knee. *Clin Orthop Relat Res.* 2000;375:185-192.
33. Sasaki T, Yasuda K. Clinical evaluation of the treatment of osteoarthritic knees using a newly designed wedged insole. *Clin Orthop Relat Res.* 1987;(221):181-187.
34. Wolfe SA, Brueckmann FR. Conservative treatment of genu valgus and varum with medial/lateral heel wedges. *Indiana Med.* 1991;84:614-615.
35. Tohyama H, Yasuda K, Kaneda K. Treatment of osteoarthritis of the knee with heel wedges. *Int Orthop.* 1991;15:31-33.
36. Keating EM, Faris PM, Ritter MA, Kane J. Use of lateral heel and sole wedges in the treatment of medial osteoarthritis of the knee. *Orthop Rev.* 1993;22:921-924.
37. Foster NE, Thomas E, Barlas P, et al. Acupuncture as an adjunct to exercise based physiotherapy for osteoarthritis of the knee: randomised controlled trial. *BMJ.* 2007;335:436.
38. Scharf HP, Mansmann U, Streitberger K, et al. Acupuncture and knee osteoarthritis: a three-armed randomized trial. *Ann Intern Med.* 2006;145:12-20.
39. Berman BM, Singh BB, Lao L, et al. A randomized trial of acupuncture as an adjunctive therapy in osteoarthritis of the knee. *Rheumatology (Oxford).* 1999;38:346-354.
40. Williamson L, Wyatt MR, Yein K, Melton JT. Severe knee osteoarthritis: a randomized controlled trial of acupuncture, physiotherapy (supervised exercise) and standard management for patients awaiting knee replacement. *Rheumatology (Oxford).* 2007;46:1445-1449.
41. Manheimer E, Lim B, Lao L, Berman B. Acupuncture for knee osteoarthritis: a randomised trial using a novel sham. *Acupunct Med.* 2006;24:S7-S14.
42. Witt CM, Jena S, Brinkhaus B, Liecker B, Wegscheider K, Willich SN. Acupuncture in patients with osteoarthritis of the knee or hip: a randomized, controlled trial with an additional nonrandomized arm. *Arthritis Rheum.* 2006;54:3485-3493.
43. White A, Foster NE, Cummings M, Barlas P. Acupuncture treatment for chronic knee pain: a systematic review. *Rheumatology (Oxford).* 2007;46:384-390.
44. Harlow T, Greaves C, White A, Brown L, Hart A, Ernst E. Randomised controlled trial of magnetic bracelets for relieving pain in osteoarthritis of the hip and knee. *BMJ.* 2004;329:1450-1454.
45. Pittler MH, Brown EM, Ernst E. Static magnets for reducing pain: systematic review and meta-analysis of randomized trials. *CMAJ.* 2007;177:736-742.
46. Hochberg MC, Altman RD, Brandt KD, et al. Guidelines for the medical management of osteoarthritis. part II. osteoarthritis of the knee. American College of Rheumatology. *Arthritis Rheum.* 1995;38:1541-1546.
47. Jordan KM, Arden NK, Doherty M, et al. EULAR recommendations 2003: an evidence based approach to the management of knee osteoarthritis: report of a task force of the standing committee for international clinical studies including therapeutic trials (ESCISIT). *Ann Rheum Dis.* 2003;62:1145-1155.
48. Gabriel SE, Jaakkimainen L, Bombardier C. Risk for serious gastrointestinal complications related to use of nonsteroidal anti-inflammatory drugs: a meta-analysis. *Ann Intern Med.* 1991;115:787-796.
49. Hippisley-Cox J, Coupland C. Risk of myocardial infarction in patients taking cyclo-oxygenase-2 inhibitors or conventional non-steroidal anti-inflammatory drugs: population-based nested case-control analysis. *BMJ.* 2005;330:1366.
50. Graham DJ, Campen D, Hui R, et al. Risk of acute myocardial infarction and sudden cardiac death in patients treated with cyclo-oxygenase 2 selective and nonselective non-steroidal anti-inflammatory drugs: nested case-control study. *Lancet.* 2005;365:475-481.
51. Johnsen SP, Larsson H, Tarone RE, et al. Risk of hospitalization for myocardial infarction among users of rofecoxib, celecoxib, and other NSAIDs: a population-based case-control study. *Arch Intern Med.* 2005;165:978-984.
52. Helin-Salmivaara A, Virtanen A, Vesalainen R, et al. NSAID use and the risk of hospitalization for first myocardial infarction in the general population: a nationwide case-control study from finland. *Eur Heart J.* 2006;27:1657-1663.
53. Chan AT, Manson JE, Albert CM, et al. Nonsteroidal antiinflammatory drugs, acetaminophen, and the risk of cardiovascular events. *Circulation.* 2006;113:1578-1587.
54. Jackson DW, Evans NA, Thomas BM. Accuracy of needle placement into the intra-articular space of the knee. *J Bone Joint Surg Am.* 2002;84-A:1522-1527.
55. Esenyel C, Demirhan M, Esenyel M, et al. Comparison of four different intra-articular injection sites in the knee: a cadaver study. *Knee Surg Sports Traumatol Arthrosc.* 2007;15:573-577.
56. Balazs EA, Denlinger JL. Viscosupplementation: a new concept in the treatment of osteoarthritis. *J Rheumatol Suppl.* 1993;39:3-9.
57. Palacio LE, Vitanzo PC. Viscosupplementation. In: Freedman M, Morrison WB, Harwood MI, eds. *Minimally Invasive Musculoskeletal Pain Medicine.* New York, NY: Informa Healthcare; 2007:53-67.
58. Caborn D, Rush J, Lanzer W, Parenti D, Murray C, Synvisc 901 Study Group. A randomized, single-blind comparison of the efficacy and tolerability of hylan G-F 20 and triamcinolone hexacetonide in patients with osteoarthritis of the knee. *J Rheumatol.* 2004;31:333-343.
59. George E. Intra-articular hyaluronan treatment for osteoarthritis. *Ann Rheum Dis.* 1998;57:637-640.
60. Brandt KD, Smith GN Jr, Simon LS. Intraarticular injection of hyaluronan as treatment for knee osteoarthritis: what is the evidence? *Arthritis Rheum.* 2000;43:1192-1203.

61. Guidolin DD, Ronchetti IP, Lini E, Guerra D, Frizziero L. Morphological analysis of articular cartilage biopsies from a randomized, clinical study comparing the effects of 500-730 kDa sodium hyaluronate (hyalgan) and methylprednisolone acetate on primary osteoarthritis of the knee. *Osteoarthritis Cartilage.* 2001;9:371-381.
62. Moreland LW. Intra-articular hyaluronan (HA) and hylans for the treatment of osteoarthritis: mechanisms of action. *Arthritis Res Ther.* 2003;5:54-67.
63. Bellamy N, Campbell J, Robinson V, Gee T, Bourne R, Wells G. Viscosupplementation for the treatment of osteoarthritis of the knee. *Cochrane Database Syst Rev.* 2006;(2):CD005321.
64. Recommendations for the medical management of osteoarthritis of the hip and knee: 2000 update: American College of Rheumatology subcommittee on osteoarthritis guidelines. *Arthritis Rheum.* 2000;43:1905-1915.
65. Torrance GW, Raynauld JP, Walker V, et al. A prospective, randomized, pragmatic, health outcomes trial evaluating the incorporation of hylan G-F 20 into the treatment paradigm for patients with knee osteoarthritis (part 2 of 2): economic results. *Osteoarthritis Cartilage.* 2002;10:518-527.
66. Raynauld JP, Torrance GW, Band PA, et al. A prospective, randomized, pragmatic, health outcomes trial evaluating the incorporation of hylan G-F 20 into the treatment paradigm for patients with knee osteoarthritis (part 1 of 2): clinical results. *Osteoarthritis Cartilage.* 2002;10:506-517.
67. Leopold SS, Warme WJ, Pettis PD, Shott S. Increased frequency of acute local reaction to intra-articular hylan GF-20 (synvisc) in patients receiving more than one course of treatment. *J Bone Joint Surg Am.* 2002;84-A:1619-1623.
68. Ozturk C, Atamaz F, Hepguler S, Argin M, Arkun R. The safety and efficacy of intraarticular hyaluronan with/without corticosteroid in knee osteoarthritis: 1-year, single-blind, randomized study. *Rheumatol Int.* 2006;26:314-319.
69. Altman RD, Moskowitz R. Intraarticular sodium hyaluronate (hyalgan) in the treatment of patients with osteoarthritis of the knee: a randomized clinical trial. Hyalgan Study Group. *J Rheumatol.* 1998;25:2203-2212.
70. Huskisson EC, Donnelly S. Hyaluronic acid in the treatment of osteoarthritis of the knee. *Rheumatology (Oxford).* 1999;38:602-607.
71. Jubb RW, Piva S, Beinat L, Dacre J, Gishen P. A one-year, randomised, placebo (saline) controlled clinical trial of 500-730 kDa sodium hyaluronate (hyalgan) on the radiological change in osteoarthritis of the knee. *Int J Clin Pract.* 2003;57:467-474.
72. Karlsson J, Sjogren LS, Lohmander LS. Comparison of two hyaluronan drugs and placebo in patients with knee osteoarthritis: a controlled, randomized, double-blind, parallel-design multicentre study. *Rheumatology (Oxford).* 2002;41:1240-1248.
73. Leopold SS, Redd BB, Warme WJ, Wehrle PA, Pettis PD, Shott S. Corticosteroid compared with hyaluronic acid injections for the treatment of osteoarthritis of the knee: a prospective, randomized trial. *J Bone Joint Surg Am.* 2003;85-A:1197-1203.
74. Wobig M, Bach G, Beks P, et al. The role of elastoviscosity in the efficacy of viscosupplementation for osteoarthritis of the knee: a comparison of hylan G-F 20 and a lower-molecular-weight hyaluronan. *Clin Ther.* 1999;21:1549-1562.

# 5

# Surgical Alternatives to Total Knee Arthroplasty

*Hany Bedair, MD and David Backstein, MD, MEd, FRCSC*

Total knee replacement has a finite survival, and for this reason surgeons delay replacement surgery as long as possible. Nonoperative measures are instituted first, but surgical intervention is often required because of progression of the disease. Nonarthroplasty options can enable the patient to function longer with the native knee and/or to delay the need for total knee arthroplasty (TKA). Arthroscopic débridement is effective for treatment of mechanically symptomatic meniscal tears in the degenerative knee. Cartilage techniques have been developed to address loss of articular cartilage. Osteotomy is ideal for young patients with one compartment disease and knee malalignment. Unicondylar TKA enables more normal knee kinematics with only one compartment being replaced.

## Arthroscopic Débridement

The arthroscopic treatment of arthritis of the knee was first described in the 1930s, initially consisting of a lavage with simple instruments.[1] As arthroscopic instrumentation has been refined, treatment of arthritis of the knee consists of lavage, removal of loose bodies, and débridement of meniscal tears and chondral flaps.

### Patient Selection

There has been a well-established record of this type of procedure relieving symptoms of arthritis in appropriately selected individuals.[2-5] Those who benefit most from arthroscopic débridement are patients with a short duration of mechanical symptoms of locking and catching, minimal malalignment, and lack of severe radiographic changes.[4,6]

### Results

Moseley et al published a highly contentious prospective study in 2002 reporting that arthroscopic treatment of arthritis of the knee was no different from placebo.[7] This study was plagued, however, with problems of study design and inclusion criteria, namely an all male veterans' administration patient population without inclusion criteria limitations (as listed above) that would predict favorable results. A similar prospective study with more strict inclusion criteria comparing physical therapy and arthroscopic débridement with physical therapy alone reported that 75% of patients improved, 14% were unchanged, and 11% were worse.[8]

### Summary

These studies tend to indicate that in a properly selected patient population, arthroscopic débridement and lavage maintains a role in the treatment of arthritis of the knee. The procedure holds no merit in the patient with bone-on-bone erosion and the absence of mechanical symptoms. It should be reserved for patients with mild arthritis and symptoms of meniscal tear such as locking, popping, and catching.



Parvizi J, Klatt B.
*Essentials in Total Knee Arthroplasty* (pp 33-42).

Table 5-1

**OUTERBRIDGE CLASSIFICATION**

|  |  |
|---|---|
| • Grade 1 | Cartilage softening and swelling, normal thickness |
| • Grade 2 | Fissures appear in cartilage, loss of cartilage thickness is less than 50% |
| • Grade 3 | Crabmeat appearance of cartilage, loss of cartilage thickness is more than 50% but not full thickness |
| • Grade 4 | Exposed subchondral bone, full thickness cartilage loss |

# CARTILAGE RESTORATION

Articular cartilage is an avascular and aneural tissue without lymphatic supply. After initial formation, the cartilage has limited intrinsic regenerative properties. Because it lacks vascular and lymphatic supply, there is no access from the body to produce a regenerative response to injury. Superficial damage to articular cartilage does not initiate an inflammatory response. The body's repair response in tissue cannot start without this initial inflammatory stimulus. Injuries in cartilage that are deep enough to penetrate the subchondral bone allow the release of inflammatory repair cells, namely fibroblasts and mesenchymal stem cells, from the subchondral vasculature.[9] Several surgical strategies have been described to promote an intrinsic repair of cartilage injury. The most commonly used is the arthroscopic subchondral microfracture technique described by Steadman et al, which relies on the formation of fibrocartilage to fill-in articular cartilage defects.[10] Other commonly used approaches to repair cartilage injuries rely upon the transfer of healthy cartilage from areas of normal cartilage into the injured site. The two most common techniques are the autologous chondrocyte implantation (ACI) and osteochondral autogenous grafting.

## Patient Selection

The ideal patient for cartilage restoration procedures is younger than the age of 50 years who has an isolated, focal Outerbridge grade III or IV lesion (Table 5-1). The opposing articular cartilage should not be degenerated beyond Outerbridge grade I or II. Limb malalignment and ligamentous instability are considered contraindications.

A diagnostic arthroscopy is considered an essential component to patient evaluation for any of these procedures to determine the grade and size of the lesion as well as to define any other concomitant pathology. The upper limit of the defects that can be filled by osteochondral autografting is approximately 4 $cm^2$ and is mainly a function of limited donor sites. Successful ACI procedures have been described in lesions up to 12 $cm^2$. Lesions of the patellofemoral compartment tend to not do as well with cartilage restoration techniques.

## Surgical Technique

### MICROFRACTURE

A standard arthroscopic set-up is used. The subchondral plate is débrided of loose cartilage flaps with an arthroscopic shaver and ringed curettes to prepare a clean bed for the cartilage regeneration. An awl is used to penetrate approximately 4 mm into the subchondral bone at intervals of 3 to 4 mm to allow the efflux of blood into the repair bed that carries fibroblasts and mesenchymal stem cells. Continuous passive motion and limited weight bearing appears to improve the formation of fibrocartilage.[10]

### AUTOLOGOUS CHONDROCYTE TRANSPLANTATION

This technique harvests nonweight-bearing cartilage from the knee, grows cartilage cells in the laboratory, and then replants them into the area of cartilage defect. Results have shown promise and since that time, this procedure has been performed in thousands of patients worldwide.[11]

Cartilage is arthroscopically harvested from either the intercondylar notch or nonweight-bearing portions of the superior medial or lateral femoral condyles. No donor site morbidity has been reported when properly performed. This tissue is then processed in the laboratory where chondrocytes are extracted from the harvested articular cartilage. The cells are then proliferated in cell culture in vitro for 2 weeks. At the second operation, an arthrotomy is performed and the cartilage lesion is débrided to clean, stable vertical edges down to subchondral bone without penetrating the subchondral plate. The bed should be dry and free of blood. A periosteal flap that is 1 to 2 mm larger than the defect is harvested from the proximal medial tibia and sewn onto the defect with the cambium side facing the subchondral bone. This is secured with 6-0 absorbable sutures at 5-mm intervals; the gaps are sealed with fibrin glue. The expanded chondrocytes are then injected under the periosteal flap into the defect and the flap is sealed.[12] Continuous passive motion is started almost immediately. Protective weight bearing is continued for 6 weeks and gradually increased to full weight bearing at 3 months. Return to running is started at 9 months.

#### Osteochondral Mosaicplasty

Osteochondral autogenous grafting is a technique used to transplant osteochondral plugs from nonweight-bearing zones of the knee to fill cartilage defects. An arthrotomy is performed to gain access to the donor and graft sites. The defects are cleaned to sharp edges. Cylindrical osteochondral plugs are harvested from the medial border of the medial femoral condyle. Specialized tools and chisels are used to harvest plugs of approximately 25 mm in length and 5 mm in diameter. The accepting chondral bed is prepared similarly, creating a cylindrical defect into which the plugs are press-fitted. The gaps are subsequently filled with fibrocartilage.[13]

### Results

The results of cartilage restoration procedures vary widely and are highly dependent on the cartilage lesion, patient selection, and technical expertise. For the arthroscopic microfracture technique, Steadman et al reported a success rate of 80% at 7 years.[14] The centers with the greatest experience with the ACI procedure have reported postoperative results at 4-year average follow-up that demonstrated 90% good to excellent results and a patient self-assessment improvement of 89% when this technique was used for isolated femoral condyle lesions measuring less than 12 cm.[2,15] Osteochondral autograft transplantation has also yielded promising results, with "excellent" clinical results having been reported in 85% to 90% of patients.[16]

### Summary

Cartilage restoration procedures have yielded promising results in young patients with isolated focal cartilaginous lesions. These techniques provide reliable alternatives to arthroplasty in the appropriate patient population who have pain and disability that is attributable to localized cartilage defects.

## Partial Knee Replacement

### Unicondylar Knee Arthroplasty

Early experience with the unicondylar knee arthroplasty (UKA) yielded unfavorable results with high failure rates from poor pain relief and need for early revision.[17] Although implant design has undergone modest improvements (eg, the use of polyethylene thicker than 6 mm), the evolution of recent success with this style of implant largely stems from improved patient selection criteria. The advantages of UKA over osteotomy are a higher rate of initial success, fewer early complications, concomitant intra-articular débridement, and simultaneous treatment of bilateral knees. When compared to TKA, UKA preserves both cruciates, leading to nearly normal knee kinematics, higher patient satisfaction with the knee "feeling more normal," and preservation of bone stock.[18,19]

#### Patient Selection

There are 2 populations for which a UKA appears to be most beneficial.[20] First, the middle-aged patient with unicompartmental disease for whom a TKA may be premature and who finds osteotomy a less attractive option for issues related to cosmesis, immobilization, and prolonged partial weight bearing may benefit from this procedure. This provides the patient with a nearly normal functioning knee for some period of time with the realization that this will likely not be a definitive procedure with the need for revision or conversion to TKA; the preservation of bone stock theoretically facilitates this conversion. The second population of patients that may benefit from this procedure is the octogenarians who will likely not outlive the lifetime of the implant, for whom the implant will serve as their first and definitive arthroplasty. This choice will provide these patients with less blood loss, faster surgery, and faster recovery. Those patients in their 7th and 8th decades may be better served with a TKA, having a greater chance of avoiding any revision arthroplasty during their lifetime. In addition, it is generally accepted that young, active males are best served with an osteotomy rather than any arthroplasty.

Preoperative evaluation of potential UKA candidates is crucial to a successful procedure. As with any procedure addressing a single compartment, the presence of any inflammatory arthridities by definition is a contraindication.

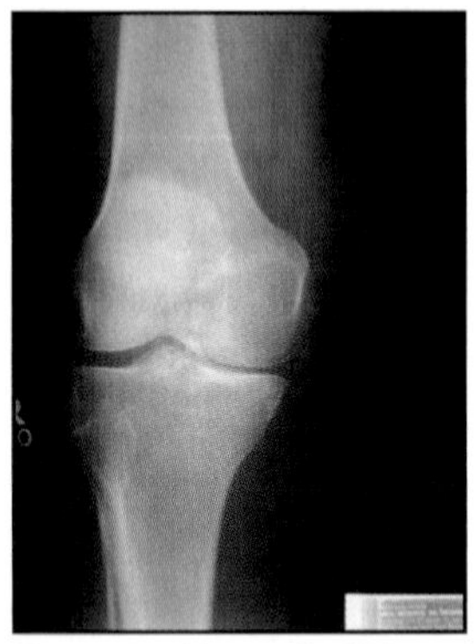

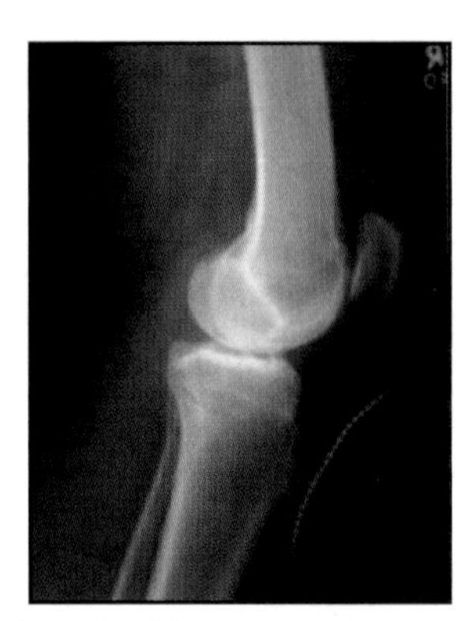

**Figure 5-1.** X-rays of a UKA candidate. Note the isolated degenerative changes in the medial compartment. The lateral x-ray does not show anterior subluxation of the tibia.

Varus deformities greater than 10 degrees, valgus deformities greater than 5 degrees, and flexion contractures greater than 15 degrees are relative contraindications.[21] Anterior tibial subluxation on the lateral radiograph and posterior wear pattern implies incompetence of the anterior cruciate ligament (ACL). The absence of an ACL is a contraindication to UKA because this tends to lead to ligamentous instability and opposite compartment wear.[22] Although few authors may accept UKA in the ACL-deficient, low-demand, sedentary patient, most would advise a simultaneous or staged ACL reconstruction and UKA to treat this combination of pathologies. Physical examination of the competency of the ACL is mandatory. Radiographic findings in the ACL-deficient knee tend to reveal lateral tibial subluxation on the AP radiograph and wear on the posterior one-third of the tibial plateau on the lateral radiograph whereas ACL-competent knees are more inclined to have wear on the anterior and middle third of the tibia. Mild chondromalacia in the opposite compartment or the patellofemoral articulation may be acceptable, but severe wear with eburnated bone in either articulation is a strong contraindication. This may be determined through the inspection of radiographs, magnetic resonance imaging (MRI), arthroscopy, or at the time of arthrotomy. Body weight remains a controversial issue with some studies reporting inferior results with patients weighing greater than 80 kg and others showing no correlation between weight and outcomes.[23,24] It appears that this procedure should be carefully considered in those patients who have significant weight problems (Figure 5-1).

## Surgical Technique

In general, surgical techniques are specific to individual implant systems, but there are several technical points that are applicable to most designs. First, overcorrection should be avoided.[25] Most authors recommend undercorrecting the mechanical axis by a few degrees to impart the majority of the force onto the implant and avoid overloading the unresurfaced side. In the varus knee, osteophytes commonly occur in the notch where the medial aspect of the lateral femoral condyle impinges on the lateral tibial spine. These must be removed because they are a common source of postoperative pain. Medial and lateral soft tissue release should be unnecessary. Removal of peripheral osteophytes will commonly correct any angular deformity. Those deformities requiring more extensive releases are likely poor candidates in the first place. Bone resections should be conservative to facilitate any future revisions. The anterior flange of the femoral component should be made flush with the trochlea to avoid disrupting the patellofemoral articulation. The tibial component should be sized appropriately to widely distribute the weight across the tibial plateau to avoid subsidence through the metaphyseal bone. Finally, multiple pin fixation of jigs onto the proximal tibia should be avoided because this has been found to be related to stress fractures and potential tibial component subsidence.[26]

## Results

Heterogeneity in study design, inclusion criteria, and outcome measures have made the long-term results of UKA difficult to evaluate and has plagued many early studies investigating the use of this procedure. It can be stated, however, that there appears to be good survivorship of these implants for the first 10 years after surgery in appropriately selected patients. The results do deteriorate in the second decade, but this is confounded by relatively small numbers of patients surviving greater than 10 years after surgery. Two large studies using currently accepted inclusion criteria were recently reported with 2 different styles of implants, one a mobile-bearing UKA and the other a metal-backed fixed bearing UKA. The first study using the Oxford (Biomet) UKA, a mobile-bearing system, reported a 95% 10-year survival rate in 94 implanted devices.[27] The second study, using the Miller-Gallante (Zimmer) metal-backed prosthesis, reported 98% 10-year survival and 95.7% 13-year survival in 49 knees.[28] The most common reason for late failure was progression of opposite compartment arthritis and patellofemoral degeneration. A large study of 516 unicondylar knee arthroplasties performed by 23 surgeons using 9 different implants reported slightly less impressive results with a 5- and 10-year survivorship of 92.6% and 88.6%, respectively.[29] The reporting of second decade results is uncommon and of small numbers of surviving patients with problems related to inclusion criteria and implant design. Three such studies report a 15-year follow-up survivorship of 79%, 88%, and 90% (Figure 5-2).[23,30,31]

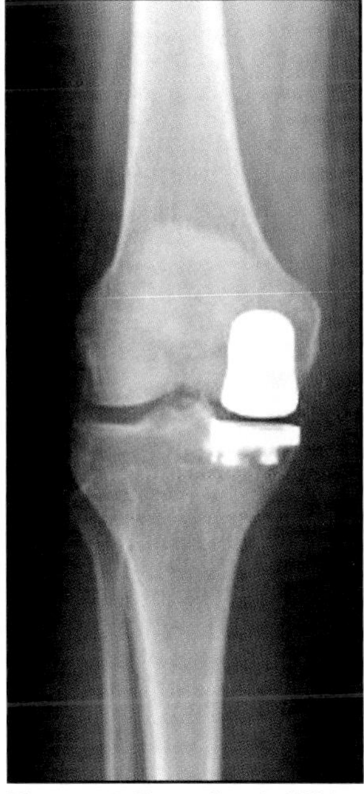

**Figure 5-2.** X-ray of medial UKA.

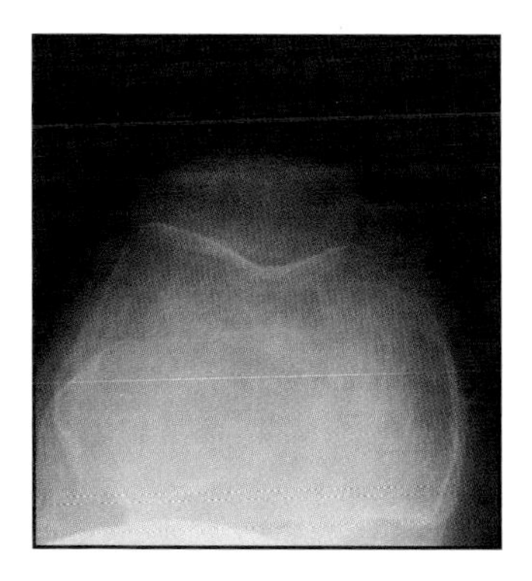

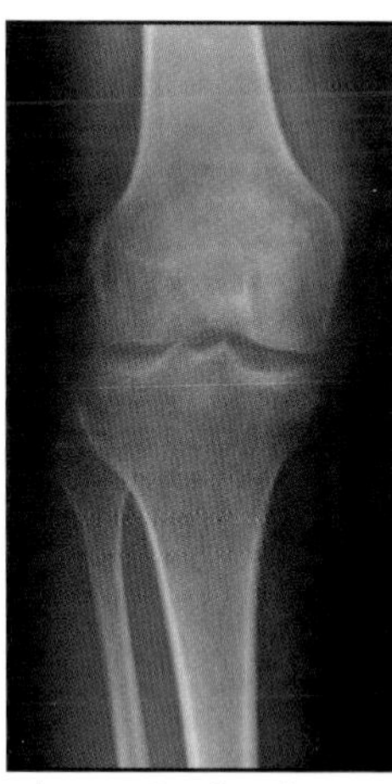

**Figure 5-3.** X-ray of patellofemoral degenerative disease. Patella is bone on bone in the trochlear groove.

### Summary

UKA appears to be a good alternative treatment for unicompartmental arthritis in the middle-aged patient as a temporizing procedure prior to a TKA and in the elderly patient as a definitive procedure. Improvements in patient selection criteria appear to have had the greatest impact on the recently observed promising results and must be strictly followed to maximize the chances of a good outcome. Not overcorrecting the deformity is also an important factor in making UKA more successful. The refinement of implant designs with thicker polyethylene and modern sterilization techniques will likely only improve the results of these implants into the second decade of use.

## Patellofemoral Arthroplasty

Patients with isolated patellofemoral disease who have failed all conservative treatment may be good candidates for arthroplasty of the patellofemoral joint. This treatment option has yielded good results for patients younger than the age of 55, whereas most patients over this age seem to fare better with a TKA.[32]

### Patient Selection

Indications for arthroplasty include grade IV chondrosis with severe pain; functional limitations; discomfort with prolonged sitting, stair use, or squatting secondary to osteoarthritis; posttraumatic chondrosis; and patellofemoral dysplasia. Patellofemoral arthroplasty should be avoided in those patients with significant malalignment or maltracking because this will lead to early failure; however, this cohort of patients may benefit from arthroplasty after the correction of these problems. This procedure should be avoided in those with grade III or IV changes in the tibiofemoral joint.[33] Patients with grade I or II changes in the tibiofemoral joint who have isolated anterior knee pain with classic symptoms of patellofemoral disease may still benefit from patellofemoral arthroplasty (Figure 5-3).

### Surgical Technique

Technical aspects of this procedure include an arthrotomy to expose the knee joint, which should be inspected thoroughly. The trochlear component should be slightly externally rotated with respect to the epicondylar axis of the knee. The component should be recessed slightly below the articular surface and should cover the entire trochlea without overhanging the medial/lateral border or extending distally into the tibiofemoral articulation. The patella is resurfaced similarly as in a TKA.[34]

### Results

The long-term clinical results have been successful. Early failures are usually secondary to errors in patient selection, failing in those who have malalignment or maltracking preoperatively.[33] The number one reason for late failure is progression of tibiofemoral arthritis. Long-term failures of the patellofemoral implant appear to be closely related to the design of specific implants (Figure 5-4).[35,36]

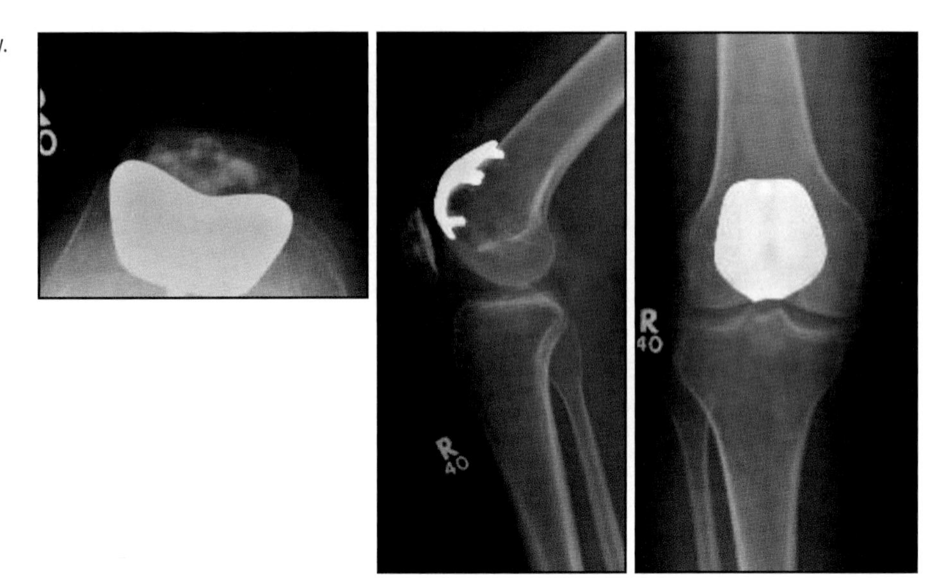


**Figure 5-4.** X-rays of patellofemoral arthroplasty.

## Summary

Younger patients with disabling arthrosis isolated to the patellofemoral joint may be good candidates for patellofemoral arthroplasty. Success of this procedure relies upon proper patient selection as well as improved prosthetic designs.

# Osteotomies of the Knee

In a varus or valgus knee with unicompartmental arthritis, an osteotomy can transfer the forces to the uninvolved joint space. The literature has documented a good rate of success with these techniques.[37] In addition, osteotomies are now used as an adjuvant to ligamentous reconstruction procedures, cartilage transplantation, or allografts. Although use of TKA and unicondylar knee replacement in younger patients has become more popular, there are limitations to these techniques. The use of TKA in the young is associated with shorter survival until revision.[38] The use of UKA is more limited in cases of deformity to less than 10 degrees of varus or 5 degrees of valgus and a flexion contracture less than 15 degrees. Osteotomies about the knee continue to remain an option for isolated medial or lateral compartment arthrosis in the young active patient.

## Patient Selection

The success of a realignment osteotomy about the knee is predicated on appropriate patient selection. This procedure is indicated for patients who are physiologically young, have high activity demands, and have isolated, localized pain to a single compartment. An age cut-off of between 50 and 60 years has been proposed; however, the patient's general level of health and activity may be a better guideline by which to include one as a candidate. Beyond the age of 60, most surgeons would recommend TKA or UKA.

Inflammatory arthritides, including chondrocalcinosis, are contraindications. Arthrosis and/or a prior meniscectomy in the compartment intended for weight bearing is an absolute contraindication. Relative contraindications include lack of motion beyond a 90 degree arc, obesity, tibiofemoral subluxation, and severe ligamentous instability. The most favorable results have been realized in knees with degenerative arthritis secondary to deformity rather than compartmental wear.

A thorough neurovascular examination of the involved extremity is required. Examination of the ipsilateral hip is mandatory and any pathology of the hip must be addressed prior to a realignment osteotomy. Those patients with a lateral thrust and high adductor moments about the knee tend to have inferior results.[39] The requirement of flexion beyond 90 degrees and a flexion of contracture of less than 10 to 15 degrees has been established only by convention. Although concomitant mild patellofemoral arthrosis is acceptable, moderate to advanced arthritis of this articulation is a contraindication. The outcomes in obese patients who exceed 1.3 times their ideal body weight are poor owing to technical difficulties during surgery and postoperative immobilization.[40] Overweight patients with a more sedentary lifestyle may benefit more from prosthetic arthroplasty.

Standard standing anteroposterior, lateral, posterior-anterior flexion weightbearing, and Merchant view radiographs are required to determine the radiographic location of the pathology and should be compared to the contralateral side. Full-length standing films from hip to ankle are required to assess the mechanical and anatomic axes of the lower extremity. The normal anatomic axis, determined by the angle formed by lines drawn down the anatomic axes of the femur and tibia, is normally 5 to 7 degrees of valgus. The weight-bearing line, a line from the center of the hip to the center of the ankle, normally passes just slightly medial to the center of the knee. The angle of the mechanical axis, a line drawn from the center of the hip to the center of the knee and from the center of the knee to the center of the ankle, is typically 1.2 degrees of varus, corresponding to approximately 60% of the force across the knee being borne by the medial compartment.

## Surgical Technique

One of the most common reasons for failure after osteotomy is either undercorrection or overcorrection, thus emphasizing the importance of preoperative planning. The direction and magnitude of angulation may dictate the optimal type of osteotomy. In general, valgus deformities are best treated with supracondylar femoral osteotomies (a "varus-producing femoral osteotomy") and varus deformities are best treated with high tibial osteotomies (a "valgus-producing tibial osteotomy"). The choice of opening versus closing wedge osteotomies is generally a surgeon's preference. Traditionally, closing wedge osteotomies are performed (lateral closing wedge tibial osteotomies for varus deformities and medial closing wedge femoral osteotomies for valgus deformities). Medial tibial opening wedge osteotomies have recently become more popular with advances in plating and grafting techniques. Dome osteotomies may allow for greater correction without adversely affecting the joint line obliquity, but they are technically more challenging. Osteotomies on both sides of the joint may be required for large or complex deformities that may result in joint line obliquity greater than 10 degrees.

The goals of a varus-producing osteotomy are different from those of a valgus-producing osteotomy. In most cases of a valgus deformity, the goal is to restore the mechanical axis through the center of the knee with a varus-producing distal femoral osteotomy. For the more common varus deformity, the goal is to position the mechanical axis so that it passes through a point that is 62% the width of tibial plateau measured from medial to lateral. This overcorrection accounts for dynamic forces that almost always establish an adductor moment across the knee. Although the precise goal for the mechanical axis angle postoperative is a source of debate, the best results seem to be with an angle of between 3 and 6 degrees of valgus.[41]

For most standard osteotomies, the weight-bearing line method is appropriate to determine the size of the wedge to be removed (for closing wedge) or introduced (for opening wedge). The angle formed by a line drawn from the center of the hip to a desired point on the joint line (50% tibial width for valgus and 62% for varus deformities) and a line drawn from this point to the center of the ankle determines the angle of correction. This angle is then drawn on the radiograph with the apex of the wedge 1 cm from the tibial cortex. The base of the triangle is the size of the opening or closing wedge. Slack collateral ligaments may also contribute to the apparent angular deformity. One degree of correction angle should be subtracted for each millimeter of tibiofemoral separation to avoid overcorrection. In addition, radiographic magnification must be taken into account.

The "rule of thumb" method, which estimates that 1 mm of angulation is produced by 1 mm of wedge height, is only accurate for a proximal tibia measuring 56 mm in width and should not be used. Because most tibias are wider than 56 mm, this method consistently underestimates the size of the wedge and thus leads to undercorrection of the deformity. Computer software exists that may assist with more complicated deformities. This analysis can optimize the angular correction by using both femoral and tibial osteotomies while avoiding joint line obliquity.

### Lateral Closing Wedge Osteotomy

Lateral closing wedge osteotomies of the proximal tibia are performed in the supine position with either a lateral-based incision or a longer longitudinal midline incision to facilitate future arthroplasty.[42,43] Subperiosteal dissection is performed along the anterior compartment and then posteriorly behind the tibia where a retractor is placed to protect the neurovascular bundle. To allow for proper closure of the tibial osteotomy, a fibular osteotomy is performed at the junction of its middle and distal thirds, or more commonly, the inner one-third of the proximal tibiofibular joint is resected. A guide pin is placed 2 cm distal and parallel to the joint line and stopped 1 cm lateral to the medial tibial cortex. An osteotomy made within 2 cm of the joint line may risk fracture of the plateau. A second guide pin is then inserted through the lateral cortex at the previously calculated wedge height. This is angled to intersect with the first pin 1 cm lateral to the medial tibial cortex. This creates a hinge along the medial cortex. Pin position is confirmed with fluoroscopy. A saw or osteotome is used to make the cuts distal to the proximal pin and proximal to the distal pin. The wedge removed should be larger posteriorly owing to the triangular shape of the tibia in cross-section. If the wedge thickness is equal both anteriorly and posteriorly, an anterior slope will be imparted to the tibial plateau; this may be desired in those patients with ACL deficiencies. A slow, gentle, constant valgus moment is placed across the knee

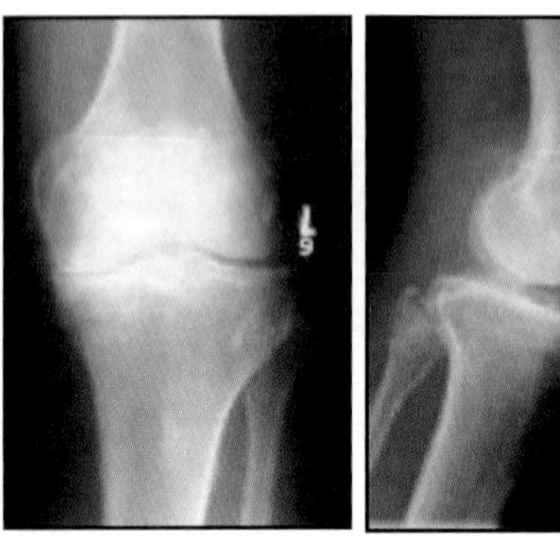
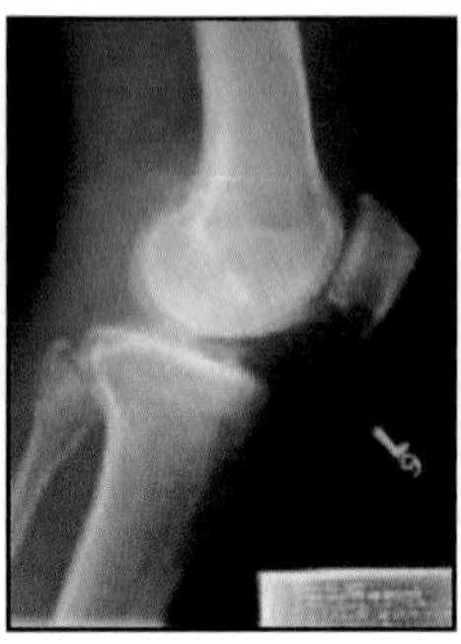
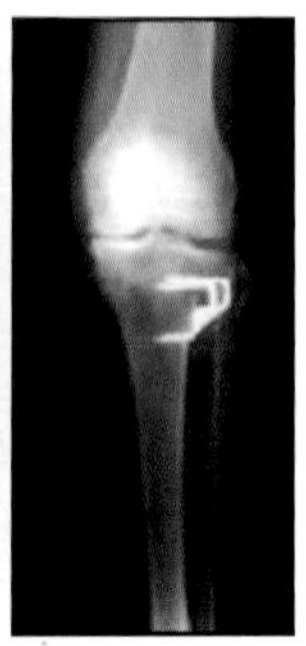

**Figure 5-5.** X-ray of lateral closing wedge osteotomy of the tibia.

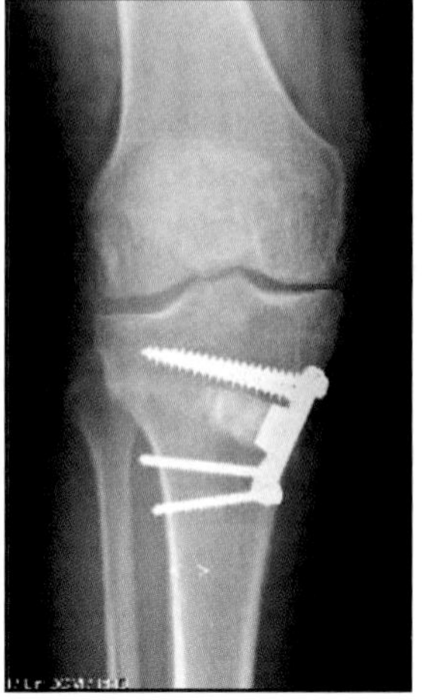
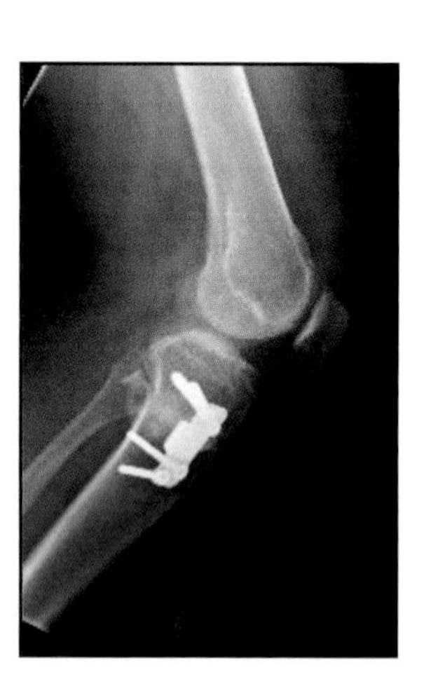

**Figure 5-6.** X-ray of medial wedge opening osteotomy of the tibia.

to close the osteotomy. Traditionally, the closure is fixed with staples inserted in a manner to encourage compression across the osteotomy site; this method of fixation requires immobilization, limited motion, and prolonged protected weight bearing, which seems to contribute to patellar tendon scarring and subsequent patella baja (Figure 5-5).[44] Rigid fixation with plates and screws allow for a quicker increase in range of motion exercises and weight-bearing advancement. This appears to reduce the complications related to patella baja.[45]

### Medial Opening Wedge Osteotomy

Medial opening wedge osteotomies of the proximal tibia may have some potential advantages over the lateral closing wedge osteotomy. The magnitude of correction can be adjusted intraoperatively and the desired sagittal slope can be easily changed. In addition, a fibular osteotomy is not needed and potential risk of iatrogenic injury to the peroneal nerve is reduced. There is, however, an increased risk of nonunion, increased time for restricted weight bearing, as well as the need for bone grafting. Some authors recommend allograft to fill smaller wedge defects, but for those greater than 7.5 mm in size, an autologous iliac crest bone graft may be needed. An incision is made between the posteromedial border of the tibia and the tibial tubercle extending 5 to 10 cm distal to the joint line. Subperiosteal dissection is used to elevate the pes anserine and medial collateral ligament and then posteriorly behind the tibia where a retractor is placed to protect the neurovascular bundle. A guide pin is inserted at an angle along a line connecting the fibular head and superior border of the tibial tubercle to ensure sufficient bone proximal to the osteotomy while protecting the patellar tendon insertion. The osteotomy is performed with a saw distal to the guide pin stopping just short of the lateral cortex. The lateral cortex can then be perforated with multiple passes of drill bit to ensure the lateral cortex is not violated, acts as a hinge, yet protects from fracture of the tibial plateau. Calibrated wedges are then slowly inserted to open the wedge, taking enough time to prevent fracture. The sagittal slope can be changed with specially designed wedges. The osteotomy site is fixed with a plate and screws, with most authors preferring a specialty step plate to maintain the height of the opening (Figure 5-6). Cancellous screws are used proximal to the osteotomy and cortical screws distally. The defect is then packed with bone graft. The osteotomy site can also be kept open through the use of external fixation. This may allow for gradual distraction and multiplanar corrections.

### Distal Femoral Osteotomy

Distal femoral osteotomies are much less common. They are generally indicated for valgus deformities for which a proximal tibial osteotomy would result in an unacceptable obliquity of the joint line (greater than 10 degrees). In a manner similar to that for the proximal tibia, the distal femur osteotomy may be a medial closing wedge or a lateral opening wedge. In either scenario, rigid fixation is mandatory as the forces across the distal femur are tremendous. Traditionally, medially closing wedge osteotomies have been fixed with an AO blade plate. More recently, distal femoral locking plates have been used both medially and laterally for closing and opening wedge osteotomies, respectively.

## Results

The results of high tibial osteotomies are variable with a trend toward poorer results with longer follow-up. It is clear, however, that the results are quite good in those procedures performed for the appropriate indications and with technical accuracy. With conversion to TKA as an end point, survival at 5, 10, and 15 years was reported as 94%, 85%, and 68%, respectively, in one study.[46] A meta-analysis of 19 publications reporting results of tibial osteotomies revealed an overall 5-year good or excellent result of 75.3%.[37] Subgroup analyses based on postoperative alignment revealed a 75% failure rate in undercorrected knees, with a 100% survivorship at 11.5 years with adequate alignment.[41] This underscores that accurate correction of malalignment is crucial to successful long-term clinical outcomes.

Distal femoral osteotomy results have similarly been favorable in appropriately selected patients, with one study reporting a 10-year survivorship of 87%.[47] Complications in distal femoral osteotomies have traditionally been higher compared to those of proximal tibial osteotomies with increased rates of nonunion, hardware failure, and undercorrection.[48]

### Complications

Neurologic injury is a devastating complication of tibial osteotomy and may be related to direct nerve injury, compression, postoperative edema, or hematoma. The incidence of these complications is markedly lower in opening wedge osteotomies, underscoring the need for careful dissection and appropriate placement of fibular osteotomies for lateral closing wedge procedures. Vascular injury is rare but most involve the popliteal artery. Great care must be taken with the posterior dissection and the passage of saw blades. Cadaveric studies have shown that flexion of the knee provides no protective benefit. Compartment syndrome is a known complication; placing drains in all wounds is highly recommended and vigilance in postoperative care is necessary. Intra-articular fracture is rare but can occur, commonly with proximal tibial fragments less than 2 cm and/or overly aggressive, rapid manipulation. All fractures must be reduced and stabilized.

Delayed union rates are 4 times higher in osteotomies performed below the tibial tubercle. Those made above the tubercle also have 2% to 4% nonunion rates compared to 4% to 19% in those made below the tubercle. Patellar tendon scarring and patella baja are common complications. The use of rigid fixation and early motion has aided in decreasing this problem. Pre-existing patella baja will likely be made worse with the use of an opening wedge osteotomy and thus a lateral closing wedge procedure is strongly encouraged.

Failure to adequately correct the deformity leads to pain, accelerated wear in the weight-bearing compartment, and premature conversion to TKA. TKA following an osteotomy presents surgical problems with previous incisions, patella baja, difficult exposure, and longer surgical times. The long-term results, however, do not appear to be adversely affected.

## Summary

Osteotomy for the treatment of unicompartmental degenerative joint disease of the knee has a long track record. Young, active patients who are considered too young or too physically demanding for a TKA may benefit from this procedure. The technical aspects of this treatment procedure, including preoperative planning and intraoperative execution, are critical for durable long-term success.

## References


1. Burman M, Finkelstein H, Mayer L. Arthroscopy of the knee joint. *J Bone Joint Surg.* 1934;16:255-268.
2. Sprague NF, 3rd. Arthroscopic débridement for degenerative knee joint disease. *Clin Orthop Relat Res.* 198;160:118-123.
3. Gross DE, Brenner SL, Esformes I, Gross ML. Arthroscopic treatment of degenerative joint disease of the knee. *Orthopedics.* 1991;14(12):1317-1321.
4. Ogilvie-Harris DJ, Fitsialos DP. Arthroscopic management of the degenerative knee. *Arthroscopy.* 1991;7(2):151-157.
5. Livesley PJ, Doherty M, Needoff M, Moulton A. Arthroscopic lavage of osteoarthritic knees. *J Bone Joint Surg Br.* 1991;73(6):922-926.
6. Salisbury RB, Nottage WM, Gardner V. The effect of alignment on results in arthroscopic débridement of the degenerative knee. *Clin Orthop Relat Res.* 198;198:268-272.
7. Moseley JB, O'Malley K, Petersen NJ, et al. A controlled trial of arthroscopic surgery for osteoarthritis of the knee. *N Engl J Med.* 2002;347(2):81-88.
8. Merchan EC, Galindo E. Arthroscope-guided surgery versus nonoperative treatment for limited degenerative osteoarthritis of the femorotibial joint in patients over 50 years of age: a prospective comparative study. *Arthroscopy.* 1993;9(6):663-667.
9. Insall J. The Pridie débridement operation for osteoarthritis of the knee. *Clin Orthop Relat Res.* 197;101:61-67.
10. Steadman JR, Rodkey WG, Rodrigo JJ. Microfracture: surgical technique and rehabilitation to treat chondral defects. *Clin Orthop Relat Res.* 200;391 Suppl:S362-S369.
11. Brittberg M, Lindahl A, Nilsson A, Ohlsson C, Isaksson O, Peterson L. Treatment of deep cartilage defects in the knee with autologous chondrocyte transplantation. *N Engl J Med.* 1994;331(14):889-895.
12. Petersen L. International experience with autologous chondrocyte transplantation. In: Scott WN, ed. *Insall and Scott Surgery of the Knee.* Vol 1. 4th ed. Philadelphia, PA: Churchill Livingstone; 2006:367-379.
13. Hangody LS, Duska I, Kaposi Z. Autlogous osteochondral transplantation: the "mosaicplasty" technique. In: Scott WN, ed. *Insall and Scott Surgery of the Knee.* Vol 1. 4th ed. Philadelphia, PA: Churchill Livingstone; 2006:391-396.
14. Steadman JR, Briggs KK, Rodrigo JJ, Kocher MS, Gill TJ, Rodkey WG. Outcomes of microfracture for traumatic chondral defects of the knee: average 11-year follow-up. *Arthroscopy.* 2003;19(5):477-484.

15. Peterson L, Minas T, Brittberg M, Nilsson A, Sjogren-Jansson E, Lindahl A. Two- to 9-year outcome after autologous chondrocyte transplantation of the knee. *Clin Orthop Relat Res.* 200;374:212-234.
16. Szerb I, Hangody L, Duska Z, Kaposi NP. Mosaicplasty: long-term follow-up. *Bull Hosp Jt Dis.* 2005;63(1-2):54-62.
17. Laskin RS. Unicompartmental tibiofemoral resurfacing arthroplasty. *J Bone Joint Surg Am.* 1978;60(2):182-185.
18. Newman JH, Ackroyd CE, Shah NA. Unicompartmental or total knee replacement? Five-year results of a prospective, randomised trial of 102 osteoarthritic knees with unicompartmental arthritis. *J Bone Joint Surg Br.* 1998;80(5):862-865.
19. Cobb AG, Kozinn SC, Scott RD. Unicondylar or total knee replacement: the patient's preference. *J Bone Joint Surg Br.* 1989;72:166.
20. Fitz WS. *Insall and Scott Surgery of the Knee.* Vol 2. 4th ed. Philadelphia: Churchill Livingstone; 2006.
21. Laskin RS. Unicompartmental knee replacement: some unanswered questions. *Clin Orthop Relat Res.* 2001;392:267-271.
22. Engh GA, Ammeen D. Is an intact anterior cruciate ligament needed in order to have a well-functioning unicondylar knee replacement? *Clin Orthop Relat Res.* 2004;428:170-173.
23. Tabor OB Jr, Tabor OB. Unicompartmental arthroplasty: a long-term follow-up study. *J Arthroplasty.* 1998;13(4):373-379.
24. Berend KR, Lombardi AV Jr, Adams JB. Obesity, young age, patellofemoral disease, and anterior knee pain: identifying the unicondylar arthroplasty patient in the United States. *Orthopedics.* 2007;30(5 Suppl):19-23.
25. Hernigou P, Deschamps G. Alignment influences wear in the knee after medial unicompartmental arthroplasty. *Clin Orthop Relat Res.* 200;423:161-165.
26. Brumby SA, Carrington R, Zayontz S, Reish T, Scott RD. Tibial plateau stress fracture: a complication of unicompartmental knee arthroplasty using 4 guide pinholes. *J Arthroplasty.* 2003;18(6):809-812.
27. Murray DW, Goodfellow JW, O'Connor JJ. The Oxford medial unicompartmental arthroplasty: a ten-year survival study. *J Bone Joint Surg Br.* 1998;80(6):983-989.
28. Berger RA, Meneghini RM, Jacobs JJ, et al. Results of unicompartmental knee arthroplasty at a minimum of ten years of follow-up. *J Bone Joint Surg Am.* 2005;87(5):999-1006.
29. Gioe TJ, Killeen KK, Hoeffel DP, et al. Analysis of unicompartmental knee arthroplasty in a community-based implant registry. *Clin Orthop Relat Res.* 200;416:111-119.
30. Weale AE, Newman JH. Unicompartmental arthroplasty and high tibial osteotomy for osteoarthrosis of the knee: a comparative study with a 12- to 17-year follow-up period. *Clin Orthop Relat Res.* 1994;302:134-137.
31. Squire MW, Callaghan JJ, Goetz DD, Sullivan PM, Johnston RC. Unicompartmental knee replacement: a minimum 15 year followup study. *Clin Orthop Relat Res.* 199;367:61-72.
32. Parvizi J, Stuart MJ, Pagnano MW, Hanssen AD. Total knee arthroplasty in patients with isolated patellofemoral arthritis. *Clin Orthop Relat Res.* 200;392:147-152.
33. Leadbetter WB, Ragland PS, Mont MA. The appropriate use of patellofemoral arthroplasty: an analysis of reported indications, contraindications, and failures. *Clin Orthop Relat Res.* 200;436:91-99.
34. Lonner J. Patellofemoral arthroplasty. In: Scott WM, ed. *Insall and Scott Surgery of the Knee.* Vol 2. 4th ed. Philadelphia, PA: Churchill Livingstone; 2006.
35. Tauro B, Ackroyd CE, Newman JH, Shah NA. The Lubinus patellofemoral arthroplasty. A five- to ten-year prospective study. *J Bone Joint Surg Br.* 2001;83(5):696-701.
36. Lonner JH. Patellofemoral arthroplasty: pros, cons, and design considerations. *Clin Orthop Relat Res.* 2004;428:158-165.
37. Virolainen P, Aro HT. High tibial osteotomy for the treatment of osteoarthritis of the knee: a review of the literature and a meta-analysis of follow-up studies. *Arch Orthop Trauma Surg.* 2004;124(4):258-261.
38. Robertsson O, Knutson K, Lewold S, Lidgren L. The Swedish Knee Arthroplasty Register 1975-1997: an update with special emphasis on 41,223 knees operated on in 1988-1997. *Acta Orthop Scand.* 2001;72(5):503-513.
39. Prodromos CC, Andriacchi TP, Galante JO. A relationship between gait and clinical changes following high tibial osteotomy. *J Bone Joint Surg Am.* 1985;67(8):1188-1194.
40. Coventry MB, Ilstrup DM, Wallrichs SL. Proximal tibial osteotomy: a critical long-term study of eighty-seven cases. *J Bone Joint Surg Am.* 1993;75(2):196-201.
41. Hernigou P, Medevielle D, Debeyre J, Goutallier D. Proximal tibial osteotomy for osteoarthritis with varus deformity: a ten to thirteen-year follow-up study. *J Bone Joint Surg Am.* 1987;69(3):332-354.
42. Coventry MB. Osteotomy of the upper portion of the tibia for degenerative arthritis of the knee: a preliminary report. *J Bone Joint Surg Am.* 1965;47:984-990.
43. Leone JH. Osteotomy in the sports knee. In: Scott WM, ed. *Insall and Scott Surgery of the Knee.* Vol 2. 4th ed. Philadelphia, PA: Churchill Livingstone; 2006.
44. Westrich GH, Peters LE, Haas SB, Buly RL, Windsor RE. Patella height after high tibial osteotomy with internal fixation and early motion. *Clin Orthop Relat Res.* 1998;354:169-174.
45. Windsor RE, Insall JN, Vince KG. Technical considerations of total knee arthroplasty after proximal tibial osteotomy. *J Bone Joint Surg Am.* 1988;70(4):547-555.
46. Hernigou P, Ma W. Open wedge tibial osteotomy with acrylic bone cement as bone substitute. *Knee.* 2001;8(2):103-110.
47. Wang JW, Hsu CC. Distal femoral varus osteotomy for osteoarthritis of the knee. *J Bone Joint Surg Am.* 2005;87(1):127-133.
48. Mathews J, Cobb AG, Richardson S, Bentley G. Distal femoral osteotomy for lateral compartment osteoarthritis of the knee. *Orthopedics.* 1998;21(4):437-440.

# 6

# The History of Modern Total Knee Arthroplasty

*Jennifer K. Bow, MD, FRCSC and Javad Parvizi, MD*

Total knee arthroplasty (TKA) is one of the most common and successful procedures in modern orthopedics. It is also a relatively new procedure that has undergone as many evolutionary changes to arrive at the procedures in use today. This evolution, however, is far from complete. This chapter will focus on the history of the development of the modern TKA, from its crude beginnings through to today's computer-navigated surgeries, with special attention to the early TKA designs that have spawned the great multitude of prostheses currently on the market. For a timeline of the development of TKA design, see Table 6-1.

## History of Surgical Knee Arthroplasty: 1861 to the 1970s

The first successful knee arthroplasty described in the literature was a resection arthroplasty performed by Ferguson in 1861.[1] The successful 5-year results from this case "put an end to 'the factious opposition of persons who knew nothing on the subject, and yet declared that no good result could be obtained unless ankylosis occurred, and that this was so rare that the operation must therefore be considered unadvisable.'"[1] Options for end-stage knee disease included amputation; arthrodesis; and attempts at arthrolysis, arthroplasty, or transplant.[2] Arthrolysis was performed through a large open incision, the soft tissues released or lengthened, then the joint closed, with or without subsequent dislocation of the joint. Resection arthroplasty and interposition arthroplasty involved removing bone and cartilage, with interposition of some autogenous or allogeneic material to prevent fusion of the bony surfaces in the case of interposition arthroplasties. Total joint transplant from another person (using amputated limbs or the joints of patients recently dead) was also tried experimentally and clinically without great success.[3,4] Although each of these methods was tried, none were reproducibly successful.

The interpositional materials used for arthroplasty included living biologic materials, such as autogenous pedicled fascial flaps,[5] fascia lata,[6-8] prepatellar fat pad[9] and skin,[10] absorbable biologic materials, such as chromized pig bladder (Baer's membrane)[11] or silver-treated fascia (Allison and Brook's membrane),[2] and "various sorts of inorganic nonabsorbable material, such as plates of magnesium, silver, gold, celluloid, zinc, rubber, etc. The results, however, of the use of non-absorbable inorganic material have been such that it has been almost completely discarded."[2] Orthopedic surgeons were on a quest for an interpositional material that could be sterile, would not induce a significant foreign body reaction, and would be absorbed by the body after a granulomatous reaction had occurred within the synovial cavity. No such ideal material was found, and the success rates of interpositional arthroplasties remained unreliable; thus, arthrodesis remained the procedure of choice for painful knees. Ankylosed knees that were left in a reasonably functional position were left as such because taking down the ankylosis could not yield a reliably satisfactory result. In 1918, Henderson from the Mayo Clinic reported on the



Parvizi J, Klatt B.
*Essentials in Total Knee Arthroplasty* (pp 43-54).

Table 6-1

## Timeline for the Development of Modern Total Knee Arthroplasty

| *Date* | *Development* | |
|---|---|---|
| 1861 | First successful excision knee arthroplasty reported by Ferguson | |
| Early 1900s | Interpositional knee arthroplasties performed using fat, skin, fascia lata, chromized pig bladder, silver-treated fascia | |
| 1938 | Boyd designs the first metallic (vitallium) interpositional knee arthroplasty<br><br>Moeys designs the first knee "alloplasty," a hinge design made of stainless steel that was implanted with good results in dogs, but never tried in humans | |
| 1951 | Walldius hinge total knee design shows promising results | |
| 1954 | Shiers reports on his hinged implant | |
| 1958, 1960 | MacIntosh and McKeever design tibial hemiarthroplasties with concave surfaces that are able to correct varus and valgus deformities by tensioning the cruciate and collateral ligaments | |
| 1963 | Young prosthesis incorporates valgus inclination at the knee and offers left- and right-sided options | |
| 1967 | Smith-Peterson femoral cap hemiarthroplasty becomes MGH Femoral Condylar Replacement | |
| | ANATOMIC | FUNCTIONAL |
| 1968 | Gunston produces Polycentric knee prosthesis | Freeman and Swanson introduce the Imperial College London Hospital (ICLH) prosthesis |
| 1970 | Kodama-Yamamoto knee is introduced | Duocondylar knee prosthesis and Unicondylar unicompartmental arthroplasty designed by Walker, Insall, Ranawat, and Inglis |
| 1971 | ***FDA approves PMMA cement*** | |
| 1971 | | Geomedic knee introduced |
| Early 1970s | Townley introduces the Anatomic knee | Eftekhar introduces the first prosthesis to use a metal component with modular polyethylene of various thicknesses |
| 1973 | | Total Condylar (TC) knee designed by Insall, Ranawat, Scott and Walker |
| 1974 | | Murray develops the Variable Axis knee, the first exchangeable modular polyethylene |
| 1977 | | Buechel and Pappas introduce first mobile-bearing TKA as part of the New Jersey Knee System (later became LCS) |
| 1979 | Hungerford and Kenna introduce porous-coating to TKA in the PCA knee | The first CAM mechanisms to account for PCL function were introduced in the Insall-Burstein PS knee and the Kinematic PS knee |
| 1980 | | Freeman-Samuelson TKA introduced, a modification of the ICLH design |
| 1990s 2000s | An enormous increase in functional and anatomic designs from many manufacturers | |

TKA = total knee arthroplasty; PS = posterior-stabilized; ICLH = Imperial College London Hospital; PCA = Porous Coated Anatomic; PMMA = polymethylmethacrylate

experience of 51 surgeons with 117 knee arthroplasties for various conditions of which 15% had good results, 25% had fair results, and 60% had poor results.[12] The knee was the joint that gave surgeons the most difficulty with its reconstruction, while at the time, the elbow, jaw, and hip each delivered more promising results. The problem in the knee was that resection of too much bone rendered the knee unstable, while not excising sufficient bone resulted in poor motion and ankylosis.

Surgeons were still attracted to the concept of interpositional arthroplasty, however, and continued to experiment with interpositional materials. Nylon as an interpositional membrane enjoyed some popularity for a time, with results reported as 83% satisfactory in chronic arthritis patients.[13] Even as late as 1968, interpositional arthroplasties were being performed using novel interpositional materials with reasonably good results, in response to the limited flexion permitted by the hinged metallic arthroplasties of that time.[14] The first metallic interpositional arthroplasty was designed by Boyd out of vitallium (cobalt-chromium alloy) in 1938 and implanted by Campbell who reported a satisfactory result on his preliminary cases in 1940.[15]

Several metallic hemiarthroplasties were designed for both the tibia and the femur to act as a type of resurfacing metallic arthroplasty for one side of the joint or the other. These included the MacIntosh hemiarthroplasty,[16] which consisted of semicircular prostheses with a concave proximal surface and a serrated distal surface to fix the prosthesis to the tibia. These were designed to resurface one or the other tibial plateau, and using these, MacIntosh was able to correct painful valgus and varus deformities by tensioning the cruciate and collateral ligaments with prostheses of various thicknesses. The prostheses were originally made of acrylic, then later out of vitallium. The McKeever prosthesis was very similar, with a T-shaped fin on the distal aspect as its mode of fixation.[17] Both of these implants enjoyed success rates well above the interpositional arthroplasty success rates of the time of 52%.[8] The MacIntosh prosthesis boasted a "good" result rate of 70%,[16] while the McKeever prosthesis showed a 97% success rate at 6 months in the hands of McKeever.[17]

On the femoral side, the femur was originally molded by Smith-Peterson to produce a femoral cap hemiarthroplasty, which initially showed disappointing results;[18] however, when an intramedullary stem was added for fixation, the success rate for the procedure was 63%.[19] This modified prosthesis was named the Massachusetts General Hospital Femoral Condylar replacement. Several other prostheses also emerged using either metal or acrylic to cap the distal femur.

Stainless steel was used for the first knee "alloplasty," designed by Moeys in 1938, which functioned as a hinge between the tibia and femur, with the tibial and femoral portions of the prosthesis set within the intramedullary canals of the respective bones.[20] This prosthesis was implanted into dogs and showed promising results, although it was never used in humans. Walldius designed an acrylic resin hinge arthroplasty for the knee in 1951. Initial results with this prosthesis showed 64% excellent results, 10% good results, and 26% failures.[21] The Walldius prosthesis was then formed out of stainless steel with a Teflon coating, and later to a cobalt-chromium roller. The design was modified again in 1958 to include a trochlear flange for the patellar articulation and longer femoral and tibial stems.[22] It remained an uncemented design. McKee developed a prosthesis very similar to the Walldius prosthesis. He obtained good success with it and later changed the prosthesis to include tri-fin femoral and tibial stems that were inserted into cement.[22] In 1954, Shiers reported preliminary results with his newly designed prosthesis.[23] It was a relatively long-stemmed tibial component with a posteriorly placed roller attached to the femoral stemmed component with a locking bolt. It was originally an uncemented design, which was later cemented due to problems with component loosening and fracture of the metal stems. Unfortunately, the loosening remained a problem despite the cemented technique, and performing an arthrodesis on the failed cemented arthroplasties proved to be difficult due to the large amount of bone that had been removed to implant the prosthesis.[24]

In 1963, Young reported on his results with his prosthesis.[25] His prosthesis included stemmed femoral and tibial components that were locked together with a bolt, locking screw, and washer. It had an uncemented design, so spikes were placed on the flat portions of the tibial and femoral components to project into the cancellous metaphyseal bone and prevent rotation around the intramedullary stem. Screws were also placed through flanges on the metaphysis to prevent distraction of the intramedullary stems within the bone canal. What was ingenious about this prosthesis, however, was the 15 degrees of valgus that was built into the femoral component. This was the first prosthesis to incorporate the valgus angle of the normal knee into its design, and the first TKA prosthesis that had a right- or left-sided femoral component. Up until this point, the hinges had been universal, for use on either the right or left sides, with no angulation at the knee. The results for this prosthesis were, however, disappointing. Of 19 prostheses inserted, there were 8 good results, 4 fair results, and 7 failures (4 due to infection, 1 due to skin slough, and 2 due to aseptic loosening).[25] Many other hinge designs (including the GUEPAR [Figure 6-1] and Stanmore knees) were advanced during this time; however, all of the designs continued to have unacceptably high rates of loosening and mechanical failure. The hinge designs began to incorporate less restraint, and a sloppy hinge consisting of a ball and socket joint attached to the tibia and femur via intramedullary stems became popular for a while (the Attenborough and Kinematic Rotating Hinge designs), and these types of hinges are still in use today for patients with ligamentous disruption or significant bone loss.[22]

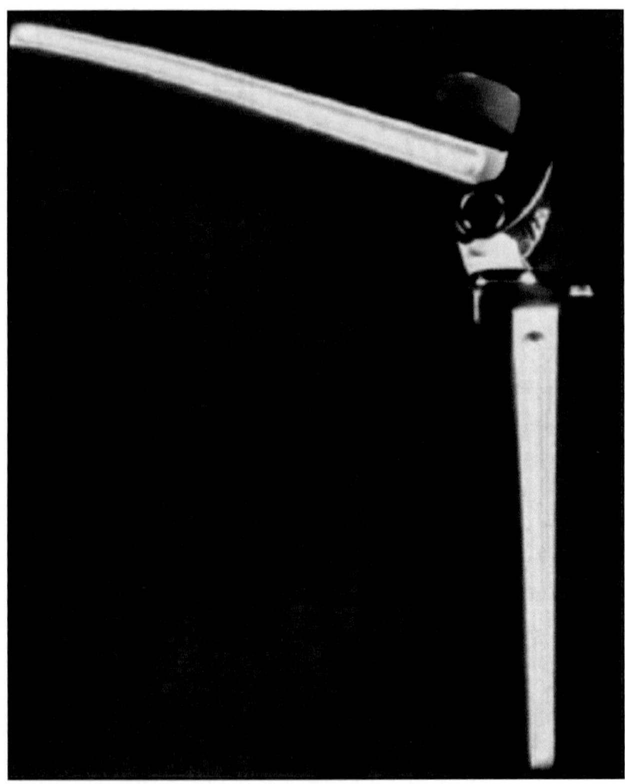

**Figure 6-1.** GUEPAR prosthesis. (Insall JN et al. A comparison of four models of total knee-replacement prostheses. *J Bone Joint Surg Am.* 1976;58(6):754-65. Reprinted with permission from The Journal of Bone and Joint Surgery, Inc.)

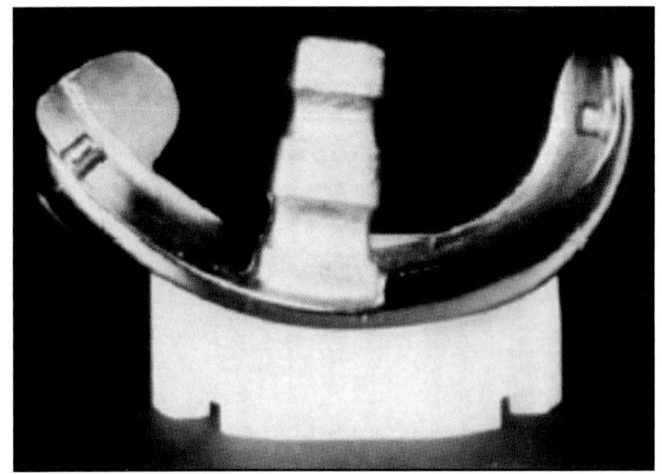

**Figure 6-2.** Unicondylar prosthesis. (Insall JN et al. A comparison of four models of total knee replacement prostheses. *J Bone Joint Surg Am.* 1976;58(6):754-65. Reprinted with permission from The Journal of Bone and Joint Surgery, Inc.)

## The Evolution of the Modern Total Condylar Prostheses

In large part because of the success of total hip arthroplasty in the 1960s with Sir Charnley's low friction arthroplasty design, the use of polyethylene as a prosthetic material, as well as the Food and Drug Administration (FDA) approval of polymethylmethacrylate (PMMA) as bone cement, the stage was set for the emergence of resurfacing arthroplasties for the knee.[26] Two schools of thought were to emerge: one dedicated to anatomic reconstruction of the knee joint, and one dedicated to the reconstruction of the knee's function while sacrificing the anatomical detail that made the knee such a difficult joint to reconstruct and maintain both mobility and stability.

### The Anatomic Perspective

The anatomic school of thought was embraced by Gunston, who produced the first resurfacing anatomic knee replacement after working in Charnley's laboratory in 1968.[27] His polycentric knee prosthesis was composed of 2 metal semicircular prostheses that slotted into the femoral condyles and 2 polyethylene concave runners that resurfaced the tibial plateaus. The cruciate and collateral ligaments, as well as the patella and the trochlear groove, were left intact. The arthroplasty gained stability by tensioning the ligaments (cruciates and collaterals) and soft tissues. This prosthesis produced very good results for the time, with only 2 of 22 initial cases requiring reoperation.[27] This approach spawned many similar prostheses including the Marmor, Manchester, Liverpool, Unicondylar (Figure 6-2) and Duocondylar (Figure 6-3). The Oxford and St. George Sled prostheses are some descendents of this type of approach.

Yamamoto introduced an anatomic prosthesis of his design, the Kodama-Yamamoto knee, in 1970. His design included a femoral mold and a minimally constrained single piece of polyethylene on the tibial side, with a central cutout for retaining the cruciate ligaments. The design was uncemented and secured with fins on the femoral side and 2 anterior staples on the tibial side. The prosthesis went through 2 modifications, Mark I and Mark II, with excellent results in 83% of patients on review of the patients with the Mark II prosthesis.[28]

Charles Townley also designed an anatomic TKA named the Anatomic knee. He worked on his designs in his own workshop and built his design on the basis of careful observation of natural knee and cadaver anatomy. His prosthesis featured a decreased radius of curvature of the femoral component in the anteroposterior direction than the mediolateral direction. This allowed for rollback during flexion and for minimal constraint. The cruciate ligaments

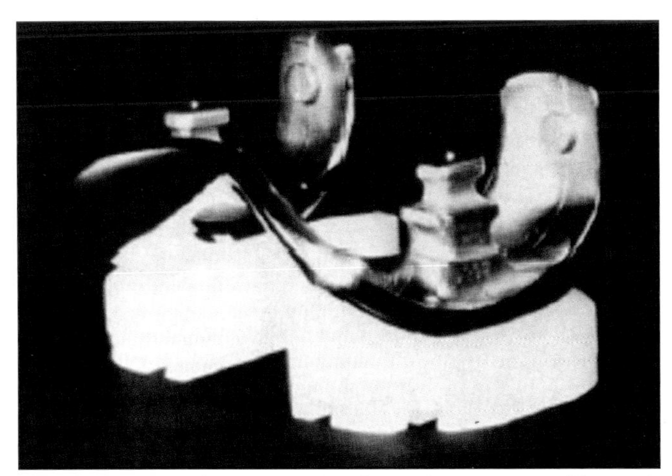

**Figure 6-3.** Duocondylar prosthesis. (Insall JN et al. A comparison of four models of total knee replacement prostheses. *J Bone Joint Surg Am.* 1976;58(6):754-65. Reprinted with permission from The Journal of Bone and Joint Surgery, Inc.)

were preserved and were relied upon to provide stability to the knee. He also included left- and right-sided anterior flanges for patellofemoral joint resurfacing. His knee design is currently marketed as the Total Knee Original, and his design has inspired many other TKA implants, including the Synatomic knee, AMK, Cloutier knee, Orthomet knee, Axiom knee, Natural knee, and the Porous Coated Anatomic (PCA).[26]

## The Functional Perspective

The functional school of thought had its origins back in the days of the interpositional arthroplasties. In 1944, Haas observed, "Instead of trying to imitate nature, and seeking a high and seemingly unattainable goal, it has appeared better to the author to divorce himself completely from the traditional concepts, and to reshape the new joint from a physiological rather than from an anatomical viewpoint."[29] Haas was speaking of an interpositional arthroplasty with which he had good success by shaping the bone ends into a simple hinge design with minimal bony contact, which upon use, allowed the body to remodel, assuming a more physiologic shape and without the ankylosis seen in many knee arthroplasties. The functional resurfacing arthroplasty subscribers looked to the function of the knee joint in order to simplify the surgical technique as well as their prosthesis designs.

Freeman and Swanson used this technique to create the Imperial College London Hospital (ICLH) prosthesis in the late 1960s.[30] This prosthesis used a cobalt-chromium femoral resurfacing cap that was cemented in place with the aid of jigs, and a polyethylene tibial surface that was cemented in place and held with 2 additional staples to ensure the stability of the tibial tray while the cement hardened. The prosthesis required the sacrifice of the cruciate ligaments and gained stability by the tensioning of the collateral ligaments using a tensor device then placing a polyethylene tibial component of sufficient thickness in order to maintain this tension. The roller-in-trough design maximized contact area between the femoral and tibial components and reduced the posterior rollback seen in knees with posterior cruciate ligament (PCL) intact. The other key concept in their design was the use of 90-degree bone cuts with large cancellous bone surfaces on which to apply the prosthetic components. Freeman introduced the concept of spacers to determine the flexion and extension gaps,[26] using a technique similar to MacIntosh's previous concept of tensioning the ligaments. The first design did not resurface the patella or the trochlea; these modifications were added in 1974. The original design likewise did not include a tibial eminence or a groove in the femoral component, which allowed some mediolateral instability.[31] These were added in 1980 and the resulting prosthesis, the Freeman-Samuelson TKA, remains on the market today.

In 1970, Walker, Insall, Ranawat, and Inglis at the Hospital for Special Surgery (HSS) developed the Duocondylar knee (see Figure 6-3), which was an anatomic design fashioned after Gunston's original design but with the femoral condylar resurfacing metal joined by an anterior bar. A Unicondylar knee (see Figure 6-2) was also designed that was essentially half of the Duocondylar knee without the anterior bar. This design could be used when only one compartment of the knee was involved by arthritis. Both of these designs required the cruciate ligaments to be intact. Experience with this device caused Insall, Ranawat, Scott and Walker to design the Total Condylar (TC) knee in 1973. The TC knee was composed of a polyethylene tibia that covered the entire surface of the tibia, with a tibial eminence and double-dished design, a femoral component that resurfaced both condyles with radii of curvature matching the natural knee and had an anterior grooved flange for the patella, as well as a domed polyethylene patellar component.[32] Ritter modified the design with cutouts in the polyethylene tibial component to preserve both cruciates or simply the PCL, giving rise to the Cruciate Condylar and Posterior Cruciate Condylar knees, respectively. Later on, Ranawat further modified the TC design to produce the Press Fit Condylar (PFC) Modular and the PFC Sigma knees. Insall modified the TC design to produce the TC II, which contained a tibial post that engaged the femoral notch to prevent hyperextension and to provide a small amount of posterior rollback in order to produce greater

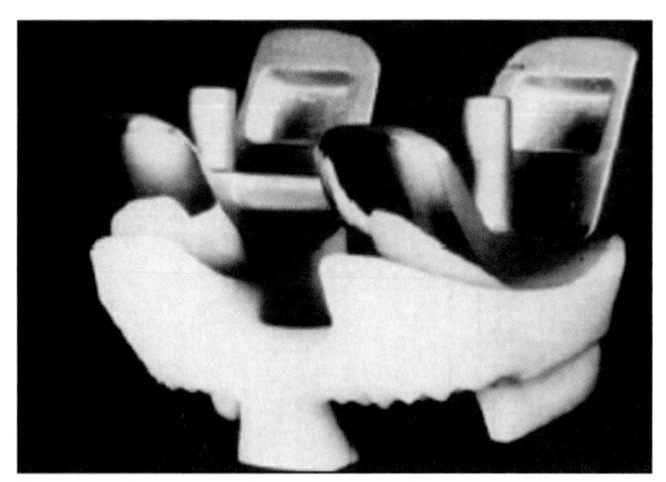

**Figure 6-4.** Geometric prosthesis. (Insall JN et al. A comparison of four models of total knee-replacement prostheses. *J Bone Joint Surg Am.* 1976;58(6):754-65. Reprinted with permission from The Journal of Bone and Joint Surgery, Inc.)

flexion. These implants were only used for a short period because of tibial component loosening. Upon analysis of the retrieved prostheses, it was determined that the cause of failure had been edge loading of the femoral prosthesis on the tibial component due to hand polishing of the femoral component leading to the removal of too much material on the femoral side.[26] A formal cam mechanism was introduced in the Insall-Burstein TC knee, and the design propagated as the Insall-Burstein TC II knee, the Optetrak Posterior-Stabilized (PS) knee, and the Advance PS knee. A different cam mechanism was designed by Walker and was used in the Kinematic, Kinematic II, Kinemax, and Kinemax Plus knees by Howmedica. Both cam mechanisms had the effect of a functional PCL, to allow greater knee flexion and prevent knee hyperextension.

The Geomedic knee was designed by a Howmedica engineer, Averill, who conceived of a dual-conforming bearing consisting of spheres on both the femoral and tibial components, joined by anterior bridges to allow retention of both cruciates. This created a sloppy hinge with maximal contact between the bearings to decrease the contact stress on the polyethylene. They later recruited a panel of surgeons to the design team, and the resulting design was named the Geometric[33] (Figure 6-4). These prostheses had a problem with tibial loosening and later designs produced by Zimmer increased the sagittal radius of the tibial component to reduce the constraint, as well as added a peg for improved tibial fixation.[26] These implants included the Geotibial and Geopatellar. Eventually, this design morphed into the Multi-Radius PS, the Miller-Gallante, and the Nexgen knees.

Eftekhar was the first surgeon to use a metal-backed tibial component with various thicknesses of polyethylene as a bearing surface. His first design used long intramedullary stems for both the femoral and tibial components. This was the Eftekhar Mark I. In the Eftekhar Mark II, the stems were removed and the components cemented, thus becoming a condylar-type replacement. This was also the first modular condylar knee with a 1.5-mm cobalt-chromium tibial component and inserts of 6, 10, and 15 mm that could be inserted and press-fit at the time of surgery.[34] In 1974, Murray likewise introduced a prosthesis, the Variable-Axis Knee, that allowed polyethylene modularity with different thicknesses able to be implanted at the time of surgery. This prosthesis locked the polyethylene liner into the metal tibial tray with a metal pin. He envisioned a useful application of such modularity—the ability to change the polyethylene insert at a later surgery for cases of wear.[26]

In 1977, another innovation in TKA design was advanced by Buechel and Pappas—the mobile-bearing TKA. They attempted to reduce constraint in their TKA design by introducing additional degrees of freedom of motion. Their design, called the bicruciate-retaining meniscal-bearing tibial component, consisted of spherical tibiofemoral-bearing surfaces in curved tracts. They also introduced a cruciate-sacrificing design with a rotating polyethylene platform. These designs were both part of the New Jersey Knee System. The original designs were cemented, and later models had a bone ongrowth surface and were termed low contact stress (LCS) knees.

Porous coating as a method of implant fixation was introduced to TKA design by Hungerford, Kenna, and Krackow in 1979 with the development of the PCA knee. The design was similar to Townley's Anatomic knee but had a 1.5-mm thick porous coating of cobalt-chromium beads. Previous cementless designs had required pegs or fins for fixation. This was the first implant to encourage bone ongrowth.[35]

The rapid development of TKA designs over the course of the 1960s and 1970s laid the foundation for the concepts behind all of our current prostheses. This explosion of creativity not only solved many of the problems inherent in knee arthroplasty, but also opened the door to new problems that will require even more creative solutions.

## Advances in the Materials for Total Knee Arthroplasty

The ability to manufacture the tibial polyethylene bearings through direct-molding of polyethylene, as opposed to machining the polyethylene, was another advance that allowed lower wear rates of the polyethylene-bearing material.[26] The discovery that polyethylene shows faster wear rates after sterilization through gamma irradiation in air[36] likewise allowed optimization of wear characteristics to avoid this method. Recently, it has also been shown that polyethylene bearings show poor wear properties the longer the component sits on the shelf (the concept of shelf-life). A shelf-life of 5 years or less correlates with better wear characteristics of the tibial component.[37] New materials are being introduced for use in total knees. Highly cross-linked polyethylene has evolved during the past decade and has been used with success in total hip arthroplasty. Although some designs utilize this material in TKA, it is not known if highly cross-linked polyethylene will have better wear characteristics than conventional polyethylene in the knee or not. Part of this issue relates to the fact that mechanism of wear in the hip and knee is different and another is the reduced mechanical properties of polyethylene with increased degree of cross linking.

Another advance seen in the materials used in TKA implant production was the hot isostatic pressing of the cobalt-chromium alloys after they had been cast. This produced a stronger implant with a finer articular surface, which reduced abrasive wear, thus increasing the lifespan of the prosthesis.[26] New metals have also been introduced for use in TKA. Oxinium is a material that is the result of a process that allows oxygen to absorb into zirconium metal. This changes the surface from a metal to ceramic. The surface is harder with less surface irregularity, and it is believed that this surface reduces polyethylene wear. A unique attraction of this material is the lack of metal particle release. Hence, oxinium knee is ideally suited for patients with suspected or proven metal (nickel) allergy.

Another material that is new to TKA is porous tantalum. Porous tantalum has excellent biocompatibility and a low modulus of elasticity, which may allow for more physiologic load transfer and preservation of the bone surrounding the metal implant. Porous tantalum allows for bone ingrowth into the metal. This novel material is useful for metal augments on revision TKA prostheses to make up for lost bone, for patellar augmentation when insufficient bone exists to resurface the patella, and for a novel form of fixation of the implants themselves.[38,39] With only short-term studies available, the outcome of tantalum prosthesis and augments in revision knee arthroplasty remains largely unknown.

## Newer Design Concepts

Developments continue in the field of TKA. Improvements in technique and implant should be welcomed with caution, as not every change is ultimately an improvement. Criteria for examining each improvement should be adopted by the surgeon. The following design objectives for a prosthesis were discussed by Freeman and colleagues in 1973[40]:

- A salvage procedure should be readily available
- The chance of loosening should be minimized (the femoral and tibial components should be incompletely constrained relative to each other, the friction between the components should be minimized, any hyperextension-limiting arrangement should be progressive and not sudden in nature, the components should be fitted to bone in a manner to spread the load over the largest possible bone-prosthesis interface)
- The rate of production of wear debris should be minimized
- The debris that is produced should be as innocuous as possible
- The probability of infection occurring should be minimized
- The consequences of any infection that should occur should be minimized
- A standard insertion procedure should be available that will allow the desired alignment to be obtained in previously deformed or unstable knees
- The prosthesis when implanted should offer movement from 5 degrees of hyperextension to at least 90 degrees of flexion
- Some freedom of rotation (particularly in flexion) and adduction or abduction should be provided
- Excessive movements in any direction should be resisted by force systems that include the soft tissues and do not loosen or break the bone-prosthesis junctions
- It is unwise to depend on the functioning of the cruciate ligaments for the correct functioning of the prosthesis
- The prosthesis should permit the removal of the intercondylar tissues in the knee and should restore cruciate function
- It is desirable to make the tibiofemoral replacement able to accommodate the patella itself or a prosthetic

posterior surface to the patella in those patients who need it

- The cost of the prosthesis should be minimized

Changes are being made to implants to accommodate greater degrees of motion. These so called "high flexion" knee implants have become popular, yet no data exists to show improved motion. There is also concern that the changes made decrease the longevity of these implants. It will take 15 to 20 years until the real answer is known.

Increased interest has also flourished in the field of mobile-bearing implants. Mobile-bearing implants are now available for revision of failed TKAs. The mobile-bearing revision system has also been introduced with metaphyseal sleeves to reconstruct bone loss. Both of these ideas are new and long-term results have not been studied.

Another recent idea in TKA design is the introduction of Gender Solutions knee by Zimmer Inc, which attempts to more accurately match the female knee anatomy. Women have a higher Q angle, with a more valgus knee. The "female knee" accounts for women's increased Q angle with an increased angulation of the femoral trochlear groove of 3 degrees, allowing for better patellar tracking. The prosthesis also has a thinner femoral anterior flange to avoid overstuffing the anterior knee since the female knee has less bone anteriorly than the male counterpart. Women also have an increased aspect ratio of the distal femur of 0.9, in comparison to the male 0.8.[41] To account for this, surgeons often downsize the femoral component when operating on a female patient to minimize overhang of the prosthesis, which risks notching the anterior femoral cortex or opening the flexion gap. The Gender Solutions knee has an aspect ratio of 0.9 to more accurately match the shape of the female distal femur. Although this concept deserves further exploration, many remain skeptical and believe that gender knee is an extension of size matching. In the early days of knee replacement, the size options for all systems were limited. Most systems now offer a wide variety of sizes, so it is easier to match native bone sizes with implants.

## Changes in Knee Arthroplasty Surgery

It is not only the prostheses and materials that have undergone rapid changes over the past century. There have been great innovations in operative technique as well as postoperative protocols that have been very effective at reducing complications and improving patient outcomes following surgery.

Infection was the most common complication following surgery in the early days of arthroplasty.[12] It remains one of the most devastating complications of TKA today. The use of sterile instruments and implants, meticulous sterile technique, preoperative prophylactic antibiotics,[42] antibiotic-impregnated cement,[43] laminar flow air circulation in the operating theater,[44] limiting the traffic of personnel in and out of the room during surgery, and early treatment of any symptoms suspicious for infection have significantly reduced the infection rates for TKA, with many institutions publishing infection rates less than 1%.[45]

Anesthesia for TKA has evolved considerably. TKA is now performed mostly under regional anesthesia, with all its proven benefits such as reduced blood loss, better pain control, and reduced cardiopulmonary and thromboembolic complications.[46,47] In addition, patients are screened preoperatively for cardiac and medical comorbidities, and their risk factors managed perioperatively to improve patient outcomes. This affects not only the cardiac morbidity of the surgery, but also helps to decrease the wound complication rates and infections (ie, by diabetes management, nutritional support). The operations are also considerably shorter today than they were 50 years ago because the instrumentation has improved and the experience of the surgical and nursing personnel has increased substantially for this procedure. The shorter intraoperative time allows for less blood loss, a decreased risk of infection, and less cardiopulmonary morbidity for the procedure.

The incisions used for TKA have also changed significantly over the years. In the early part of the 20th century, a U-shaped incision ending distal to the tibial tubercle with the limbs of the U extending out past the collateral ligaments was the standard incision.[2,6] A tibial tubercle osteotomy was also commonly performed for exposure.[2,6] This type of incision likely also contributed to the high infection rate and was the cause of certain TKA failures due to skin slough or failure of the skin to heal. The move to a long medial parapatellar approach to the knee was an important improvement to the surgical technique.[9] In modern day, there is controversy over minimally invasive surgery for total joint arthroplasty. Minimally invasive techniques in TKA surgery include a limited medial parapatellar incision and arthrotomy with subluxation but not eversion of the patella. A subvastus approach to the knee joint may also be used, with proponents stating that pain control, quadriceps function, and range of motion are better in the short term after a minimally invasive approach.[48,49] Skeptics of the minimally invasive approach argue that the prostheses are more likely to be malpositioned without the anatomic landmarks visible, and correct implant placement is the most important surgical factor in ensuring a good TKA result. At the time of writing, minimally invasive approaches in TKA have not shown a clear advantage over the medial parapatellar approach, which would still be considered the gold standard in this regard.

Instrumentation for TKA has evolved substantially since the time of the first condylar arthroplasties. The pioneers in the field such as Insall and Freeman made their own instruments for insertion of their arthroplasty devices.[26] Today, there are a multitude of prostheses on the market, each with their own specific instrumentation and jigs. Most of the jigs and guides have become user-friendly and are specific both to the prosthesis as well as the surgical technique being used. Likewise, the removal of the prostheses has been made much easier by the manufacture of specific removal tools for the various implants.

The instrumentation for TKA continues to evolve. Computer navigation is being used more frequently as a means of determining the position of the bone cuts and the placement of the prosthesis and is also an excellent tool for aligning the implants along the mechanical axis of the leg, irrespective of other deformities in the limb that may impede the use of intramedullary alignment devices.[50] It is now also being used to measure joint range of motion and knee stability. Although the computer navigation does offer improvements in the accuracy and reproducibility of the implant positioning, this has not yet translated into improved clinical outcomes for patients or into better wear characteristics of the bearing surfaces.[51] It remains to be seen whether this improved accuracy will correlate with a long-term clinical benefit. One benefit of computer navigation is to allow correct placement of TKA prosthetics through minimal incision surgical techniques; the computer in this case may act as the surgeon's frame of reference for prosthetic placement when the usual intraarticular landmarks cannot be visualized.[52] Other uses of computers for TKA will likely be found in the future, and robots are already being conceived to aid in the surgical practice of TKA.[53]

The postoperative protocol for TKA has undergone substantial changes from the early days until the present. Early postoperative regimens often had patients confined to bed for 3 weeks or more, with the leg bandaged and not allowing any exercise of the limb. Weight bearing was often not commenced before 6 weeks, and patients could expect a hospital stay of 1 month or longer. Today, patients are no longer being kept nonweight bearing following TKA and are encouraged to begin weight bearing on the first postoperative day. Physiotherapy begins from day 1, performing active and passive range of motion immediately. Pain control is much better managed in present times, and patients can expect a cocktail of postoperative analgesics as well as regional blocks or epidurals. Patients often leave the hospital 3 days postoperatively, and sometimes sooner. Thromboprophylaxis is the standard of care. All of these innovations have contributed to decreasing the morbidity and mortality associated with TKA.

The patient population served by TKA has also changed throughout the course of the procedure's history. At the turn of the century, arthroplasty was used on select patients with knee disease due to traumatic injuries, tuberculosis, septic arthritis, often gonococcal in nature, and rheumatoid arthritis. Today, tuberculous disease of the joints is seen rarely in developed nations, and septic arthritis and traumatic injuries are usually treated aggressively to preserve the joint as much as possible. The patient populations seen most commonly as candidates for TKA today are those with osteoarthritis and rheumatoid arthritis.

## Expanding Indications for Total Knee Arthroplasty

All of these improvements in TKA have made the procedure safer and more successful than at any other point in history. Because of this, the indications for TKA are broadening, and more patients can now be considered candidates for the procedure. Previously, TKAs were not performed in young and active patients because it was believed that they would wear out the implants. Likewise, TKAs were not advised for the elderly because it was believed that they could not withstand such invasive surgery nor the rehabilitation. Patients with multiple joint rheumatoid involvement were discouraged from undergoing the surgery because they would continue to have handicaps. Today, TKAs are more durable than ever and patients are encouraged to maintain a relatively active lifestyle postoperatively. The advances in anesthesia have meant that the elderly can survive and benefit from the surgery. Those with multiple joint involvement may undergo multiple procedures to maximize their function in spite of their disease.

The revision of failed TKAs is also a significant improvement that has occurred over the past 50 years. Previously, failed TKAs were treated with arthrodesis or amputation because there were no other options available. Today, it would be the rare case that would require such a drastic surgery because revision implants are available that can make up for bone defects as well as ligamentous deficiencies. These revision implants also provide the option of TKA for patients with difficult deformities who would not have been considered for TKA prior to the innovation of these implants.

## Summary

TKA, as a surgical procedure, has undergone an amazing evolution over the past 100 years. As the indications for TKA continue to expand, and as the implants and surgical techniques become more refined, patients will continue to demand better function, more durability, and a more "natural" feel from their TKA. In response to these demands, we can expect to see continued evolution of the TKA for many years to come.

## References


1. Ferguson M. Excision of the knee joint: recovery with a false joint and a useful limb. *Med Times Gazette.* 1861;1:601.
2. Allison N, Brooks B. Arthroplasty: experimental and clinical methods. *J Bone Joint Surg Am.* 1918;s2-16:83-93.
3. Herndon CH, Chase SW. Experimental studies in the transplantation of whole joints. *J Bone Joint Surg Am.* 1952;34:564-578.
4. Lexer E. Joint transplantations and arthroplasty. *Surg Gynec Obstet.* 1925;40:782-809.
5. Murphy JB. Arthroplasty of ankylosed joints. *Trans Am Surg Assoc.* 1913;31:67-137.
6. Putti V. Arthroplasty of the knee joint. *J Bone Joint Surg Am.* 1920;2(9):530-534.
7. Albee FH. Original features in arthroplasty of the knee with improved prognosis. *Surg Gynec Obstet.* 1928;47:312.
8. Miller A, Friedman B. Fascial arthroplasty of the knee. *J Bone Joint Surg Am.* 1952;34:55-63.
9. Campbell WC. Arthroplasty of the knee: report of cases. *J Bone Joint Surg Am.* 1921;3:430-434.
10. Brown JE, McGaw WH, Shaw DT. Use of cutis as an interposing membrane in arthroplasty of the knee. *J Bone Joint Surg Am.* 1958;40:1003-1018.
11. Baer WS. Arthroplasty with the aid of animal membrane. *J Bone Joint Surg Am.* 1918;s2-16:171-199.
12. Henderson MS. What are the real results of arthroplasty? *J Bone Joint Surg Am.* 1918;s2-16:30-33.
13. Kuhns JG, Potter TA, Hormell RS, Elliston WA. Nylon membrane arthroplasty of the knee in chronic arthritis. *J Bone Joint Surg Am.* 1953;35:929-936.
14. Yamada K, Shinno N. Arthroplasty of the knee: a follow-up study of fifty-four cases treated by operative reconstruction of the sliding apparatus of the knee. *J Bone Joint Surg Am.* 1969;51:1480-1488.
15. Campbell WC. Interposition of vitallium plates in arthroplasties of the knee: preliminary report. *Am J Surg.* 1940;47(3):639-641.
16. MacIntosh DL. Hemiarthroplasty of the knee using a space occupying prosthesis for painful varus and valgus deformities. *J Bone Joint Surg Am.* 1958;40:1431.
17. McKeever DC. Tibial plateau prosthesis. *Clin Orthop.* 1960;18:86-95.
18. Potter TA, Weinfeld MS, Thomas WH. Arthroplasty of the knee in rheumatoid arthritis and osteoarthritis: a follow-up study after implantation of the McKeever and MacIntosh prostheses. *J Bone Joint Surg Am.* 1972;54:1-24.
19. Jones WN. Mold Arthroplasty of the Knee. Paper read at the Annual Meeting of The American Academy of Orthopaedic Surgeons; San Francisco, CA; January 1967.
20. Moeys EJ. Metal alloplasty of the knee joint: an experimental study. *J Bone Joint Surg Am.* 1954;36:363-367.
21. Walldius B. Arthroplasty of the knee using acrylic prosthesis. *Acta Orthop Scand.* 1953;23(2):121-131.
22. Shetty AA, Tindall A, Ting P, Heatley FW. The evolution of total knee arthroplasty. Part II: the hinged knee replacement and the semi-constrained knee replacement. *Curr Orthop.* 2003;17:403-407.
23. Shiers LG. Arthroplasty of the knee: interim report of a new method. *J Bone Joint Surg Br.* 1960;42:31-39.
24. Arden GP. Computer aided analysis of total knee replacement. *Ann Rheum Dis.* 1983;42(4):415-420.
25. Young HH. Use of a hinged vitallium prosthesis for total knee arthroplasty: a preliminary report. *J Bone Joint Surg Am.* 1963;45:1627-1642.
26. Robinson RP. The early innovators of today's resurfacing condylar knees. *J Arthroplasty.* 2005;20(1)s1:2-26.
27. Gunston FH. Polycentric knee arthroplasty: prosthetic simulation of normal knee movement. *J Bone Joint Surg Br.* 1971;53(2):272-277.
28. Yamamoto S, Nakata S, Kondoh Y. A follow-up study of an uncemented knee replacement: the results of 312 knees using the Kodama-Yamamoto prosthesis. *J Bone Joint Surg Br.* 1989;71(3):505-508.
29. Haas J. Functional arthroplasty. *J Bone Joint Surg Am.* 1944;26(2):297-306.
30. Freeman MAR, Swanson SAV, Todd RC. The classic: total replacement of the knee using the Freeman-Swanson knee prosthesis. *Clin Orthop Rel Res.* 2003;416:4-22.
31. Goldberg VM, Henderson BT. The Freeman-Swanson ICHL total knee arthroplasty: complications and problems. *J Bone Joint Surg Am.* 1980;62:1338-1344.
32. Insall J, Ranawat CS, Scott WN, Walker P. Total condylar knee replacement: Preliminary report. *Clin Orthop.* 1976;120:148-154.
33. Riley LH Jr. Geometric total knee replacement: operative considerations. *Orthop Clin North Am.* 1973;4:561-573.
34. Eftekhar NS. Total knee-replacement arthroplasty: results with the intramedullary adjustable total knee prosthesis. *J Bone Joint Surg Am.* 1983;65:293.
35. Hungerford DS, Kenna RV, Krackow KA. The porous-coated anatomic total knee. *Orthop Clin North Am.* 1982;13:103.
36. Collier JP, Sperling DK, Currier JH, et al. Impact of gamma sterilization on clinical performance of polyethylene in the knee. *J Arthroplasty.* 1996;11:377-389.

37. Bohl JR, Bohl WR, Postak PD, Greenwald AS. The Coventry Award: the effects of shelf life on clinical outcome for gamma sterilized polyethylene tibial components. *Clin Orthop Rel Res.* 1999;367:28-38.

38. Nasser S, Poggie RA. Revision and salvage patellar arthroplasty using a porous tantalum implant. *J Arthroplasty.* 2004;19(5):562-572.

39. Levine B, Sporer S, Della Valle CJ, Jacobs JJ, Paprosky W. Porous tantalum in reconstructive surgery of the knee: a review. *J Knee Surg.* 2007;20(3):185-194.

40. Freeman MAR, Swanson SAV, Todd RC. Total replacement of the knee using the Freeman-Swanson knee prosthesis. *Clin Orthop Rel Res.* 1973;94:153-170.

41. Booth RE Jr. Sex and the total knee: gender-sensitive designs. *Orthopedics.* 2006;29(9):836-840.

42. Marculescu CE, Osmon DR. Antibiotic prophylaxis in orthopedic prosthetic surgery. *Infect Dis Clin North Am.* 2005;19(4):931-946.

43. Bourne RB. Prophylactic use of antibiotic bone cement: an emerging standard—in the affirmative. *J Arthroplasty.* 2004;19(4 Suppl 1):69-72.

44. Kakwani RG, Yohannan D, Wahab KH. The effect of laminar air-flow on the results of Austin-Moore hemiarthroplasty. *Injury.* 2007;38(7):820-823.

45. Peersman G, Laskin R, Davis J, Peterson M. Infection in total knee replacement: a retrospective review of 6489 total knee replacements. *Clin Orthop Relat Res.* 2001;(392):15-23.

46. Delis KT, Knaggs AL, Mason P, Macleod KG. Effects of epidural and general anesthesia combined versus general anesthesia alone on the venous hemodynamics of the lower limb: a randomized study. *Thromb Haemost.* 2004;92(5):1003-1011.

47. Hollmann MW, Wieczorek KS, Smart M, Durieux ME. Epidural anesthesia prevents hypercoagulation in patients undergoing major orthopedic surgery. *Reg Anesth Pain Med.* 2001;26(3):215-222.

48. Laskin RS. Minimally invasive total knee replacement using a mini-mid vastus incision technique and results. *Surg Technol Int.* 2004;13:231-238.

49. Laskin RS, Beksac B, Phongjunakorn A, et al. Minimally invasive total knee replacement through a mini-midvastus incision: an outcome study. *Clin Orthop Relat Res.* 2004;428:74-81.

50. Decking R, Markmann Y, Fuchs J, Puhl W, Scharf HP. Leg axis after computer-navigated total knee arthroplasty: a prospective randomized trial comparing computer-navigated and manual implantation. *J Arthroplasty.* 2005;20(3):282-288.

51. Decking R, Markmann Y, Mattes T, Puhl W, Scharf HP. On the outcome of computer-assisted total knee replacement. *Acta Chir Orthop Traumatol Cech.* 2007;74(3):171-174.

52. Stulberg SD. Minimally invasive navigated knee surgery: an American perspective. *Orthopedics.* 2005;28(10 Suppl):s1241-s1246.

53. Shi F, Zhang J, Liu Y, Zhao Z. A hand-eye robotic model for total knee replacement surgery. *Med Image Comput Comput Assist Interv.* 2005;8(Pt 2):122-130.

# 7

# Indications for Total Knee Arthroplasty

*Harvey E. Smith, MD and Craig J. Della Valle, MD*

Osteoarthritis in the United States has an estimated annual cost of 65 billion dollars[1] in terms of both medical expenses and lost days from work. In the United States, the incidence and prevalence of osteoarthritis are increasing for reasons that have yet to be fully identified. An estimated 27 million adults in the United States have clinical osteoarthritis,[2] and the prevalence of osteoarthritis in the United States is anticipated to rise to 59 million people (18% of the population) by 2020.[3,4] Osteoarthritis of the knee has an incidence reported to range from 164 to 240 per 100,000 person-years.[3,5] The demographic of individuals over the age of 65 is increasing, and both the incidence and prevalence of osteoarthritis correlate with population age.[1,6] As a population, the average body mass index (BMI) is increasing, and weight has been demonstrated to correlate with the development of knee osteoarthritis.[7,8] Medical advances in magnetic resonance imaging (MRI)[9] as well as increased patient awareness may also contribute to earlier presentation and diagnosis. The combination of an increasing elderly demographic, increasing BMI, and increased awareness and diagnostic sensitivity suggests that osteoarthritis will become an even larger problem in the coming decades.[10]

The diagnosis of osteoarthritis likely encompasses what is increasingly suspected to be many different disease processes with a common endpoint of articular cartilage loss and joint destruction. The etiology is multifactorial and suspected to include a genetic component,[3,11-13] anatomic predisposition to disease progression due to limb alignment,[3,8,14-16] occupation and lifestyle,[1] medical comorbidities,[17] and age.[6]

Most cases of osteoarthritis are currently classified as idiopathic; other commonly reported causes are inflammatory arthritis, anatomic deformity, traumatic injury, hemophilia, avascular necrosis, and Paget's disease. Deformity of the knee may be either congenital or acquired; irrespective of etiology, the altered anatomic axis results in medial or lateral shift of the mechanical axis, with resultant disproportionate loading and shear forces in the respective compartment.[18] Cross-sectional studies have demonstrated a correlation between joint injury and the subsequent development of osteoarthritis.[3,19] Trauma to the joint may result in subsequent arthritis due to direct cartilage injury, ligamentous or muscular injury altering joint stability and biomechanics, or fracture deformity altering the natural joint alignment.

Although the etiology is multifactorial, the clinical course of osteoarthritis is well described. Injury or degeneration of the collagen matrix decreases its efficacy in constraining the proteoglycans; unconstrained, the hydroscopic proteoglycans swell, while at the same time lose their stiffness to compressibility.[20] This decreased stiffness to compressibility decreases the ability of the solid matrix to dissipate the energy of compressive loads through the frictional drag of water molecules through the matrix.[21-26] Consequently, a higher proportion of the load is transmitted to the solid matrix, resulting in increased solid matrix destruction. The end result is loss of cartilage and subsequent collapse of the joint space.



Parvizi J, Klatt B.
*Essentials in Total Knee Arthroplasty* (pp 55-60).

# The Decision for Operative Management

Total knee arthroplasty (TKA) is arguably one of the most successful operations in terms of patient satisfaction, improvement in function, success rate of the procedure, and alleviation of pain and suffering. Given the success of the procedure, there is surprisingly little agreement among physicians regarding indications for the procedure.[27] Cross et al[27] in a review of the literature found poor levels of consensus among rheumatologists, family practitioners, internists, and orthopedists regarding clinical agreement for proceeding with or referring a patient for TKA. This is confounded by the variety of physician specialties to which the patient may present for initial evaluation. Patients may present for initial evaluation to a family medicine physician, rheumatologist, internist, or orthopedic surgeon. Similarly, a review of the literature by Kane et al[28] demonstrated that the scientific quality of current evidence is too weak to make specific recommendations about indications.

The lack of a defined algorithm or a decision-tree that delineates exact criteria for TKA is indicative not of the procedure (the literature is clear that patients' function measured by either physician-reported or patient-reported indices is consistently and reproducibly improved by TKA and there is reliable alleviation of pain[28-32]) but of the varied nature of disease presentation.

A broad spectrum of diseases may present with knee pain due to a variety of pathologies with a common endpoint of joint destruction with pain and loss of function. It is the responsibility of the orthopedist to confirm with physical examination and imaging studies that the patient's pain and loss of function are amenable to surgical management. Imaging studies should include standing weight-bearing anteroposterior views, 45-degree flexion weight-bearing posteroanterior views, lateral view, and Merchant view.[20] Classic technique requires long alignment view to plan mechanical axis correction, but this image is not always included in a standard series. Although subchondral edema on MRI has been postulated to portend more rapid progression of disease,[9] MRI imaging is not at this time considered part of the standard imaging series. Issues that must be considered are how the patient's quality of life is affected, timing of potential surgery, and a clear discussion of relative risks and benefits so that the patient may make an informed decision. Relative issues that must be considered are the age of the patient (younger patients have a higher risk of subsequent revision surgery due to implant failure whereas older patients generally have a higher prevalence of comorbidities), medical comorbidities that may increase perioperative morbidity and affect surgical outcome, patient activity level, and postoperative expectations. In part due to the high rate of immediate success of the procedure, it is incumbent upon the orthopedist to at times temper the enthusiasm of the patient and referring physician for surgery in favor of nonoperative measures.

A trial of nonoperative treatment is warranted in almost all cases for patients presenting for evaluation of the arthritic knee. TKA has risks that, although low in incidence, may be severe. Pain and loss of function are generally the symptoms that lead to referral for evaluation, and an attempt to ameliorate these symptoms may forestall surgical intervention entirely in some cases or delay it by several years. Although the ultimate lifespan of current implant technology remains to be determined, it is intuitively desirable to delay surgery if an acceptable quality of life for the patient can be obtained via nonoperative measures, particularly in younger patients.

Nonoperative management of arthritis[33] includes anti-inflammatory medications, acetaminophen, the use of an assist device, activity modification, physical therapy, intra-articular injections of hyaluronic acid derivatives,[34,35] and corticosteroid injections.[36,37] Hyaluronic acid derivatives have been shown in some studies to alleviate symptoms sufficiently to delay progression to knee replacement surgery by a median of 2.1 years.[35] An unloader brace may provide some relief for patients with a disease affecting predominantly the medial compartment.[38] Although nonoperative management may offer varying degrees of symptomatic alleviation, there remains no established method to repair or replace articular cartilage. Consequently, although nonoperative therapies may alleviate the symptoms of disease, no validated method has been shown to reverse the disease process; most patients will have progression of disease and symptoms. The role of the orthopedist is to ascertain when the patient feels the pain and detriment to his or her quality of life is significant enough to eschew nonoperative management in favor of arthroplasty.

## Patient-Specific Considerations

By definition of its elective nature, TKA has no absolute indications. There are, however, many relative patient-specific factors to consider in developing a treatment plan.

The first patient-modifying factor to consider is age. With earlier generation knee replacements there was concern regarding the longevity of the implant, and the assumption that a relatively young (less than 60 years of age) patient would likely need a revision procedure. Given the loss of bone stock with polyethylene wear, presumed increased activity of younger patients, and concerns about a substantial probability of at least one revision procedure, orthopedists historically viewed younger age as a relative contraindication to TKA. The development of polyethylene-bearing surfaces with improved wear characteristics and improved confidence in the longevity of the newer generation implants has resulted in an increasing number of younger patients undergoing knee replacement. To date, the results in these younger cohorts have been comparable to older patients.[39,40] From a therapeutic perspective, restoring function to individuals in their younger years with arthritis has a profound effect on their quality of life and is intuitively more desirable than requiring patients live with disability and pain until they have reached what has been considered a more appropriate age, particularly in the younger patient with inflammatory polyarthropathies.[41] It should be stressed, however, that results in younger (less than 50 years of age) cohorts are generally of a preliminary nature and include relatively small numbers of patients.

Older patients (defined in various studies ranging from over 65 years of age to 90 years of age) have higher acute complication rates relative to younger patients[42-45] but overall outcomes that are generally comparable to younger patients.[46,47] These results suggest that the overall health status and lifestyle of the patient need to be considered over chronological age, and advanced age may not be a contraindication for a patient with acceptable medical risk for whom joint replacement will improve quality of life.

Any major medical comorbidity adversely affects surgical risks; an inclusive discussion of all such comorbidities is beyond the scope of this chapter, but it is imperative that every patient has a thorough preoperative medical evaluation. Due to its increasing prevalence and association with obesity, diabetes mellitus merits specific mention. Type II diabetes is recognized at such an increasing rate that some have termed it an epidemic.[48] The diabetic patient is at higher risk for wound infection[49-52] and has lower functional scores compared to matched controls.[52,53]

For optimal results, TKA necessitates patient compliance with postoperative physical therapy and range of motion exercises. Patients with dementia or psychological factors that the physician believes would result in poor compliance with postoperative care should be considered a population in which knee replacement may be contraindicated. Similarly, patients involved in competitive sports or manual laborers need to be educated on the expectation that they must substantially modify their activity postoperatively; a patient that is unwilling to modify his or her activity may not be an appropriate candidate. The heavy laborer may be better suited with nonoperative management until he or she is able to change his or her job requirements or consider a knee arthrodesis. Patients receiving workman's compensation have been shown to have significantly worse outcomes compared to matched controls with respect to subjective findings.[54]

Obese patients have shown similar improvements after TKA when compared to nonobese patients.[55-57] Morbidly obese patients have been demonstrated to have a higher rate of perioperative complications, particularly wound drainage, infections, and medial collateral ligament avulsion.[58-60] Nutritional status should also be assessed preoperatively, because obese patients as a population have a higher incidence of malnutrition, particularly with respect to protein stores.

TKA for the treatment of post-traumatic arthritis presents several technical challenges for which the surgeon should be prepared. Due to either sequelae of the injury mechanism or prior surgical procedures on the joint, there may be a compromised soft tissue envelope and prior surgical incisions. Preoperative consultation with a plastic surgeon may be warranted, and the soft tissue envelope should be closely monitored postoperatively for any early signs of tissue ischemia. Any post-traumatic deformities or soft tissue contractures may complicate soft tissue balancing. A higher rate of infection has been noted when TKA is performed in the setting of prior surgeries for trauma, and some have advocated preoperative joint aspiration in this setting to exclude infection.[61,62]

Deficiency of the extensor mechanism, neuropathic arthropathy, severe peripheral vascular disease, and a compromised soft tissue envelope are relative contraindications to TKA.[63,64] Total knee replacement in the setting of neuropathic arthropathy has a higher rate of complication and failure,[65] and the surgeon must be prepared to address significant bone defects and associated soft tissue imbalances; implants and techniques used in complex revisions may be necessary.[66]

Extensor mechanism deficiency is problematic as the altered force vectors result in knee instability. Extensor mechanism reconstruction has been reported with both allograft[67-69] and connective tissue prosthesis.[70] Extensor mechanism reconstruction has been demonstrated to improve functional status with a patient satisfaction approaching 90%, but persistent extensor lag is common.[71] These factors are summarized in Table 7-1.

Active infection and inability of the patient to medically tolerate the procedure are absolute contraindications to TKA.[63,64] A history of prior infection[72] necessitates exclusion of any current infection by laboratory evaluation (complete blood count, C-reactive protein, and erythrocyte sedimentation rate)[73] and joint aspiration.

Table 7-1

**RELATIVE AND ABSOLUTE CONTRAINDICATIONS TO TOTAL KNEE ARTHROPLASTY**

| *RELATIVE CONSIDERATIONS* | | *REFERENCES* |
|---|---|---|
| Age < 55 | Newer implants comparable results to older cohorts | Gill et al[39]<br>Gioe et al[40] |
| Adolescent | May be indicated with debilitating polyarthropathy | Cage et al[41]<br>Parvizi et al[66] |
| Workman's compensation | Worse outcomes than matched controls | Mont et al[54] |
| Obesity | Increased perioperative complications<br>Long-term results comparable to nonobese | Patel et al[58]<br>Miric et al[59]<br>Winiarsky et al[60]<br>Deshmukh et al[55]<br>Stickles et al[56]<br>Amin et al[57] |
| Post-traumatic arthritis | Higher rate of infection if prior open reduction internal fixation | Saleh et al[61]<br>Roffi and Merritt[62] |
| Extensor mechanism deficiency | Instability<br>Extensor lag with reconstruction | Emerson et al[67]<br>Emerson et al[68]<br>Burde and Sweeney[69]<br>Sherief et al[70]<br>Burnett et al[71] |
| Neuropathic arthropathy | Higher rate failure<br>Technically challenging | Kim et al[65]<br>Parvizi et al[66] |
| History prior infection | Must exclude current infection<br>Higher postoperative infection rate | Lee et al[72]<br>Greidanus et al[73] |
| *ABSOLUTE CONTRAINDICATIONS* | | |
| Active infection | | |
| Inability to tolerate procedure | | |
| Inability to comply with postoperative care | | |

TKA provides consistently good results and has been demonstrated to reproducibly alleviate pain from arthritis, correct deformity, and restore function. Due to the wide spectrum of conditions that may contribute to degeneration of the knee, a defined algorithm of when to operate does not exist. The expected long-term results of the operation, including the potential need and complexity of any revision procedures, will vary based on patient-specific and disease-specific factors. It is the responsibility of the orthopedist to weigh the patient-specific factors and consider the impact of disease on the patient's quality of life so that an informed decision can be made in concert with the patient on when to proceed to operative management.

## REFERENCES

1. Garstang SV, Stitik TP. Osteoarthritis: epidemiology, risk factors, and pathophysiology. *Am J Phys Med Rehabil.* 2006;85: S2-11; quiz S2-4.
2. Lawrence RC, Felson DT, Helmick CG, et al. Estimates of the prevalence of arthritis and other rheumatic conditions in the United States: part II. *Arthritis Rheum.* 2007;58:26-35.
3. Sharma L, Kapoor D, Issa S. Epidemiology of osteoarthritis: an update. *Curr Opin Rheumatol.* 2006;18:147-156.
4. Lawrence RC, Helmick CG, Arnett FC, et al. Estimates of the prevalence of arthritis and selected musculoskeletal disorders in the United States. *Arthritis Rheum.* 1998;41:778-799.
5. Wilson MG, Michet CJ Jr, Ilstrup DM, et al. Idiopathic symptomatic osteoarthritis of the hip and knee: a population-based incidence study. *Mayo Clin Proc.* 1990;65:1214-1221.

6. Oliveria SA, Felson DT, Reed JI, et al. Incidence of symptomatic hand, hip, and knee osteoarthritis among patients in a health maintenance organization. *Arthritis Rheum.* 1995;38:1134-1141.
7. Felson DT, Anderson JJ, Naimark A, et al. Obesity and knee osteoarthritis. The Framingham Study. *Ann Intern Med.* 1988;109:18-24.
8. Sharma L, Lou C, Cahue S, et al. The mechanism of the effect of obesity in knee osteoarthritis: the mediating role of malalignment. *Arthritis Rheum.* 2000;43:568-575.
9. Felson DT, McLaughlin S, Goggins J, et al. Bone marrow edema and its relation to progression of knee osteoarthritis. *Ann Intern Med.* 2003;139:330-336.
10. Issa SN, Sharma L. Epidemiology of osteoarthritis: an update. *Curr Rheumatol Rep.* 2006;8:7-15.
11. Neame RL, Muir K, Doherty S, et al. Genetic risk of knee osteoarthritis: a sibling study. *Ann Rheum Dis.* 2004;63:1022-1027.
12. Loughlin J. The genetic epidemiology of human primary OA: current status. *Expert Rev Mol Med.* 2005;7:1-12.
13. Zhang W, Doherty M. How important are genetic factors in osteoarthritis? Contributions from family studies. *J Rheumatol.* 2005;32:1139-1142.
14. Felson DT, Goggins J, Niu J, et al. The effect of body weight on progression of knee osteoarthritis is dependent on alignment. *Arthritis Rheum.* 2004;50:3904-3909.
15. Lohmander LS, Felson D. Can we identify a "high risk" patient profile to determine who will experience rapid progression of osteoarthritis? *Osteoarthritis Cartilage.* 2004;12 (Suppl A):S49-S52.
16. Hunter DJ, Niu J, Felson DT, et al. Knee alignment does not predict incident osteoarthritis: the Framingham osteoarthritis study. *Arthritis Rheum.* 2007;56:1212-1218.
17. Gabriel SE, Crowson CS, O'Fallon WM. Comorbidity in arthritis. *J Rheumatol.* 1999;26:2475-2479.
18. Sharma L, Song J, Felson DT, et al. The role of knee alignment in disease progression and functional decline in knee osteoarthritis. *JAMA.* 2001;286:188-195.
19. Gelber AC, Hochberg MC, Mead LA, et al. Joint injury in young adults and risk for subsequent knee and hip osteoarthritis. *Ann Intern Med.* 2000;133:321-328.
20. Cole BJ, Harner CD. Degenerative arthritis of the knee in active patients: evaluation and management. *J Am Acad Orthop Surg.* 1999;7:389-402.
21. Maroudas AI. Balance between swelling pressure and collagen tension in normal and degenerate cartilage. *Nature.* 1976;260:808-809.
22. Maroudas A, Ziv I, Weisman N, et al. Studies of hydration and swelling pressure in normal and osteoarthritic cartilage. *Biorheology.* 1985;22:159-169.
23. Maroudas A, Venn M. Chemical composition and swelling of normal and osteoarthrotic femoral head cartilage. II. Swelling. *Ann Rheum Dis.* 1977;36:399-406.
24. Venn M, Maroudas A. Chemical composition and swelling of normal and osteoarthrotic femoral head cartilage. I. Chemical composition. *Ann Rheum Dis.* 1977;36:121-129.
25. Bank RA, Soudry M, Maroudas A, et al. The increased swelling and instantaneous deformation of osteoarthritic cartilage is highly correlated with collagen degradation. *Arthritis Rheum.* 2000;43:2202-2210.
26. Basser PJ, Schneiderman R, Bank RA, et al. Mechanical properties of the collagen network in human articular cartilage as measured by osmotic stress technique. *Arch Biochem Biophys.* 1998;351:207-219.
27. Cross WW 3rd, Saleh KJ, Wilt TJ, et al. Agreement about indications for total knee arthroplasty. *Clin Orthop Relat Res.* 2006;446:34-39.
28. Kane RL, Saleh KJ, Wilt TJ, et al. The functional outcomes of total knee arthroplasty. *J Bone Joint Surg Am.* 2005;87:1719-1724.
29. Furnes O, Espehaug B, Lie SA, et al. Early failures among 7,174 primary total knee replacements: a follow-up study from the Norwegian Arthroplasty Register 1994-2000. *Acta Orthop Scand.* 2002;73:117-129.
30. Robertsson O, Scott G, Freeman MA. Ten-year survival of the cemented Freeman-Samuelson primary knee arthroplasty. Data from the Swedish Knee Arthroplasty Register and the Royal London Hospital. *J Bone Joint Surg Br.* 2000;82:506-507.
31. Robertsson O, Dunbar M, Pehrsson T, et al. Patient satisfaction after knee arthroplasty: a report on 27,372 knees operated on between 1981 and 1995 in Sweden. *Acta Orthop Scand.* 2000;71:262-267.
32. Robertsson O, Knutson K, Lewold S, et al. The Swedish Knee Arthroplasty Register 1975-1997: an update with special emphasis on 41,223 knees operated on in 1988-1997. *Acta Orthop Scand.* 2001;72:503-513.
33. Gartlan J, Nelson M, Jones G. Osteoarthritis management of the knee: treatment options post the NSAID cardiotoxicity controversy. *Aust Fam Physician.* 2007;36:717-718.
34. Waddell DD. Viscosupplementation with hyaluronans for osteoarthritis of the knee: clinical efficacy and economic implications. *Drugs Aging.* 2007;24:629-642.
35. Waddell DD, Bricker DC. Total knee replacement delayed with Hylan G-F 20 use in patients with grade IV osteoarthritis. *J Manag Care Pharm.* 2007;13:113-121.
36. Bellamy N, Campbell J, Robinson V, et al. Intraarticular corticosteroid for treatment of osteoarthritis of the knee. *Cochrane Database Syst Rev.* 2006:CD005328.
37. Schumacher HR, Chen LX. Injectable corticosteroids in treatment of arthritis of the knee. *Am J Med.* 2005;118:1208-1214.
38. Hewett TE, Noyes FR, Barber-Westin SD, et al. Decrease in knee joint pain and increase in function in patients with medial compartment arthrosis: a prospective analysis of valgus bracing. *Orthopedics.* 1998;21:131-138.
39. Gill GS, Chan KC, Mills DM. 5- to 18-year follow-up study of cemented total knee arthroplasty for patients 55 years old or younger. *J Arthroplasty.* 1997;12:49-54.
40. Gioe TJ, Novak C, Sinner P, et al. Knee arthroplasty in the young patient: survival in a community registry. *Clin Orthop Relat Res.* 2007;464:83-87.

41. Cage DJ, Granberry WM, Tullos HS. Long-term results of total arthroplasty in adolescents with debilitating polyarthropathy. *Clin Orthop Relat Res.* 1992;283:156-162.

42. SooHoo NF, Lieberman JR, Ko CY, et al. Factors predicting complication rates following total knee replacement. *J Bone Joint Surg Am.* 2006;88:480-485.

43. Pagnano MW, McLamb LA, Trousdale RT. Total knee arthroplasty for patients 90 years of age and older. *Clin Orthop Relat Res.* 2004;418:179-183.

44. Laskin RS. Total knee replacement in patients older than 85 years. *Clin Orthop Relat Res.* 1999;367:43-49.

45. Hosick WB, Lotke PA, Baldwin A. Total knee arthroplasty in patients 80 years of age and older. *Clin Orthop Relat Res.* 1994;299:77-80.

46. Adam RF, Noble J. Primary total knee arthroplasty in the elderly. *J Arthroplasty.* 1994;9:495-497.

47. Dinah A, Mears S. Primary total knee arthroplasty in the elderly. *Curr Opin Orthopedics.* 2008;19:63-67.

48. Mainous AG 3rd, Baker R, Koopman RJ, et al. Impact of the population at risk of diabetes on projections of diabetes burden in the United States: an epidemic on the way. *Diabetologia.* 2007;50:934-940.

49. Lai K, Bohm ER, Burnell C, et al. Presence of medical comorbidities in patients with infected primary hip or knee arthroplasties. *J Arthroplasty.* 2007;22:651-656.

50. Syahrizal AB, Kareem BA, Anbanadan S, et al. Risk factors for infection in total knee replacement surgery at hospital Kuala Lumpur. *Med J Malaysia.* 2001;56 (Suppl D):5-8.

51. Yang K, Yeo SJ, Lee BP, et al. Total knee arthroplasty in diabetic patients: a study of 109 consecutive cases. *J Arthroplasty.* 2001;16:102-106.

52. Serna F, Mont MA, Krackow KA, et al. Total knee arthroplasty in diabetic patients: comparison to a matched control group. *J Arthroplasty.* 1994;9:375-379.

53. Papagelopoulos PJ, Idusuyi OB, Wallrichs SL, et al. Long term outcome and survivorship analysis of primary total knee arthroplasty in patients with diabetes mellitus. *Clin Orthop Relat Res.* 1996;330:124-132.

54. Mont MA, Mayerson JA, Krackow KA, et al. Total knee arthroplasty in patients receiving Workers' Compensation. *J Bone Joint Surg Am.* 1998;80:1285-1290.

55. Deshmukh RG, Hayes JH, Pinder IM. Does body weight influence outcome after total knee arthroplasty? A 1-year analysis. *J Arthroplasty.* 2002;17:315-319.

56. Stickles B, Phillips L, Brox WT, et al. Defining the relationship between obesity and total joint arthroplasty. *Obes Res.* 2001;9:219-223.

57. Amin AK, Patton JT, Cook RE, et al. Does obesity influence the clinical outcome at five years following total knee replacement for osteoarthritis? *J Bone Joint Surg Br.* 2006;88:335-340.

58. Patel VP, Walsh M, Sehgal B, et al. Factors associated with prolonged wound drainage after primary total hip and knee arthroplasty. *J Bone Joint Surg Am.* 2007;89:33-38.

59. Miric A, Lim M, Kahn B, et al. Perioperative morbidity following total knee arthroplasty among obese patients. *J Knee Surg.* 2002;15:77-83.

60. Winiarsky R, Barth P, Lotke P. Total knee arthroplasty in morbidly obese patients. *J Bone Joint Surg Am.* 1998;80:1770-1774.

61. Saleh KJ, Sherman P, Katkin P, et al. Total knee arthroplasty after open reduction and internal fixation of fractures of the tibial plateau: a minimum five-year follow-up study. *J Bone Joint Surg Am.* 2001;83-A:1144-1148.

62. Roffi RP, Merritt PO. Total knee replacement after fractures about the knee. *Orthop Rev.* 1990;19:614-620.

63. Insall J. Indications and contraindications for total knee replacement. In: Insall J, ed. *Surgery of the Knee.* 2nd ed. New York, NY: Churchill Livingstone; 1993:719-721.

64. Thadani PJ, Spitzer AI. Primary total knee arthroplasty: indications and long-term results. *Curr Opin Orthopedics.* 2000;11:41-48.

65. Kim YH, Kim JS, Oh SW. Total knee arthroplasty in neuropathic arthropathy. *J Bone Joint Surg Br.* 2002;84:216-219.

66. Parvizi J, Marrs J, Morrey BF. Total knee arthroplasty for neuropathic (Charcot) joints. *Clin Orthop Relat Res.* 2003;416:145-50.

67. Emerson RH Jr, Head WC, Malinin TI. Reconstruction of patellar tendon rupture after total knee arthroplasty with an extensor mechanism allograft. *Clin Orthop Relat Res.* 1990;154-161.

68. Emerson RH Jr, Head WC, Malinin TI. Extensor mechanism reconstruction with an allograft after total knee arthroplasty. *Clin Orthop Relat Res.* 1994;303:79-85.

69. Burde C, Sweeney P. [Extensor mechanism allograft reconstruction after total knee replacement]. *Orthopade.* 2007;36:372-378.

70. Sherief TI, Naguib AM, Sefton GK. Use of Leeds-Keio connective tissue prosthesis (L-K CTP) for reconstruction of deficient extensor mechanism with total knee replacement. *Knee.* 2005;12:319-322.

71. Burnett RS, Butler RA, Barrack RL. Extensor mechanism allograft reconstruction in TKA at a mean of 56 months. *Clin Orthop Relat Res.* 2006;452:159-165.

72. Lee GC, Pagnano MW, Hanssen AD. Total knee arthroplasty after prior bone or joint sepsis about the knee. *Clin Orthop Relat Res.* 2002;404:226-231.

73. Greidanus NV, Masri BA, Garbuz DS, et al. Use of erythrocyte sedimentation rate and C-reactive protein level to diagnose infection before revision total knee arthroplasty: a prospective evaluation. *J Bone Joint Surg Am.* 2007;89:1409-1416.

# 8

# Preoperative Patient Evaluation for Total Knee Arthroplasty

*Benjamin Bender, MD; Ashok L. Gowda, BS; and Javad Parvizi, MD*

Patients presenting for orthopedic care with an arthritic knee complain primarily of pain and functional decline marked by difficulty walking, climbing stairs, and rising from a seated position. Concerns of deformity and instability may be contributing symptoms that influence the choice of treatment. Prior to surgical intervention, a thorough preoperative evaluation of the patient should be undertaken and should include a thorough history, physical examination, and appropriate imaging studies.

It has been widely recognized that a major source of failure of knee surgery is the inability to live up to unreasonable patient expectations. As a result, it is important for the surgeon to document with specificity the presenting symptoms and objective measures of knee function and performance. Tools that allow for clarification of such patient expectations can help direct care and can provide a baseline against which postintervention outcomes can be compared. General health assessment questionnaires including the Knee score, Western Ontario and McMaster Universities Osteoarthritis Index, and the Short Form 36 are being used with increasing frequency to evaluate the impact of knee arthritis and subsequent treatment. These validated measures provide information on the effect of knee procedures on the patient's general sense of well being and have been shown to offer consistent correlation with clinical outcome measures.

## History

Concurrent with expectations management, a history should be elicited through information gathered from the patient's chart and from a direct history from the patient. History questioning should be guided by an effort to distinguish knee pain from hip pain referred to the knee, peripheral vascular claudication, or other disorders. Concurrent illness, relevant history, medications, allergies, previous surgeries, and previous anesthetics should all be documented. Fundamental elements of history include the onset of pain; severity; duration; affect on functioning; night pain; noticeable catching, popping, or locking; as well as previous treatments (pharmacologic, physical, and occupational therapy) or surgeries. Additionally, the patient's occupation, hobbies, and treatment goals should be elicited.

Numerous medical comorbidities are pointed out as the risk factors for prosthetic joint infection that may lead to poor prognosis. Among the reported risk factors are rheumatoid arthritis; diabetes mellitus; poor nutritional status; obesity; concurrent urinary tract infection; steroid therapy; malignancy; prolonged operation time; hypokalemia; allogeneic blood transfusion; history of smoking; postoperative surgical site infection; prior joint surgery; and preoperative infection of teeth, skin or urinary tract.

Information gathering should also include current medications and allergies. Medications such as aspirin, nonsteroidal anti-inflammatory drugs (NSAIDs), anticoagulants, antibiotics, oral hypoglycemics, glucocorticoids, methotrexate, and anticytokines should be monitored prior to the operation. Information regarding antibiotics is important as surgery should be delayed until resolution of infection when possible. Insulin and glucocorticoids should be decreased prior to surgery and oral hypoglycemics should be held



Parvizi J, Klatt B.
*Essentials in Total Knee Arthroplasty* (pp 61-64).

the day of surgery. It is currently unclear if methotrexate should be discontinued in those who are being treated for rheumatoid arthritis, though there appears to be benefit in its continuation. Anticytokines such as TNF-alpha have been shown to have an association with increased rates of infection.

Allergy documentation should include allergic reaction to antibiotics and opioid analgesics including reaction type because these are commonly used in the perioperative and postoperative setting.

Social history regarding the patient's domestic environment and the availability of caregivers postoperatively is crucial for the discharge postoperative planning. Discharge to a rehabilitation or skilled nursing facility may be necessary if caregivers are not available or if the domestic environment is not favorable to guarantee safe, efficient rehabilitation.

## Physical Examination

Physical examination during surgical evaluation is an important aspect of any procedure. Candidates for knee surgery should undergo a comprehensive musculoskeletal exam, including observation and palpation. Physical examination should begin as soon as the patient walks into the examination room. Posture, usage of assisting devices (cane, brace), sitting down or getting up from the chair, and transfer to the examination table can all assist the clinician in the diagnosis.

Observations should be made prior to manipulation to assess gait pattern and skin changes. Gait analysis should consist of observation of an antalgic gait, knee thrust, and Trendelenburg gait that may suggest knee arthritis, ligament instability, or hip joint disease, respectively. Skin analysis should be undertaken to look for signs of infection, including swelling and rubor, scars indicating previous operations, or any psoriatic lesions in the surgical area. Inspection can reveal peripheral vascular issues such as edema or venous stasis. Any gross deformities, including varus, valgus, recurvatum, or flexion contracture, should be documented.

Once observations have been completed, the knee should be palpated for evidence of effusion, crepitus, and patellar tracking. Medial and lateral joint lines should also be palpated for evidence of meniscal pathology. Distal pulses including the dorsalis pedis (DP) and posterior tibialis (TP) should be palpated. Distal edema should be evaluated for pitting.

The concluding element of physical examination is palpation. Range of motion, muscle strength and tone, sensory and deep tendon reflex assessment, ligament stability, meniscal examination, and spine and hip examination should be thoroughly examined and documented. It is not infrequent to have hip pathology present with knee pain as the main complaint. Examination of the spine and hip are important to exclude referred pain to the knee and can be conducted with the straight leg test or hip internal rotation. The anterior and posterior drawer test, pivot shift, Lachman's test, and valgus and varus stress tests should be performed. Also, tenderness at the pes-anserinus bursa, iliotibial band, or proximal tibiofibular joint should be noted. Additionally, the presence of a distended popliteal cyst (Baker's cyst), which is associated with the osteoarthritic changes in the knee, should be detected and documented.

Subgroups of patients may need only unicondylar knee replacement. Medial compartment osteoarthritic changes without any changes in the other compartments of the knee are frequently detected in the radiographs. These patients usually present with localized medial compartment pain and the medial compartment typically is tender to palpation.

Another subgroup is patients with patellofemoral osteoarthritic changes. Generally, these patients are younger in age than the usual patient with degenerative joint disease of the knee; furthermore, these patients present with the ability to walk long distances, which the usual patient with degenerative joint disease cannot do. The only major limitation is walking up or down the stairs and getting up from a chair. Patellar grind test is positive on physical examination. These patients should be considered for patellofemoral resurfacing.

## Radiographic Evaluation

Radiographs are used for assessment and templating of the knee prior to surgery. The recommended radiographs for the evaluation of a painful knee are AP 45 degrees weight-bearing, lateral, and sky-line (Merchant view with the knee flexed 45 degrees) views. Using insufficient imaging studies to plan treatment bears great risk. Supine images of the knee that are routinely obtained in a primary care can severely underestimate the degree of arthritic changes in the knee.

Anterior posterior views should be obtained to determine femoral/tibial angle; medial and lateral joint spacing; the size, position, and integrity of the patella; and features that might indicate bipartite patella, osteochondritis dissecans, or calcification of the origin of the medial collateral ligament (MCL).

A standing long cassette AP radiograph of both limbs can be used for assessment of mechanical and anatomic axes in surgical planning. Symptoms of hip pathology should prompt AP of the pelvis and lateral x-rays of the involved hip.

Typical arthritic changes that should be noted on the radiographs are narrowing of the joint space, subchondral sclerosis, and osteophytes. Assessment as to which compartment is involved in the degenerative process should be carried out as well.

On lateral radiograph of the knee, 3 popular methods can be used to evaluate the height of the patella. The first is the Blumensaat's line; the inferior edge of the patella should lie on a line extended from the intercondylar notch with the knee flexed at 30 degrees. The second method uses the Insall-Salvati Index, which is the ratio of the length of the patellar tendon to the length of the patella itself; an index of more than 1.2 is considered to verify patella alta, but less than 0.8 verifies patella baja. The third method is the Blackburne-Peel index, which is the distance from the tibial articular surface to the inferior articular surface of the patella; it should be 0.8, more than 1.2 is considered to indicate patella alta.

MRI is warranted to assess for meniscal and ligament integrity. MRI is a sensitive tool in the recognition of pathology in the knee but is not specific for articular cartilage or bone abnormalities unless certain sequences are performed. T1-weighted fat-suppressed three-dimensional spoiled gradient-echo technique and T2-weighted fast spin-echo technique are necessary to augment precision of detection of articular cartilage lesions. Cartilage has higher signal intensity than fluid on T1-weighted images and a lower intensity on T2 images. Meniscal abnormalities diagnosed on MRI are considered to represent the dominant pathology, prompting referral for arthroscopic intervention. MRI is valuable in identifying and defining avascular lesions of the knee. It is possible to determine the extent of the lesion and the integrity of the overlying cartilage.

## Preoperative Testing

Extensive unnecessary testing results in higher cost of preoperative evaluation and often detects minor abnormalities of which many have no clinical relevance. Many studies have shown that preoperative routine testing of all patients is of limited value. Preoperatively, all patients should be seen in a preadmission clinic and consulted as to the necessary preoperative tests work-up. Tests and consults should be ordered based on history and physical examination findings. Screening tests that should commonly be ordered include complete blood count, basic chemistry panel, and coagulation studies (prothrombin time, international normalized ratio [INR], and partial thromboplastin time). Specific coagulation studies should be ordered based on the patient medical and family history (protein C and S, coagulation factors, Factor V Leiden, antithrombin III, antiphospholipid antibodies, prothrombin G20210A). A specific deep venous thrombosis (DVT) prophylaxis plan should be formed based on the findings of the coagulation test. Electrocardiogram and chest radiographs are often required depending on patient age, medical history, and anesthesia guidelines. Furthermore, urinalysis and urine culture should be ordered, and any signs of infection should be eradicated prior to the surgical procedure. Dental clearance should also be obtained. Any anomalies found in the preoperative evaluation should be documented and corrected before the procedure.

## Perioperative Care

Proper perioperative education of surgical patients is significant in guaranteeing the utmost probability of a successful patient outcome. Informing the patient leads to less anxiety and to a better understanding of what is needed to recover best. Most ambulatory surgery centers have sessions where the patient meets with nurses, anesthesia staff, physical therapists, and occupational therapists. Time is taken to give the patient a good idea of what to expect on the day of surgery and thereafter. Anesthesia staff can evaluate the patient for the proper technique and explain this in advance to comfort the patient. Pain management can also be reviewed. The patient can think of ways to make his or her home ready for the recovery period. Equipment can be issued as needed for the home environment. Plans can be formed for having family or friends available for transportation from the hospital and short-term help at home. The informed and prepared patient has less apprehension and is prepared for a faster, easier recovery.

## Summary

Preoperative evaluation of a patient prior to knee surgery is a fundamental part of every surgical procedure. Evaluation should consist of a comprehensive history as well as relevant history regarding the knee, physical exam, laboratory evaluation, radiologic evaluation, and management of patient expectations and patient education.

## Suggested Readings

Ahlberg A, Carlsson AS, Lindberg L. Hematogenous infection in total joint replacement. *Clin Orthop Relat Res.* 1978;(137):69-75.

Barie PS. Antibiotic-resistant gram-positive cocci: implications for surgical practice. *World J Surg.* 1998;22:118-126.

Berbari EF, Hanssen AD, Duffy MC, et al. Risk factors for prosthetic joint infection: case-control study. *Clin Infect Dis.* 1998;27:1247-1254.

Fitzgerald RH Jr, Nolan DR, Ilstrup DM, Van Scoy RE, Washington JA, Coventry MB. Deep wound sepsis following total hip arthroplasty. *J Bone Joint Surg Am.* 1977;59:847-855.

Hanssen AD, Osmon DR, Nelson CL. Prevention of deep periprosthetic joint infection. *Instr Course Lect.* 1997;46:555-567.

Innerhofer P, Walleczek C, Luz G, et al. Transfusion of buffy coat-depleted blood components and risk of postoperative infection in orthopedic patients. *Transfusion.* 1999;39:625-632.

Johansson K, Hupli M, Salantera S. Patient's learning needs after hip arthroplasty. *J Clin Nurs.* 2002;11:634-639.

Johansson K, Nuutila LM, Virtanen H, Katajisto J, Salantera S. Preoperative education for orthopedic patients: systematic review. *J Adv Nurs.* 2005;50:212-223.

Pellino T, Tluczek A, Collins M, et al. Increasing self-efficacy through empowerment: preoperative education for orthopedic patients. *Orthop Nurs.* 1998;17:48-51,54-59.

Prouty A, Cooper M, Thomas P, et al. Multidisciplinary patient education for total joint replacement surgery patients. *Orthop Nurs.* 2006;25(4):257-261.

Ridge RA, Goodson AS. The relationship between multidisciplinary discharge outcomes and functional status after total hip replacement. *Orthop Nurs.* 2000;19:71-82.

Shuldham C. A review of the impact of preoperative education on recovery from surgery: 1999. *Int J Nurs Stud.* 1999;36:171-177

Vessely MB, Whaley AL, Harmsen WS, Schleck CD, Berry DJ. The Chitranjan Ranawat Award: long-term survivorship and failure modes of 1000 cemented condylar total knee arthroplasties. *Clin Orthop Relat Res.* 2006;452:28-34.

Wilson MG, Kelley K, Thornhill TS. Infection as a complication of total knee-replacement arthroplasty: risk factors and treatment in sixty-seven cases. *J Bone Joint Surg Am.* 1990;72:878-883.

# 9

# Surgical Approaches to Total Knee Arthroplasty

*Gregg R. Klein, MD and Mark A. Hartzband, MD*

Total knee arthroplasty (TKA) remains the gold standard for treatment of end-stage knee arthritis. Excellent long-term results with survival from 95% to 99% at 15 years have been reported.[1,2] To perform the procedure, adequate exposure and visualization of the joint is required.

Many different surgical approaches to primary TKA have been described including the medial parapatellar, midvastus, subvastus, and lateral parapatellar. The ideal approach is one in which the surgeon can obtain adequate exposure in a reproducible manner. In addition, it is important that this exposure can be made extensile if necessary.

## Skin Incision

Many different skin incisions have been described. The most common is an anterior midline incision. This incision is commonly made directly midline, slightly medial to the midline, or midline with a slight medial curve. Generally, a straight midline incision is made centered over the patella in the medial/lateral direction. Although used less commonly today, some authors favor a medial parapatellar incision because this incision theoretically has been shown to be subjected to less tension with knee flexion[3] and favors a more cosmetically pleasing scar as it follows Langer's lines of the knee. Keeping the incision off the midline of the patella also minimizes scar pain when kneeling. Injury to the infrapatellar branch of the saphenous nerve is common with both skin incisions, resulting in numbness lateral to the incision postoperatively.[4] Sundaram et al did not find a significant difference in the cosmetic appearance of the scars or incidence of lateral skin numbness when comparing the midline and medial parapatellar skin incisions.[5]

Using a surgical marking pen, the medial, lateral, superior, and inferior borders of the patella should be marked along with the tibial tubercle (Figure 9-1A). The incision should then be marked in relation to these landmarks (Figure 9-1B). The anatomical landmarks should be marked in flexion and the incision performed in flexion. The skin over the tibial tubercle translates laterally as the knee is taken from extension to 90 degrees of flexion.[6] If the incision is planned in extension, the scar may end up directly over the tubercle at 90 degrees of flexion and may cause increased anterior knee pain. The length of the incision is dependent on the size of the patient, the preoperative deformity, soft tissue thickness, and the exposure that is necessary. It is important not to make the incision too small as this will limit the surgical exposure and thus visualization. As more experience is gained, the incision size may be shortened. In general, the incisions should extend from proximal to the superior pole of the patella to the distal aspect of the tibial tubercle. The distal aspect of the incision should be placed medial to the tibial tubercle.

Previous incisions over the knee make the choice of incision during arthroplasty more challenging. Prior transverse incisions m ay be crossed in a perpendicular manner without difficulty. Crossing transverse incisions at acute angles should be avoided to prevent avascular segments of the skin. When multiple longitudinal incisions exist, the most lateral incision that will afford proper exposure should be used



Parvizi J, Klatt D.
*Essentials in Total Knee Arthroplasty* (pp 65-72).

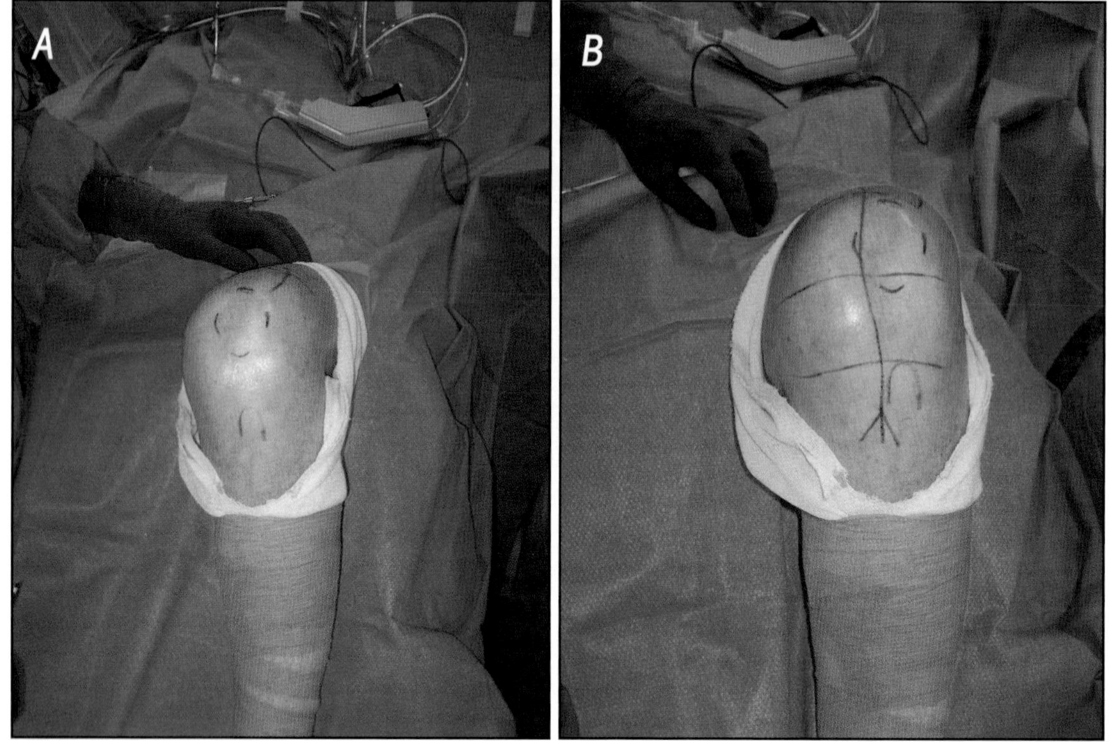


**Figure 9-1.** (A) The landmarks are marked on the skin. (B) The incision is marked.

because the blood supply from the saphenous and descending geniculate arteries is medially based.[7] However, long lateral longitudinal incisions that require making a large subcutaneous flap should be avoided. In addition, small far medial or far lateral incisions (ie, previous open meniscectomies) can be ignored if they are distant from the midline. Parallel incisions with small skin bridges should be avoided. Finally, if a lateral longitudinal incision exists but a more recent medial incision was made that healed without difficulty, the newer medial incisions may be used. If any doubt exists about soft tissue compromise or healing potential, a referral to a plastic surgeon may be necessary.

The blood supply to the skin has been well documented.[7] The skin blood supply arises from deep perforating vessels of the saphenous artery and the descending genicular artery, which anastomose just superficial to the fascia. After anastomosing at the level of the fascia, the vessels penetrate the subcutaneous fat and proceed to the epidermal layer. After the skin incision, surgical dissections should proceed straight through the subcutaneous fat directly to the extensor mechanism. Subcutaneous undermining should be minimized as there is little communication of the blood vessels in the superficial layer. Dissection deep into the fascia will preserve the subcutaneous blood supply.[8]

## Medial Parapatellar Approach

The medial parapatellar approach is the most commonly used exposure in TKA (Figure 9-2). This capsular incision is simple, reproducible, and extensile if necessary. The skin incision is made as described above and carried through the subcutaneous tissue in a single layer. The extensor mechanism, which consists of the quadriceps, patella and patellar ligament, is identified. The arthrotomy begins longitudinally at the medial quadriceps tendon. There is not a set amount of quadriceps tendon that is divided proximally because this is determined by the amount of exposure necessary. Three to 5 mm of quadriceps tendon is left attached to the vastus medialis obliquis (VMO) for later repair. The incision then proceeds distally and curves laterally around the medial aspect of the patella through the medial knee retinaculum. A few millimeters of retinaculum is left attached to the patella for later repair. The incision curves slightly laterally at the inferior aspect of the patella and then proceeds distally parallel to the patellar tendon. At the level of the proximal tibia, dissection is carried directly down to the anterior tibial cortex 5 mm medial to the tibial tubercle. Leaving a small cuff of tissue medial to the tibial tubercle will make repair of the arthrotomy easier.

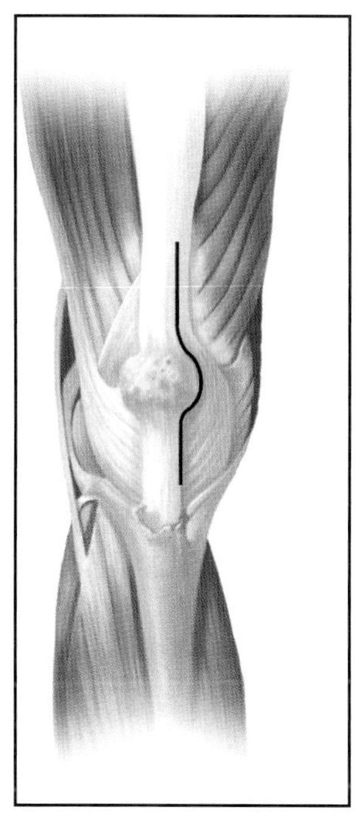

**Figure 9-2.** Medial parapatellar approach.

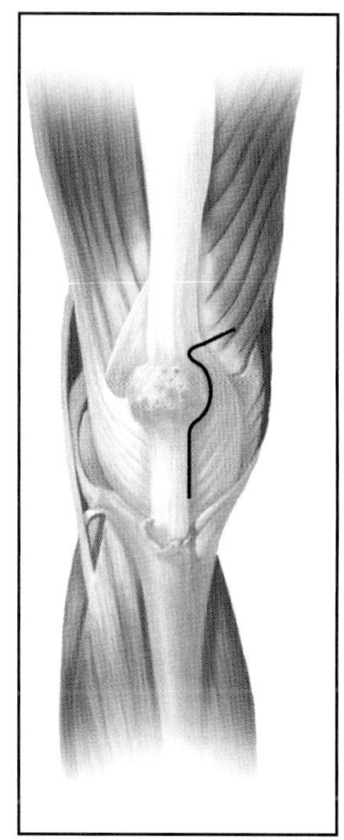

**Figure 9-3.** Midvastus approach.

A sleeve of the medial soft tissue is subperiosteally released, including the deep medial collateral ligament and medial capsule starting from the medial border of the patellar tendon and extending posteromedially. The extent of the release depends on the preoperative deformity. The distal extent of this release is approximately 8 mm below the joint line. This exposure is usually carried to the midcoronal plane of the tibia. The lateral gutter is restored by subluxing the patella laterally in extension to identify and release the patella-femoral ligament.

The infrapatellar fat pad may be excised if desired. There is controversy regarding whether excision of the fat pad results in inferior results. Meneghini et al reviewed 1055 primary total knee replacements with and without fat pad excision and found that fat pad excision had no significant effect on patellar tendon contracture, range of motion, Knee Society Score, or function scores.[9] However, knees in which the fat pad was removed were nearly twice as likely to experience postoperative pain.[9] Lemon et al compared knees in which the fat pad was excised and those in which it was retained and found that the fat pad excision group showed significant patellar tendon shortening of 4.2%.[10]

Historically, the patella is everted during TKA. More recently, authors have recommended against patellar eversion to aid in functional recovery. Walter et al prospectively compared knees in which the patella was everted during exposure and found that avoiding patellar eversion enhanced return of quadriceps function.[11] Stoffel et al used laser Doppler flowmetry to quantify patella intraosseous blood flow and found that blood flow was preserved more significantly in patients with lateral patellar retraction as compared to patellar eversion.[12]

The knee arthroplasty is then performed as desired. Arthrotomy closure has been described in both flexion and extension. It is important to reapproximate the capsular closure to prevent patella baja. Recent studies are inconclusive as to whether there is a difference between closure in flexion or extension. Masri et al prospectively randomized knees closed in flexion or extension and concluded that the degree of flexion of capsular closure did not have an effect on early rehabilitation.[13] In contrast, Emerson et al has reported that knees closed in flexion demonstrated a statistically significant increase in postoperative motion at 1 year.[14]

## Midvastus Approach

The midvastus approach was popularized by Engh and Parks in the 1990s (Figure 9-3).[15] An anterior midline incision is used and dissection is carried through the subcutaneous tissue. The extensor mechanism is identified. The arthrotomy is usually done with the knee in 60 degrees of flexion. The insertion of the VMO at the superior medial pole of the patella is identified. A finger is used to bluntly split the VMO at the superior medial pole of the patella, and the incision then extends in a superior medial direction for approximately 4 cm. It is important to maintain full thickness of the muscle in line with its fibers. The quadriceps tendon is not violated in this approach. The distal aspect of this approach is identical to the medial parapatellar approach and proceeds distally around the patella and medial to the tibial tubercle. Capsular folds are then released as necessary. The patella femoral ligament is released in a similar manner to the medial parapatellar approach.

The insertion of the VMO is preserved and the quadriceps tendon is preserved in this exposure. Eversion of the patella may be easier with this approach when compared to the subvastus approach. Reported advantages such as less lateral release and early straight leg raise are controversial. Relative contraindications included knees with less than 80 degrees of flexion, obesity, hypertrophic arthritis, and previous high tibial osteotomy.[15]

Closure is performed in 60 degrees of flexion. A suture is placed at the interval of the capsule and muscular attachment. It is generally not necessary to repair the muscle proximally.

## Subvastus Approach

The subvastus approach has been described as a more anatomic approach for TKA but is used less commonly (Figure 9-4).[16] The extensor mechanism is preserved, which theoretically may result in less postoperative quadriceps dysfunction and less need for a lateral retinacular release.

An anterior midline incision is used with dissection carried down to the extensor mechanism. The inferior border of the VMO is identified. The surgeon uses his or her finger to bluntly dissect the VMO free from the underlying periosteum and intramuscular septum. The VMO is retracted anterolaterally to identify the underlying joint capsule. The capsule is then transversely incised at the level of the midpatella and starting medially and proceeding to the medial aspect of the patella. The distal extent of the arthrotomy proceeds as previously described. The knee is then flexed and the patella is subluxed laterally while the VMO is further freed from the intermuscular septum. The fat pad is excised as desired.

After the arthroplasty is performed, the horizontal and vertical aspects of the capsular incisions are closed with interrupted resorbable sutures. There is no need to repair the VMO to the intermuscular septum. Contraindications to this approach include morbid obesity, previous knee arthrotomy, high tibial osteotomy, and revision TKA.[16]

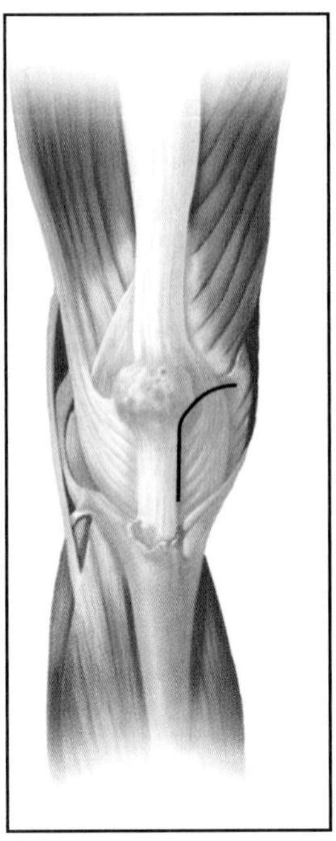

**Figure 9-4.** Subvastus approach.

## Lateral Parapatellar Approach

The lateral parapatellar approach is useful in the valgus TKA. The approach can be very helpful in fixed valgus deformities. The approach is similar to the medial approach, except that the releases come from the lateral joint line. In a valgus knee, the lateral structures need to be released to balance the knee and the medial structures are lax. This approach makes good sense. Eversion of the patella can be challenging, and exposure can be improved with cutting the patella first.

## Comparison Studies

A true consensus does not exist as to which approach is best. Multiple comparison studies of different knee approaches have been performed using the medial parapatellar approach as the gold standard.

White et al[17] compared 109 patients who underwent bilateral TKA with a medial parapatellar approach on one side and a midvastus approach on the other. All other surgical aspects, including implant choice and physical therapy protocols, were identical. The authors found that the midvastus approach resulted in less postoperative pain, a quicker time to straight leg raise, and a lower incidence of lateral retinacular release. However, the clinical results at 6 months were identical.

Keating et al[18] prospectively compared 100 bilateral total knee replacements with a midvastus approach on one side and a medial parapatellar approach on the other. There were no differences in range of motion, ability to straight-leg raise, or lateral release. There were 2 postoperative hematomas and 1 manipulation in the midvastus group and no complications in the medial parapatellar group. The authors did not recommend this approach over the medial parapatellar approach.

Kelly et al[19] prospectively randomized 51 knees undergoing TKA into either a medial parapatellar or midvastus approach. The authors found no difference in functional parameters. However, there was a greater incidence of lateral release and blood loss in the medial parapatellar group. In addition, the authors found a 43% incidence of electromyographic (EMG) changes in the vastus splitting group. At the 5-year follow-up, 7 knees with abnormal EMG findings postoperatively had a normal EMG exam. Two knees had evidence of chronic changes without functional deficit. In the 2 knees with chronic changes, the muscle was split with sharp dissection, whereas the 7 knees that returned to normal were split with blunt dissection.

Matsueda and Gustilo[20] retrospectively reviewed 169 consecutive knee arthroplasties treated with a medial parapatellar approach and 167 arthroplasties treated with a subvastus approach and found no difference in functional parameters and range of motion. There was a lower rate of lateral retinacular release in the subvastus group (37%) as compared to the medial parapatellar group (67%). However, the study was performed over a 9-year period and changing technique may have resulted in this decreased lateral release rate. In addition, both procedures in this study seem to have an astoundingly high rate of lateral release.

In a prospective randomized blinded study, Roysam and Oakley[21] compared the results of a medial parapatellar approach to the subvastus approach and found that the subvastus group had a significantly earlier return of straight-leg raise, lower consumption of opiates in the first week, less blood loss and greater knee flexion at 1 week.

Weinhardt et al[22] randomized knees into either a medial parapatellar approach or a subvastus approach and found that the subvastus group attained full extension and 90 degrees of flexion earlier. However, there was not a significant difference in range of motion of function by the time patients were discharged from the hospital.

## Extensile Approaches

On occasion, an extensile approach may be needed to perform TKA. This might include patients with previous tibial osteotomy, severe contractures, and prior deformities. These extensile approaches are more commonly used in revision surgery. The extensile approach may be planned from the outset or be decided upon during TKA if exposure becomes a challenge. With experience it is possible to determine from the outset if one of these approaches will be needed, but often it is best to make the decision after exposure has been attempted. Often these extensile approach techniques are not needed once the débridement of scar has been completed. Three commonly used extensile approaches are described. The best option is the Quadriceps snip (Figure 9-5). This approach was described by Insall and affords some advantages. The repaired tendon can be treated and rehabbed like a standard TKA. Tibial tubercle osteotomy is shown in Figure 9-6. With tubercle osteotomy, the rehab is slowed as aggressive rehab may lead to a nonunion of the osteotomy. It can be a challenge to fix the tubercle with a screw because the implant will be in the proximal tibia. Wire fixation is another option but is less ideal. Patella turndown is shown in Figure 9-7. This approach is rarely used because the quad snip provides more than adequate visualization with less morbidity.

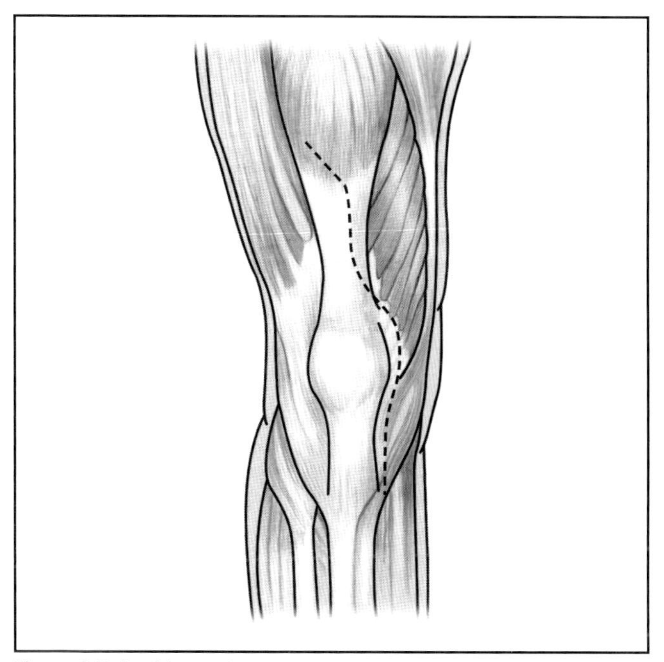

**Figure 9-5.** Quadriceps snip.

## Summary

The goal of TKA is to obtain a well-functioning arthroplasty with good long-term survivorship. Different surgical approaches have been described, and each surgical approach

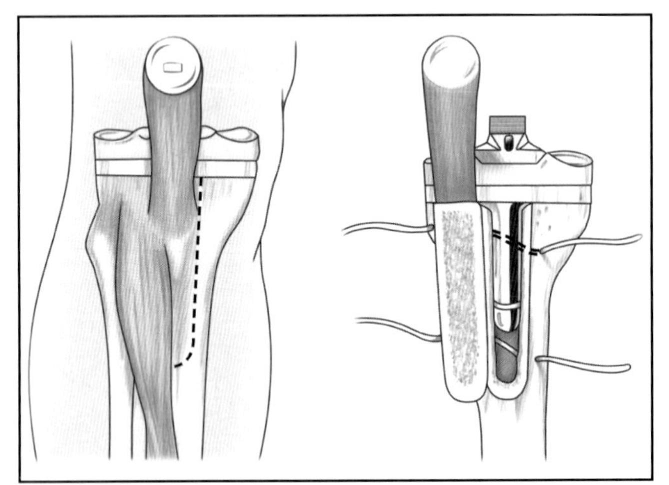

**Figure 9-6.** Tibial tubercle osteotomy/slide approach.

described has its advantages and disadvantages (Table 9-1). Obviously, there is still debate over which approach is the best, and the real test will be the long-term outcomes from each of these approaches.

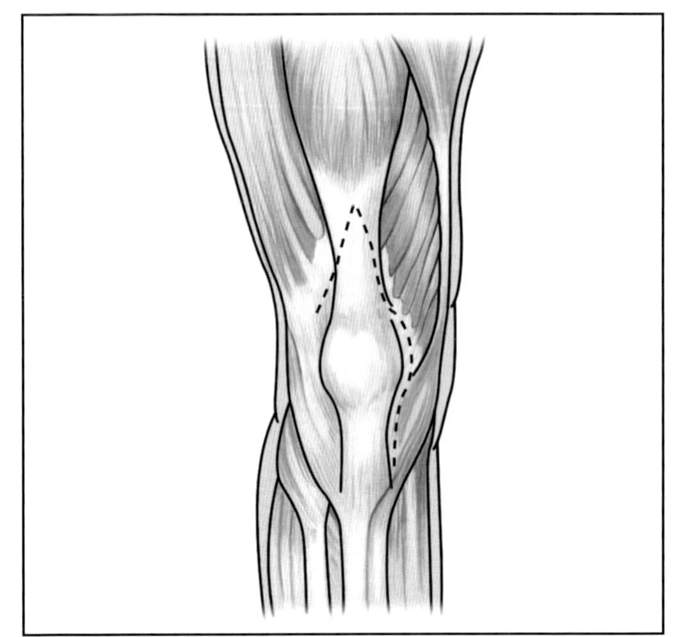

**Figure 9-7.** Patella turndown.

## References


1. Ranawat CS, Flynn WF Jr, Saddler S, et al. Long-term results of the total condylar knee arthroplasty: a 15-year survivorship study. *Clin Orthop Relat Res.* 1993;286:94-102.
2. Scuderi GR, Insall JN, Windsor RE, et al. Survivorship of cemented knee replacements. *J Bone Joint Surg Br.* 1989;71:798.
3. Johnson DP, Houghton TA, Radford P. Anterior midline or medial parapatellar incision for arthroplasty of the knee: a comparative study. *J Bone Joint Surg Br.* 1986;68:812.
4. Chambers GH. The prepatellar nerve: a cause of suboptimal results in knee arthrotomy. *Clin Orthop Relat Res.* 1972;82:157.
5. Sundaram RO, Ramakrishnan M, Harvey RA, et al. Comparison of scars and resulting hypoaesthesia between the medial parapatellar and midline skin incisions in total knee arthroplasty. *Knee.* 2007;14(5):375-378.
6. Yacoubian SV, Scott RD. Skin incision translation in total knee arthroplasty: the difference between flexion and extension. *J Arthroplasty.* 2007;22:353.
7. Haertsch PA. The blood supply to the skin of the leg: a post-mortem investigation. *Br J Plast Surg.* 1981;34:470.
8. Younger AS, Duncan CP, Masri BA. Surgical exposures in revision total knee arthroplasty. *J Am Acad Orthop Surg.* 1998;6:55.
9. Meneghini RM, Pierson JL, Bagsby D, et al. The effect of retropatellar fat pad excision on patellar tendon contracture and functional outcomes after total knee arthroplasty. *J Arthroplasty.* 2007;22:47.
10. Lemon M, Packham I, Narang K, et al. Patellar tendon length after knee arthroplasty with and without preservation of the infrapatellar fat pad. *J Arthroplasty.* 2007;22:574.
11. Walter F, Haynes MB, Markel DC. A randomized prospective study evaluating the effect of patellar eversion on the early functional outcomes in primary total knee arthroplasty. *J Arthroplasty.* 2007;22:509.
12. Stoffel KK, Flivik G, Yates PJ, et al. Intraosseous blood flow of the everted or laterally-retracted patella during total knee arthroplasty. *Knee.* 2007;14(6):434-438.
13. Masri BA, Laskin RS, Windsor RE, et al. Knee closure in total knee replacement: a randomized prospective trial. *Clin Orthop Relat Res.* 1996;331:81-86.
14. Emerson RH Jr, Ayers C, Higgins LL. Surgical closing in total knee arthroplasty: a series followup. *Clin Orthop Relat Res.* 1999;368:176-181.
15. Engh GA, Parks NL. Surgical technique of the midvastus arthrotomy. *Clin Orthop Relat Res.* 1998;351:270-274.
16. Hofmann AA, Plaster RL, Murdock LE. Subvastus (Southern) approach for primary total knee arthroplasty. *Clin Orthop Relat Res.* 1991;269:70-77.
17. White RE Jr, Allman JK, Trauger JA, Dales BH. Clinical comparison of the midvastus and medial parapatellar surgical approaches. *Clin Orthop Relat Res.* 1999;367:117-122.
18. Keating EM, Faris PM, Meding JB, et al. Comparison of the midvastus muscle-splitting approach with the median parapatellar approach in total knee arthroplasty. *J Arthroplasty.* 1999;14:29.
19. Kelly MJ, Rumi MN, Kothari M, et al. Comparison of the vastus-splitting and median parapatellar approaches for primary total knee arthroplasty: a prospective, randomized study. *J Bone Joint Surg Am.* 2006;88:715.
20. Matsueda M, Gustilo RB. Subvastus and medial parapatellar approaches in total knee arthroplasty. *Clin Orthop Relat Res.* 2000;371:161-168.

Table 9-1

**Comparison of Different Exposures for Primary Total Knee Arthroplasty**

| Approach | Advantage | Disadvantage |
|---|---|---|
| Medial parapatellar approach | Extensile<br>Easy<br>Reproducible | Detachment of VMO<br>Interruption of patellar vascular supply[23] |
| Midvastus approach | VMO insertion on patella preserved<br>Avoid quadriceps tendon incision<br>Patella blood supply less interrupted | Less extensile<br>Exposure more difficult in large patients with contractures |
| Subvastus approach | Anatomic exposure<br>Extensor mechanism not violated | Not extensile<br>Potential for neurovascular injury |

21. Roysam GS, Oakley MJ. Subvastus approach for total knee arthroplasty: a prospective, randomized, and observer-blinded trial. *J Arthroplasty.* 2001;16:454.

22. Weinhardt C, Barisic M, Bergmann EG, et al. Early results of subvastus versus medial parapatellar approach in primary total knee arthroplasty. *Arch Orthop Trauma Surg.* 2004;124:401.

23. Kayler DE, Lyttle D. Surgical interruption of patellar blood supply by total knee arthroplasty. *Clin Orthop Relat Res.* 1988;(229):221-227.

# 10

# Operating Room Set-Up

*Manny Porat, MD and William Hozack, MD*

## Preoperative Planning

Preoperative planning of the total knee arthroplasty begins prior to arrival of the patient into the hospital. The patient undergoes a thorough outpatient evaluation that includes a full set of radiographs of the knee. Additional radiographs such as long-leg standing or full femur/tibia radiographs may be available for patients with severe intra- or extra-articular deformities. The radiographs should be posted in a visible area so they can be referred to prior to and during the case. Possible valgus or varus deformities, extra-articular deformities, flexion contractures, and previous implants or hardware noted on radiographs are important considerations for the patient set-up of each case. If revision augments or stems are likely to be used, this should be recognized preoperatively and planned for. Many surgeons prefer to template prior to surgery to aid in planning, and this can be educational for a resident to understand size and position of components. Templating can provide a general estimate of sizing for the operating room (OR) team. Recognizing and planning for situations where the implant company may need to provide a small or large implant is crucial.

The history should also be reviewed for information that might affect set-up, including allergies to Betadine, tape, latex, or antibiotics. Patients with pacemakers or defibrillators may need special attention and planning. Other pertinent information to review includes previous orthopedic and nonorthopedic surgeries; medical conditions, such as rheumatoid arthritis; and bleeding disorders or possible fistulas, which might affect the patient set-up. In addition, preoperative medical notes (from the internist) and the laboratory values should be reviewed to assess the need for possible preoperative medications or treatments.

A courteous resident should appropriately introduce him- or herself to the patient prior to the surgery, check that the consent for the procedure is completed, and ensure that the appropriate extremity is clearly delineated.[1] At this time, the patient is often ready to be brought to the OR or an intermediate room for the administration of anesthesia. Patients receiving regional anesthesia will most likely have difficulty moving their lower extremities after administration of the anesthesia and may require assistance or supervision while transferring them onto the OR table. It is important to be cognizant that these patients will have sensory deficits; therefore, their lower extremities should be appropriately secured during transportation to the OR. Bony prominences need to be well padded during the case.

## Antibiotic Prophylaxis

The use of antibiotic prophylaxis has been universally recommended for all patients undergoing total knee arthroplasty. Current American Academy of Orthopedic Surgeons (AAOS) recommendations state that cefazolin or cefuroxime is the preferred antibiotic for most patients. Patients with known drug allergies to penicillin or other beta lactam drugs should receive clindamycin or vancomycin. Patients with documented colonization with methicillin-resistant *Staphylococcus aureus* (MRSA) or who come from facilities



Parvizi J, Klatt B.
*Essentials in Total Knee Arthroplasty* (pp 73-78).

with recent outbreaks of MRSA should be prophylactically treated with vancomycin.

Ideal administration time is within 1 hour prior to skin incision and prior to tourniquet inflation. Due to the increased infusion time, vancomycin should be started 2 hours prior to incision. Additional intraoperative doses of the chosen antibiotic should be given if the operation extends beyond the half life of the drug or in cases with large intraoperative blood loss. Regardless of whether drains or catheters were placed during the procedure, the antibiotics should not be continued past 24 hours from the conclusion of the operation.[2]

## Patient Set-Up

The patient should be placed in the center of the operating table with his or her head placed appropriately for anesthesia administration. Modern total knee arthroplasty is typically performed on an electric-hydraulic surgical table. In order to reduce the incidence of infection, a potentially devastating complication, surgery can be performed in a laminar flow OR.[3] In this type of room, the table should be placed within the zone of laminar airflow. A safety belt is commonly placed around the patient to secure him or her to the surgical table. At this time, confirm with the anesthesiologist that the patient is properly sedated for manipulations of the hips and lower extremities. The arms should be placed away from the patient's side and secured on a separate arm board so as to not interfere during the surgery. Patients who are under anesthesia lose the protective sensation needed to avoid pressure ulcers. Therefore, it is an important practice to pad and protect the bony prominences.

At this point, any warming blanket, socks, or additional clothing should be removed. If a Foley catheter is needed, appropriate insertion should be performed and the tubing should be secured away from the operative side so it does not contaminate the field or get pulled during the operation. Next, atraumatic hair removal from the operative site should be performed using an electric shaver, taking care not to damage the skin surface.

Most current total knee arthroplasty surgeries are performed using a midline incision.[4] However, patients undergoing total knee arthroplasty may have varying degrees of external rotation of their lower limbs. In some cases, making this traditional midline incision may be awkward if the patella is facing in extreme external rotation during a resting position. Therefore, common knee landmarks may be less accessible, making surgery more cumbersome. To rectify this problem, the surgeon can place a small bump underneath the hip of the operative side, which will return the knee to midline position for surgery. The bump can consist of operative gel pads with several rolled blankets or operative gel pads alone.

Development of postoperative deep venous thrombosis is a well-known complication of surgery. Intraoperative use of a pneumatic compression device during surgery can be considered. Another method is to give intravenous heparin just prior to tourniquet inflation.[5]

Electrocautery is often used during modern arthroplasty surgery. The "bovie" passes high frequency alternating current into the body, allowing the current to cut tissue or coagulate blood. The current machines require grounding pads to be placed on the patient. The optimal positions for the grounding pads are away from the surgical field and away from any implants that may react with the grounding pad. If the patient does not have a history of a previous hip or knee arthroplasty, a common location for the grounding pad is the contralateral thigh. In the event of bilateral knee arthroplasty, the abdomen or flank should be considered for grounding pad placement. Care should be taken to place the grounding pad as far as possible from previously implanted defibrillators or implantable cardioverter-defibrillators (ICDs).[6] A review of the literature has demonstrated several cases of electrocautery-induced ventricular tachyarrhythmias, including ventricular tachycardia (VT) or ventricular fibrillation (VF).[7] Prior to application of the pad, the skin should be dry and checked for any lacerations, erythema, or prior damage.

Knee arthroplasty is often performed using extremity tourniquets during the procedure to facilitate the ease of the operation by limiting intraoperative blood loss. Care should be taken during application of this tourniquet because it can fail or cause complications if improperly placed. First, assess the thigh by estimating its girth or measuring its circumference. The tourniquet should be placed as proximal as possible on the operative thigh to allow for potential incision extension. Prior to the tourniquet application, wrap soft cotton around the area where the tourniquet will be placed to prevent possible abrasions when inflated.[8] The tourniquet should be wrapped tightly and great care should be taken to exclude any section of the genitalia. The tubing should be facing away from the surgical field and connected to the inflation device. Once the cuff is secured, set the desired pressure and alarm time and test that the cuff works properly. Current recommendation for tourniquet pressure is 100 mm Hg above the systolic blood pressure.[9] Possible complications of tourniquets include failure during operation, skin abrasions, underlying tissue damage, and possible nerve damage (Figure 10-1).[10,11]

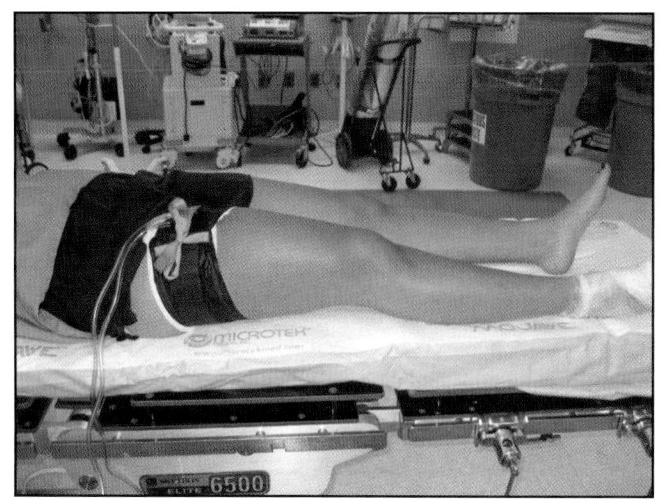


**Figure 10-1.** Proper tourniquet placement.

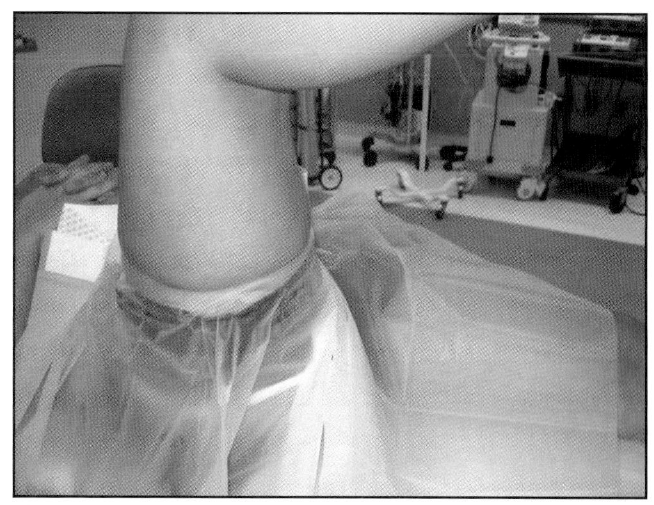

**Figure 10-2.** Proper placement of U-drape.

Attention should now be given to isolating the operative field. Many surgeons will place boundaries in anticipation of the surgical prep. Commonly used disposable boundaries are the Steri-Drapes made by 3M (St. Paul, MN). The 3M 1015 Steri-Drape, conventionally called the "U-drape," should be used to wrap the distal border of the tourniquet. This is easily accomplished with the operative lower extremity flexed to 90 degrees at the hip and 90 degrees at the knee. The drape is then wrapped around the border of the cuff starting at the midline (Figure 10-2). This marks the superior border of the prep. This procedure can also be done using a sheet. The distal border of the prep site is often delineated with a 3M 1000 Steri-Drape that covers the ankle and foot below. This can be secured to the foot with surgical tape, but it is important not to overtighten the tape because it is not meant to be a tourniquet. Plastic surgical tape has been documented to be an effective barrier to bacterial penetration onto the surgical field and should be an integral part of the draping process.[12] Now that the operative site is adequately outlined, attention can be drawn to foot bump placement.

The placement of the foot bump plays an important role during surgery because the operative knee is commonly flexed during the procedure for optimal visualization of the posterior anatomy and for insertion of components. To maintain a flexed knee position, many surgeons will place a bump at the end of the bed. The most common means to locate optimal foot bump placement is to flex the knee to 90 degrees and secure the bump at the location of the heel (Figure 10-3). Based on surgeon preference, more or less flexion can be incorporated into the placement of the foot bump. Foot holders are also available and can be used in place of the bump.

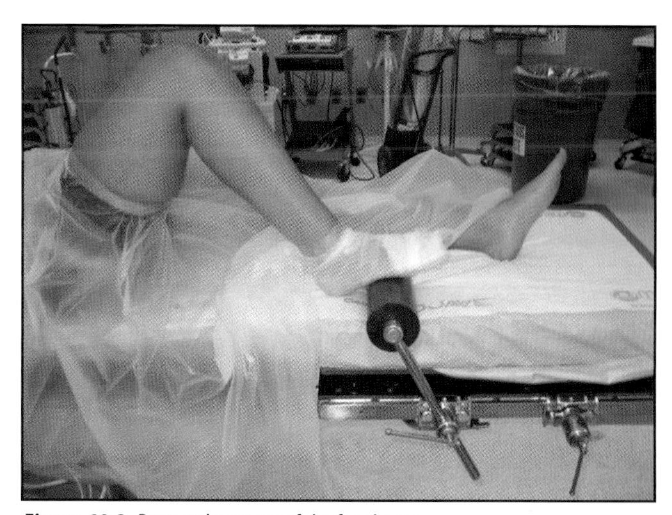

**Figure 10-3.** Proper placement of the foot bump.

## Skin Preparation

Before the knee can be cleaned, the extremity must be isolated from the non-sterile OR table beneath it. There are 2 methods to accomplish this task, one of which involves additional help. If additional help is available, the holder can grab the foot, which has a 3M 1000 Steri-Drape already wrapped around it, and hold the extremity in the air while it is being prepped. The leg holder should be fully scrubbed and gowned prior to holding because this has been shown to reduce the possibility of introducing bacteria to the surgical field.[13] If additional help is not available, the second option is to wrap the ankle with a stirrup and hang the leg by a "candy cane" rod. The candy cane should be secured to the distal end of the operating table and properly fastened with a clamp. The leg is now ready to be cleaned (Figure 10-4).

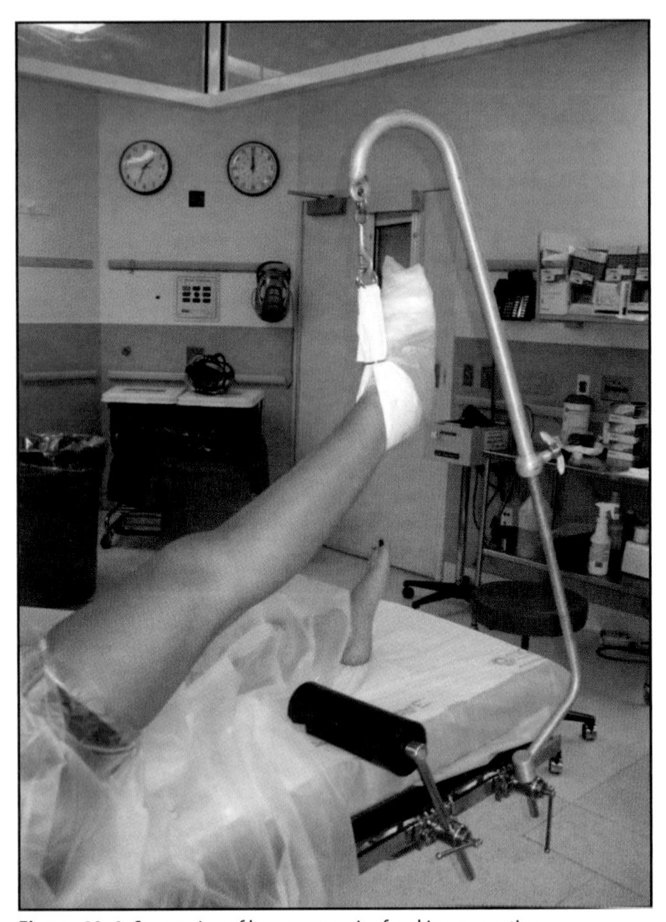

**Figure 10-4.** Suspension of lower extremity for skin preparation.

Several cleansers are available to sterilize the operative leg once it is ready for prepping. Traditionally, Betadine is used in a paint-and-scrub technique, which has shown to be both effective alone and in conjunction with an isopropyl alcohol wash. There are currently several choices on the market, including aqueous chlorhexidine, ChloraPrep (CareFusion, Leawood, KS), and DuraPrep (3M) solutions. These all-in-one solutions come in prepackaged applicators that are easily activated and have been shown to be equal in antimicrobial efficacy to the traditional paint-and-scrub technique.[14] These newer cleansers are often less cumbersome to use and leave a sticky residue on the skin that makes the Ioban (3M) adhere stronger.[15] Regardless of which solution is used, all visible areas of the skin should be cleaned to ensure maximal efficacy. A quick review of the patient's allergies is prudent to confirm that the patient does not have allergies to iodine, which could trigger a reaction with the Betadine solution.

It is recommended to start by painting the incision first and move away from the area of the incision in concentric circles. This potentially inhibits the operator from introducing contamination to the incision site from other skin areas. If the traditional paint-and-scrub technique is preferred, the entire operative leg should be covered with no less than 3 consecutive coats of Betadine. Once the Betadine is sufficiently applied, 3 coats of isopropyl alcohol should be applied. It is recommended to wait until the alcohol appears dry prior to beginning the draping process.

## Draping Process

The draping process is a critical part of beginning any surgical procedure. Proper sterile technique and diligence should be used to minimize possible sources of contamination. Staff and assistants who are involved in draping should wear 3 pairs of gloves and discard the top pair prior to initiating surgery. Typically, several people are needed to properly position and place the drapes in a sterile fashion. One scrubbed person should remove the foot from the candy cane and suspend it in the air using a sterile stockinette. It is important to be cognizant not to contaminate the gown by touching the unsterile operating table or contaminate the recently prepped extremity. The down sheet should be placed first across the bottom of the operating table and cover the nonoperative leg. Next, the impermeable sheet should be attached to the proximal part of the leg close to the tourniquet. This sheet should be wrapped circumferentially around the tourniquet along the same path as the 3M 1015 Steri-Drape. The bottom drapes should be attached in a similar fashion around the proximal thigh with the ends sprawled along the lower half of the operating table. The superior ends of the drapes are attached by their sticky ends to the top of the tourniquet and laid down horizontally across the operating table. These ends are typically given to the anesthesiologist who will often create a barrier by attaching the superior ends of the sheet to intravenous poles, allowing for access to the head and airway if needed. At this time, the stockinette can be carefully rolled down to the level of the tourniquet. The stockinette should be wrapped to the foot and distal tibia and secured properly to prevent it from loosening during the case. If this is not done properly, undesired areas of the lower extremity may be exposed during the surgery. Coban wrap (3M) is a useful tool for maintaining sterility below the level of the tibial tubercle. This material will only adhere to itself and is easily removed at the end of the case. The tibial tubercle should be easily accessible because it can be a noteworthy landmark during the procedure. At this point, the entire table should be sterile and the leg can safely be placed on the field. An additional sterile barrier can be created using a clear plastic curtain that is often attached to the ends of the laminar flow glass from the ceiling or intravenous poles. Those who apply this sterile curtain should remove their top gloves after this step.

The operative site should be covered with a stockinette at this time. Using sterile scissors, make a midline slit in the stockinette over the knee and proximal thigh while being careful not to damage the underlying skin. Create an opening in the stockinette large enough to view the superior and inferior edges of the incision. The incision should be marked. The surgeon should then remove his or her top gloves. An Ioban should then be used to completely overlap the opening that was made with the scissors and the remaining Ioban should be wrapped around the posterior aspect of the knee. The use of Ioban has been shown to reduce drape lift-off, which can be a potential source of contamination during the operation.[16] Ioban also provides a durable iodine coverage to the skin throughout the surgery. With the electrocautery and suction at the surgeon's disposal, the extremity is ready for exsanguination and tourniquet inflation. Once these are performed, the initial incision can be made and the operation can begin.

## References


1. American Academy of Orthopedic Surgeons. Joint commission guidelines. http://www3.aaos.org/member/safety/guidelines.cfm. Accessed May 14, 2010.
2. American Academy of Orthopedic Surgeons. Information statement. http://www.aaos.org/about/papers/advistmt/1027.asp. Accessed May 14, 2010.
3. Ahl T, Dalén N, Jörbeck H, Hoborn J. Air contamination during hip and knee arthroplasties: horizontal laminar flow randomized vs. conventional ventilation. *Acta Orthop Scand.* 1995;66(1):17-20.
4. Malik MH, Chougle A, Pradhan N, Gambhir AK, Porter ML Ann. Primary total knee replacement: a comparison of a nationally agreed guide to best practice and current surgical technique as determined by the North West Regional Arthroplasty Register. *R Coll Surg England.* 2005;87(2):117-122.
5. Westrich GH, Menezes A, Sharrock N, Sculco TP. Thromboembolic disease prophylaxis in total knee arthroplasty using intraoperative heparin and postoperative pneumatic foot compression. *J Arthroplasty.* 1999;14(6):651-656.
6. Nercessian OA, Wu H, Nazarian D, Mahmud F. Intraoperative pacemaker dysfunction caused by the use of electrocautery during a total hip arthroplasty. *J Arthroplasty.* 1998;13(5):599-602.
7. Lo R, Mitrache A, Quan W, Cohen TJ. Electrocautery-induced ventricular tachycardia and fibrillation during device implantation and explantation. *J Invasive Cardiol.* 2007;19(1):12-15.
8. Olivecrona C, Tidermark J, Hamberg P, Ponzer S, Cederfjäll C. Skin protection underneath the pneumatic tourniquet during total knee arthroplasty: a randomized controlled trial of 92 patients. *Acta Orthop.* 2006;77(3):519-523.
9. Ishii Y, Matsuda Y. Effect of tourniquet pressure on perioperative blood loss associated with cementless total knee arthroplasty: a prospective, randomized study. *J Arthroplasty.* 2005;20(3):325-330.
10. Tamvakopoulos GS, Toms AP, Glasgow M. Subcutaneous thigh fat necrosis as a result of tourniquet control during total knee arthroplasty. *Ann R Coll Surg Engl.* 2005;87(5):W11-W13.
11. Nercessian OA, Ugwonali OF, Park S. Peroneal nerve palsy after total knee arthroplasty. *J Arthroplasty.* 2005;20(8):1068-1073.
12. French ML, Eitzen HE, Ritter MA. The plastic surgical adhesive drape: an evaluation of its efficacy as a microbial barrier. *Ann Surg.* 1976;184:46.
13. Brown AR, Taylor GJ, Gregg PJ. Air contamination during skin preparation and draping in joint replacement surgery. *J Bone Joint Surg Br.* 1996;78:92.
14. Gilliam DL, Nelson CL. Comparison of a one-step iodophor skin preparation versus traditional preparation in total joint surgery. *Clin Orthop Relat Res.* 1990;(250):258-260.
15. Jacobson C, Osmon DR, Hanssen A, et al. Prevention of wound contamination using DuraPrep solution plus Ioban 2 drapes. *Clin Orthop Relat Res.* 2005;439:32-37.
16. Alexander JW, Aerni S, Plettner JP. Development of a safe and effective one-minute preoperative skin preparation. *Arch Surg.* 1985;120:1357.

# 11

# Surgical Principles of Total Knee Arthroplasty

*Gregory K. Deirmengian, MD and Carl A. Deirmengian, MD*

A large number of total knee arthroplasty systems are currently available. Each prosthetic system employs specific design features that attempt to optimize the biomechanics of the reconstructed knee. These designs aim to maximize range of motion, improve stability, minimize wear, and provide the patients with the "feel" of a normal knee.

Although the design features of total knee arthroplasty systems continue to develop, the basic surgical principles of soft tissue balancing and of proper component alignment and positioning remain constant. A perfectly designed prosthetic system cannot counteract the effects of components implanted with improper balance and alignment. The goal of this chapter is to describe the surgical principles used in implanting a well-aligned, well-balanced total knee arthroplasty.

## Relevant Normal Knee Anatomy and Biomechanics

An understanding of normal knee anatomy and biomechanics is essential to accomplishing the technical goals of total knee arthroplasty. The parameters reviewed below represent average values obtained from lower extremities in static alignment. In this position, the weight-bearing mechanical axis transverses the knee joint in a manner that best distributes the force. The goal of a well-balanced, well-aligned total knee arthroplasty is to distribute the forces across the joint surface evenly. Achieving this goal maximizes knee function while avoiding contact loading and minimizing the rate of wear.[1,2]

The alignment parameters of the lower extremity are typically referenced with the vertical midline axis of the body. The mechanical axis of the lower extremity represents the line of force that crosses the center of the axis of the hip and tibiotalar joints in the coronal plane, forming a 3-degree valgus angle with the vertical midline axis. The anatomic axes of the femur and tibia are formed by straight lines that traverse the center of the femoral and tibial shafts with normal anatomy. The anatomic axis of the femur normally forms a 9-degree valgus angle with the vertical midline axis and a corresponding 6-degree valgus angle with the mechanical axis of the lower extremity. It is important to note that these values are variable and are influenced by pelvic width and femoral neck offset. Because the tibia is a straight, relatively symmetrical bone and the mechanical axis traverses it centrally, the anatomic axis of the tibia normally aligns with the mechanical axis and forms the same 3-degree valgus angle with the vertical midline axis (Figure 11-1A).

The horizontal joint line axis is formed by a line that bisects the knee joint and, in normal static alignment, is perpendicular to the vertical midline axis. As such, the joint surface of the tibia forms a 3-degree varus angle with the perpendicular to the anatomic axis of the tibia. In full extension, the joint surface of the femur forms a 3-degree valgus angle with the perpendicular to mechanical axis of the lower extremity and a 9-degree valgus angle with the perpendicular to anatomic axis of the femur. In 90 degrees of flexion, the surface of the posterior femoral condyles has 3 degrees of internal rotation relative to the epicondylar axis that corresponds to the 3-degree varus angle of the tibial joint line (Figure 11-1B). The valgus angle of the knee is formed by



Parvizi J, Klatt B.
*Essentials in Total Knee Arthroplasty* (pp 79-90).

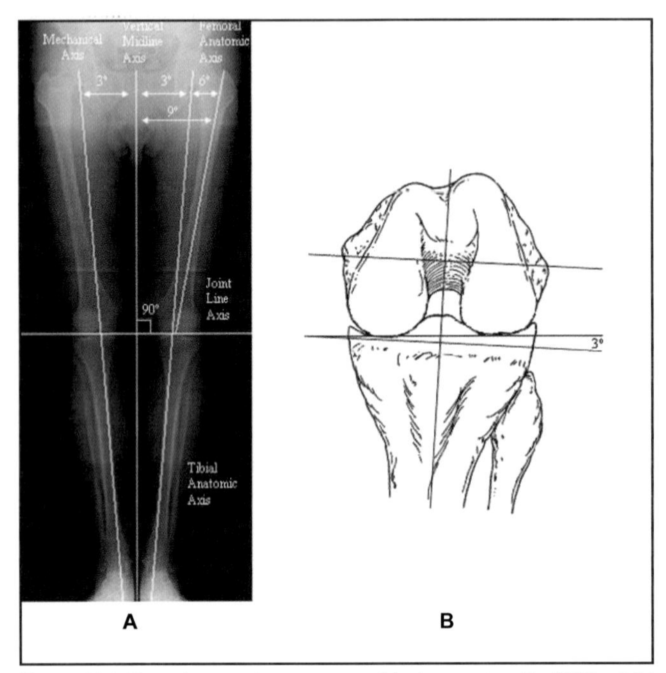


**Figure 11-1.** Normal anatomic parameters of the lower extremity. (A) The right lower extremity depicts the mechanical axis of the lower extremity, which traverses the knee slightly medial to the midline. The left lower extremity depicts the femoral and tibial anatomic axes as well as the joint line axis and demonstrates their relationships with the mechanical axis and vertical midline axis. (B) The posterior condylar axis of the femur and its relationship to the anatomic axis of the tibia is depicted. (Figure 1B is adapted from Canale ST. *Campbell's Operative Orthopaedics*. 10th ed. New York, NY: Mosby; 2003.)

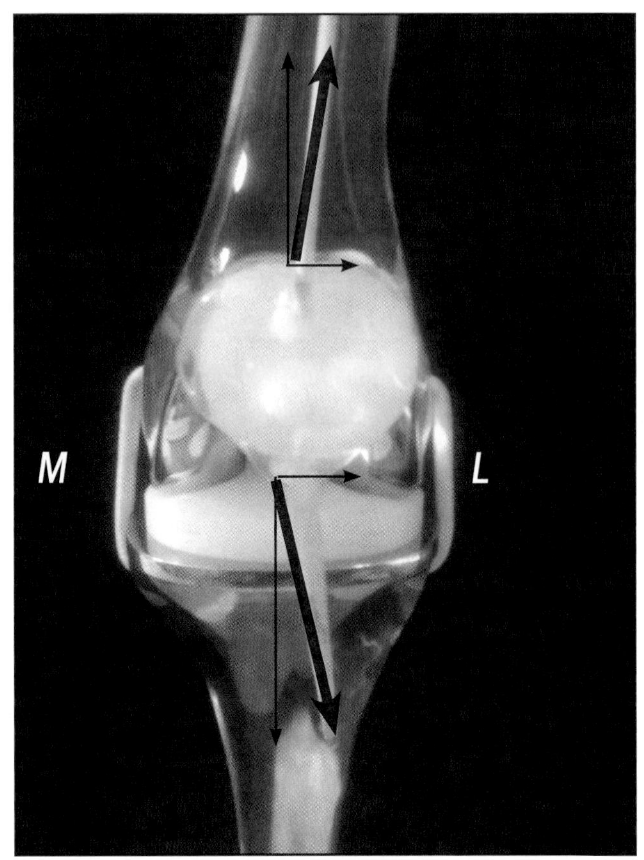


**Figure 11-2.** Model of a knee demonstrating dynamic patellofemoral biomechanics. The superior bold vector represents the line of force of the quadriceps muscle on the patella. The inferior bold vector represents the normal force of the patellar tendon on the patella. The corresponding thin arrows overlaying the 2 bold arrows represent the vertical and horizontal vector components. The "Q" angle represents the angle formed by the bold vectors. M = medial; L = lateral.

the intersection of the anatomic axes of the femur and tibia and is influenced by the tibial and femoral joint surface angles. The average valgus angle of the knee is 6 degrees. When the lower extremity anatomy and alignment parameters described above are within normal limits, the mechanical weight-bearing axis of the lower extremity crosses just slightly medial to the central axis of the knee joint.[2]

Patellofemoral tracking is influenced by the shape and orientation of the articular surfaces of the patella and femoral trochlea as well as the lines of forces of the soft tissues that attach to the patella. The "Q" angle is formed by the intersection of the lines connecting the origins and insertions of the patellar tendon and the quadriceps musculotendinous complex. Clinically, the anterior superior iliac spine is used as a palpable surrogate marker for the multiple origins of the quadriceps muscle. Each vector of force that acts on the patella can be separated into horizontal and vertical components. No matter the quantitative value, the vertical superior force vector of the quadriceps is equally matched by the vertical inferior normal force vector of the patellar tendon. As a result, the superior/inferior position of the patella is not influenced by changes in the amount of force applied by the quadriceps. On the other hand, the horizontal vector forces of the quadriceps and patellar tendon are both aimed laterally and their magnitudes are directly related to the value of the "Q" angle (Figure 11-2). Although increasing the force applied to the patella by the quadriceps encourages lateral translation of the patella, the shapes and orientation of the patella and femoral trochlea normally prevent this tendency. The horizontal motion of the patella is also influenced by the tension of its attachments to the static medial and lateral retinaculum (Figure 11-3).

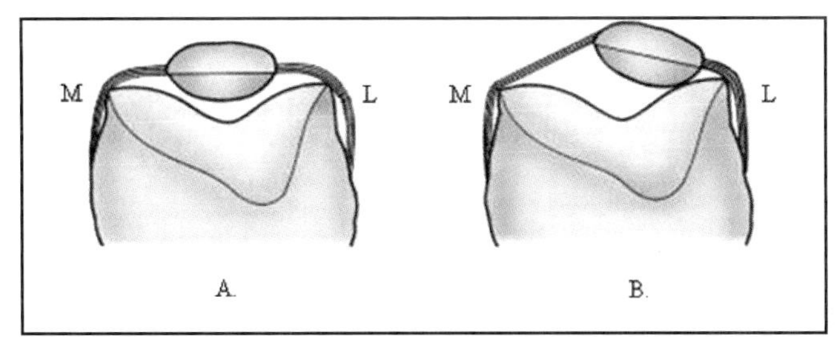


**Figure 11-3.** Pictorial demonstration of static patellofemoral biomechanics. (A) The shapes and orientations of the patella and femoral trochlea influence central patella tracking. (B) Tight relative tensioning of the lateral retinacula acts as a static lateral restraint to central patella tracking. M = medial; L = lateral. (Adapted from Scott WN. *Insall and Scott's Surgery of the Knee*. 4th ed. Philadelphia, PA: Elsevier; 2006.)

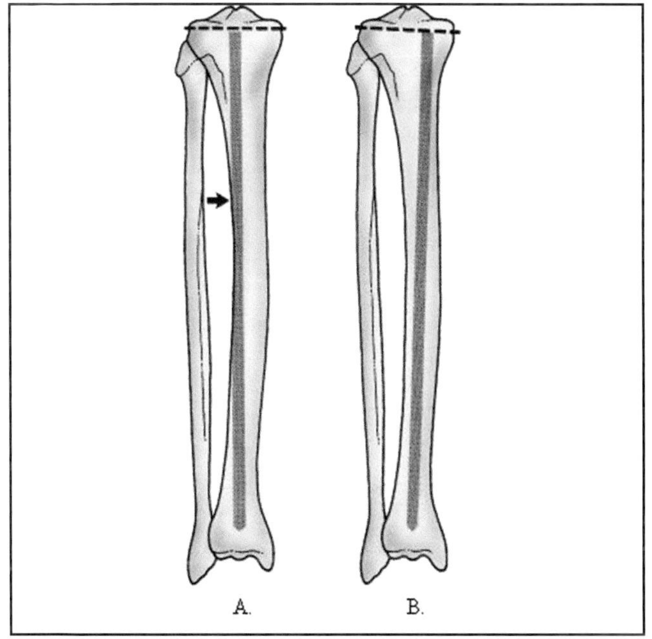


**Figure 11-4.** Influence of tibial deformity on the use of an intramedullary tibial guide. (A) With apex medial tibial bowing, normal proximal positioning of the intramedullary tibial guide leads to breaching of the lateral tibial cortex with the guide. (B) Medial deviation of the proximal tibial starting point of the intramedullary guide in order to accommodate the tibial deformity leads to a valgus tibial cut. (Adapted from Scott WN. *Insall and Scott's Surgery of the Knee*. 4th ed. Philadelphia, PA: Elsevier; 2006.)

## Surgical Principles of Tibial Preparation

Several parameters are determined by the surgeon in the preparation of the tibia, including the ultimate alignment, orientation, and rotation of the tibial component. The determination of these parameters, to a large degree, depends on the guides and jigs provided with each specific device system. To that end, the importance of understanding the details of the prosthetic system of choice cannot be overstated. An intramedullary guide, an extramedullary guide, or computer navigation guide can be used in performing the tibial cut. The guide directs the level of bone resection, the coronal alignment of the cut tibial surface, and the degree of tibial slope in the sagittal plane.

An intramedullary guide uses the tibial canal to position the cutting jig. The use of an intramedullary guide presumes the axis of the intramedullary canal matches the anatomic axis of the tibia in the coronal and sagittal planes. The advantage of an intramedullary guide is that, with normal tibia anatomy, it may minimize the effect of surgeon error in referencing the anatomic axis of the tibia. The disadvantages of an intramedullary guide are that it requires violation of the intramedullary space, which may increase the risk of fat embolism,[3-5] and it is inaccurate in cases of abnormal tibial bowing or canal offset (Figure 11-4). With an extramedullary guide, the surgeon uses external tibia landmarks to estimate the anatomic axis and align the cutting jig (Figure 11-5). The advantages of an extramedullary tibia guide are that it avoids violation of the intramedullary space and it can better estimate the anatomic axis of the tibia when abnormal bowing exists. The disadvantage of an extramedullary guide is that it introduces the factor of surgeon error with inexact judgment of tibial landmarks.[5] Although the tibial cutting guide is used to align the cutting jig, it is important to note that the orientation of the cutting slot within the jig itself also influences the orientation of the tibia cut. For example, a tibia cutting jig may be designed with a given degree of preset posterior slope (see Figure 11-5). With computer navigation, the tibial guide is placed to cut the bone in the exact position desired. The guide does not violate the femoral canal and can be adjusted to the exact desired position. After the cuts are made with the use of the computer, they can be checked for accuracy by computer guidance.

In the coronal plane, the surgeon sets the cutting guide to determine the varus-valgus alignment of the tibial cut. The anatomic approach reproduces normal anatomy by creating a 3-degree varus cut with respect to the anatomic axis of the tibia. The disadvantage of this approach results from an unavoidable margin of error that leads to some tibial cuts aligned in more or less than 3 degrees of varus. Tibial cuts malaligned with a significant varus deformity cause a focus of the weight-bearing forces within the medial compartment, leading to an increased rate of polyethylene wear and early clinical failure.[6-9] In order to avoid this result, most surgeons use the classical approach, which creates a tibial cut perpendicular to the anatomic axis of the tibia.

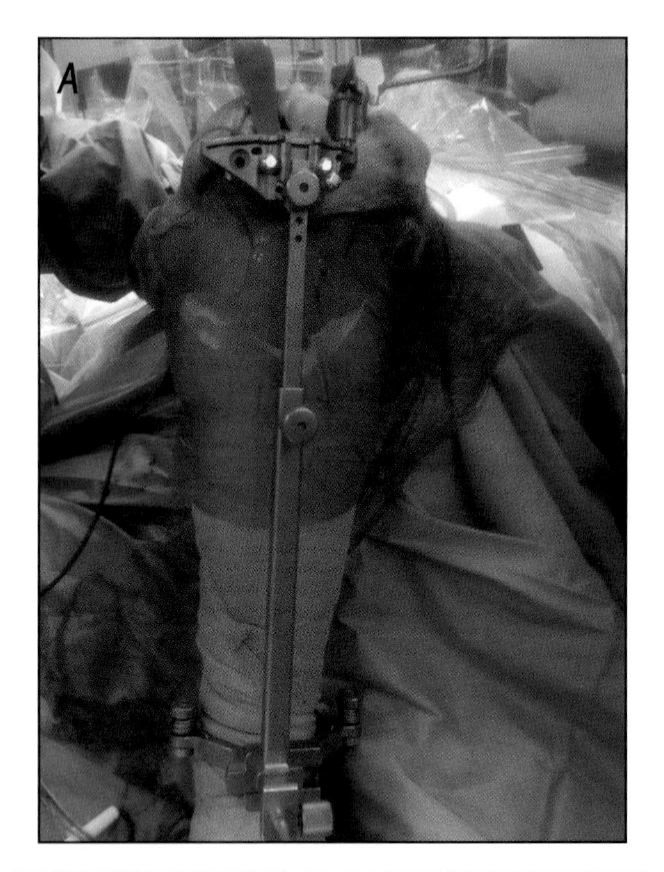


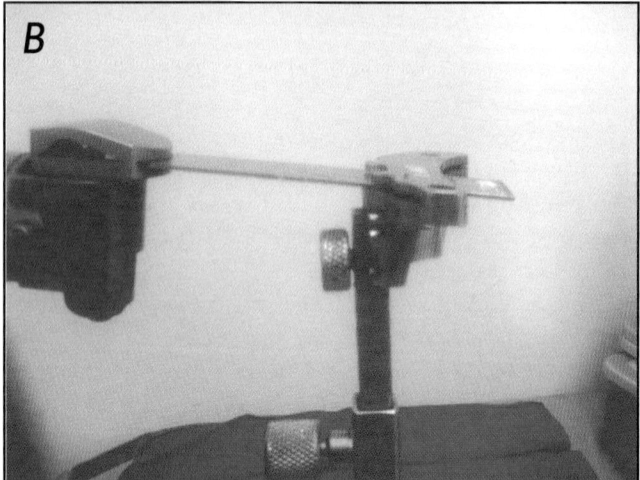


**Figure 11-5.** Extramedullary tibial guide. (A) The external tibial guide sets the orientation and position of the tibial cutting jig based on the palpable surface landmarks of the bone. (B) For this specific guide, the cutting jig is set on the extramedullary guide with a preset 7 degrees of posterior slope. Surgical instrumentation associated with other device systems may not preset intrinsic posterior slope in this manner and in these cases, the surgeon determines the degree of posterior slope based on adjustments made to the external tibial guide.

The accuracy of a perpendicular cut is easier to judge by the surgeon, decreasing the margin of error. Furthermore, a perpendicular cut shifts the margin of error outside the range of a significant varus malalignment. In the sagittal plane, a posterior slope of the tibial cut may be set from 0 to 10 degrees depending on the specifics of the prosthetic system as well as surgeon preference. Greater posterior slope of the tibia opens the flexion gap of the knee and can allow for better flexion. Although posterior slope may improve the maximum flexion and minimize the risk of a recurvatum deformity, it raises the risk of varus-valgus deformity in the coronal plane with malrotation of the component (Figure 11-6). In addition to determining the orientation of the tibial cut in the sagittal and coronal planes, the cutting guide and jig also set the level of proximal tibia resection. The level of resection aims to match the height of the tibial polyethylene with the amount of resected bone. Discordance between these values can be used for soft tissue balancing, as discussed next.

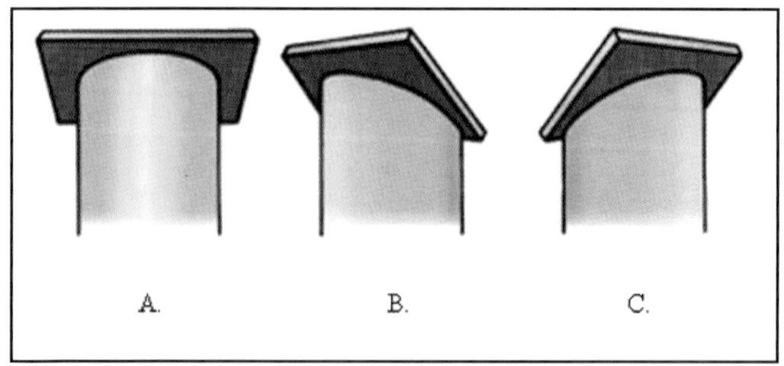


**Figure 11-6.** Influence of the posterior slope on the coronal orientation of the tibial cut. (A) With appropriate orientation and alignment, the degree of posterior slope does not influence the varus-valgus orientation of the cut in the coronal plan. (B, C) With inappropriate rotational alignment of the cutting jig, the degree of posterior slope directly leads to changes in the varus or valgus angle of the cut in the coronal plane. (Adapted from Scott WN. *Insall and Scott's Surgery of the Knee.* 4th ed. Philadelphia, PA: Elsevier; 2006.)

Once the tibial cut is completed, the size and rotational orientation of the component are determined. A finite number of tibial component sizes are available with each prosthetic system, and a perfect match with the size and shape of a given patient's tibial surface is uncommon. The most appropriately sized component seats on a rim of supportive cortical bone without overhanging the tibial surface. Undersizing of the tibial component may result in insufficient bony support with early component subsidence and failure while component oversizing creates overhang, which may cause pain and compromise appropriate soft tissue tensioning (Figure 11-7). An appropriately sized tibial component typically allows the surgeon some flexibility in determining its rotation and positioning, variables that primarily affect patellofemoral tracking. There is usually a significant medial osteophyte on the tibia with the varus knee, and these tibial osteophytes should be removed. Removing this bone will improve the balancing of the medial collateral ligament.

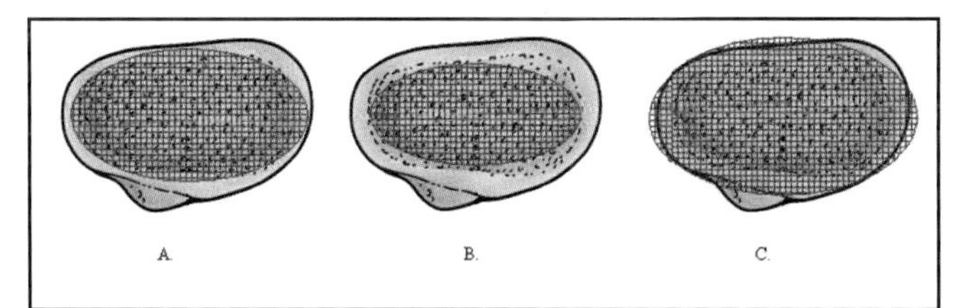


**Figure 11-7.** Placement and support of the tibial component on the cut surface of the tibia. (A) With appropriate sizing, the tibial component (red checkered oval) sits on an intact cortical rim without overhanging the cut surface of the tibia. (B) With undersizing, the tibial component sits on structurally weak medullary bone, placing the component at risk for subsidence. (C) With oversizing, the tibial component sits well supported on an intact cortical rim but overhangs the cut surface of the proximal tibia, leading to tenting of the surrounding soft tissue structures. (Adapted from Scott WN. *Insall and Scott's Surgery of the Knee.* 4th ed. Philadelphia, PA: Elsevier; 2006.)

## Surgical Principles of Femoral Preparation

In preparing the femur, the surgeon determines several parameters that affect the ultimate alignment and orientation of the femoral component. As with tibial preparation, an extramedullary guide, intramedullary guide, or computer navigation guide may be used to reference the femoral axes. Because the relevant femoral landmarks are not easily palpated, extramedullary guides are inaccurate and difficult to use. Intramedullary guides accurately estimate the anatomic axis of the femur with normal femoral anatomy and are commonly used in femoral preparation. With abnormal femoral bowing or when more proximal hardware precludes the use of an intramedullary guide, an extramedullary guide or computer navigation may be used to more accurately reference the femoral axes. Extramedullary guides and computer navigation have the advantage that they do not violate the femoral canal and may lead to decreased fat embolism.

The distal femoral cut determines the ultimate valgus angle of the femoral component. In order to maintain both symmetric soft tissue balancing in extension and the normal 6-degree valgus angle of the knee, the distal femoral cut is typically set at 5 to 7 degrees of valgus when using a classic perpendicular tibial cut. This 5 to 7 degrees is based on the average, but these values are variable and are influenced by pelvic width and femoral neck offset. The number will be different in the valgus knee, and many surgeons will set the distal cut to 4 degrees. The only certain way to determine the proper distal femoral valgus angle is to measure preoperative long alignment views or to use computer navigation. An anatomic tibial cut would necessitate an average 9-degree valgus distal femoral cut, but most surgeons no longer use the anatomic cut.

The distal cutting jig also determines the level of distal femoral resection. Maintaining the level of the joint line requires resecting the same amount of distal femoral bone that will be replaced by the distal aspect of the femoral component. Discordance between these values can be used to make soft tissue balancing adjustments in extension, but leads to elevation or depression of the joint line. In a knee with a flexion contracture greater than 10 degrees, many surgeons will resect an additional 2 mm of distal femur. This slightly elevates the joint line, but allows for restoration of full extension of the knee.

The rotation and sagittal alignment of the component are determined prior to the completion of the anterior, posterior, and chamfer cuts. In order to maintain symmetric soft tissue balancing in flexion, the rotation of the component is set in 3 degrees of external rotation relative to the posterior condylar axis when using a classic perpendicular tibial cut. Landmarks that are referenced in setting the appropriate rotation of the femoral component include the epicondylar axis, Whiteside's line, and the posterior condylar axis (Figure 11-8). Some systems use a flexion gap tensioning to set the rotation. This technique requires the surgeon to cut the tibia first. Once the distal femur is cut, the extension gap must be tensioned and balanced. The knee is then flexed to 90 degrees and the tensioner is used to set the rotation of the cutting block to establish a symmetrical gap in flexion. In the sagittal plane, the component is typically set in neutral alignment, parallel to the femoral shaft. The component can be flexed slightly in some designs. The surgeon can also choose to slightly flex the component in an attempt to decrease the size of the flexion gap. Excessive flexion will lead to a problem in cruciate-replacing knees if the anterior post impinges in extension on the box.

The size of the femoral component refers to its anteroposterior length. A finite number of femoral component sizes are available for each prosthetic system, and a perfect match with a given patient's anteroposterior femoral dimension is uncommon. As such, the femoral component must be slightly oversized or undersized and the surgeon must chose to focus this mismatch anteriorly or posteriorly (Figure 11-9).

An anterior referencing system positions the cutting jig in a manner that leads to a level of resection of anterior femoral bone that is equally replaced by the anterior aspect of the prosthesis. The posterior femoral bone resection is unequally matched by the posterior aspect of the prosthesis, but with the great variety of sizes now available, the differences are slight. The surgeon needs to be attentive to choosing the appropriate-sized implant to best match the posterior

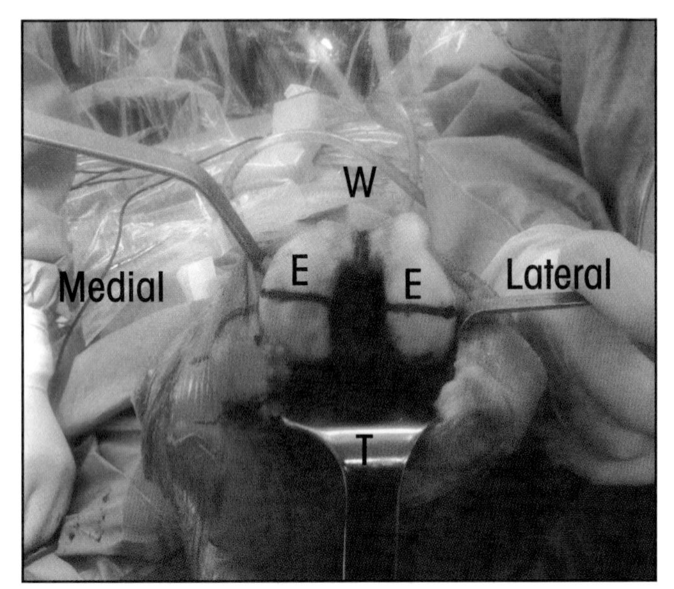


**Figure 11-8.** Rotational landmarks of the femur. Several references are used in setting the rotation of the femoral component. Three degrees of external rotation relative to the posterior condylar line creates a rectangular flexion gap with a classic tibial cut and also optimizes patellofemoral mechanics. The epicondylar axis and the axis of the tibial cut are perpendicular to Whiteside's and are 3 degrees externally rotated relative to the posterior condylar line. W = Whiteside's line, E = epicondylar axis, T = axis of the tibial cut.

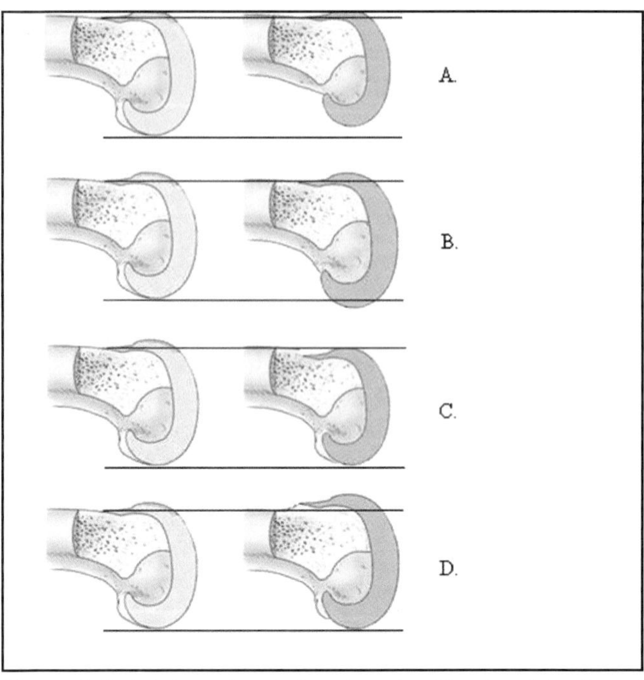


**Figure 11-9.** Anterior and posterior referencing. The size of the femoral component refers to the distance from the anterior cortex of the distal femur to the posterior aspect of the femoral condyle. The left images represent the native distal femur and the right images represent the distal femur after bone resection and replacement with the femoral component (gray). With anterior referencing (A, B), the resected anterior bone is equally matched by the anterior aspect of the femoral component. Slight undersizing of the component (A) is focused posteriorly and as a result, the resected posterior bone is under-matched by the posterior aspect of the component, leading to a loose flexion gap. Slight oversizing of the component (B) is also focused posteriorly and as a result, the resected posterior bone is overmatched by the posterior aspect of the component, leading to a tight flexion gap. With posterior referencing (C, D), the resected posterior bone is equally matched by the posterior aspect of the femoral component. Slight undersizing of the component (C) is focused anteriorly and results in femoral "notching." Slight oversizing of the component (D) is also focused anteriorly and may result in "overstuffing" of the patellofemoral joint. (Adapted from Scott WN. *Insall and Scott's Surgery of the Knee.* 4th ed. Philadelphia, PA: Elsevier; 2006.)

femoral dimensions. With an oversized component, the dimension of the posterior aspect of the component is greater than the amount of resected bone, tending toward tight soft tissue tensioning in flexion. With an undersized component, the dimension of the posterior aspect of the component is less than the amount of resected bone, tending toward loose soft tissue tensioning in flexion. If the flexion gap is loose, the implant can be flexed to tighten this space. With anterior referencing, it is crucial that the anterior cut be flush on the anterior cortex of the femur. If not directly on this cortex, an oversized implant may be required to restore the flexion gap. These larger implants are also larger in medial-lateral width, and this can lead to undesirable overhang of the femoral implant.

A posterior referencing system positions the cutting jig in a manner that leads to a level of resection of posterior femoral bone that is equally replaced by the posterior aspect of the prosthesis. As a result, the anterior femoral bone resection is unequally matched by the anterior aspect of the prosthesis. With an oversized component, the dimension of the anterior aspect of the component is greater than that of the resected bone. This results in tight patellofemoral soft tissue tensioning, also known as an "overstuffed" patellofemoral joint, which may compromise the degree of full flexion. With an undersized component, the anterior femoral cut may breach the anterior cortex of the distal femur, also known as "notching." This "notch" decreases the torsional strength of the distal femur and was thought to contribute to supracondylar femoral fractures.[10] Newer clinical studies demonstrate no increased risk of fracture with notching of the distal femur.[11] It is technically preferable to minimize any notching and to match the implant size to the native femoral size. The risk of "notching" in a posterior referencing system can be minimized by placing the component in

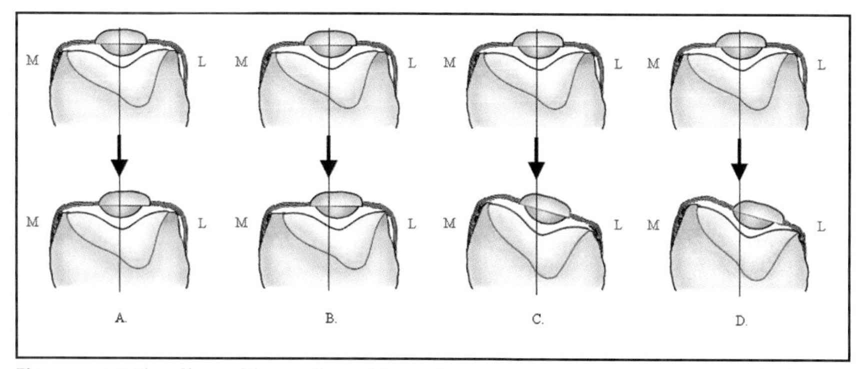


**Figure 11-10.** The effects of the patellar and femoral components on patellofemoral mechanics. The top images represent the patellofemoral articulation with neutral rotation and translation of the femoral component and neutral positioning of the patellar component. In this scenario, the center of the patella sits in line with the deepest part of the femoral component. (A) Medialization of the patellar component causes a relative lateralization of the patella, decreasing the "Q" angle. (B, C) Lateralization and external rotation of the femoral component independently direct the patella laterally, decreasing the "Q" angle. (D) Femoral and patellar component orientation and positioning are demonstrated to cause an additive effect in the lateralization of the patella, decreasing the "Q" angle and minimizing the risk of lateral maltracking. M = medial, L = lateral. (Adapted from Scott WN. *Insall and Scott's Surgery of the Knee.* 4th ed. Philadelphia, PA: Elsevier; 2006.)

slight flexion or by using a component designed with an anterior flange. These approaches are useful when femoral component downsizing is necessary.

The shape and dimensions of the remaining aspects of the femoral component are in proportion to its anteroposterior size. With an appropriately sized component, the medial-lateral dimension of the component is typically slightly less than that of the cut surface of the distal femur. In this case, the surgeon has flexibility in determining the medial-lateral orientation of the component without creating overhang. When the option is available, the component is set laterally in order to optimize patellofemoral mechanics, as described next.

## Surgical Principles of Patellofemoral Mechanics

Several techniques are used to optimize patellofemoral tracking during total knee arthroplasty. Maltracking of the patella may lead to abnormal contact loading, early patellar component wear, chronic anterior knee pain, and/or patellar instability. Because of the combined lateral horizontal force vectors of the quadriceps and patellar tendons on the patella, there is a tendency for lateral patellar translation during active quadriceps contraction (see Figure 11-2). The risk of lateral patellar maltracking can be minimized using surgical techniques aimed at decreasing the "Q" angle and at accommodating the lateral tendency of the patella through strategic positioning of the femoral component. Choices made in the alignment and positioning of the tibial, femoral, and patellar components can be used to achieve these 2 goals.[12,13]

The 3 theoretical anatomic approaches to decreasing the "Q" angle are medialization of the quadriceps origin, lateralization of the patella, and medialization of the tibial tubercle. The latter 2 approaches are the only surgically feasible means of achieving this goal. Since the patellar component is normally smaller than the undersurface of the cut patella, the surgeon typically has flexibility in its positioning. Because it is the patellar component itself rather than the patella that articulates with the trochlea of the femoral component, the patellar component indirectly influences the position of the patella in space. A component that is laterally positioned on the undersurface of the cut patella causes a relative medialization of the patella with patellofemoral articulation, and a component that is medially positioned causes a relative lateralization of the patella with patellofemoral articulation. As such, medialization of the component with patella resurfacing decreases the ultimate "Q" angle (Figure 11-10).

The rotation of the tibial component indirectly influences the position of the tibial tubercle in space (Figure 11-11). Internal rotation of the tibial component on the cut surface of the tibia causes a relative external rotation of the tibial tubercle, lateralizing the structure and increasing the "Q" angle. External rotation of the tibial component on the

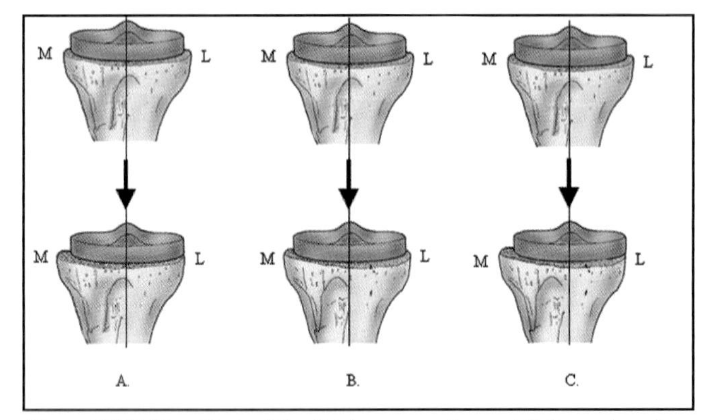


**Figure 11-11.** The effects of the tibial component on patellofemoral mechanics. The top images represent neutral rotation and translation of the tibial component. (A) Lateral positioning of the tibial component leads to a relative medialization of the tibial tubercle, decreasing the "Q" angle. (B) External rotation of the tibial component leads to a relative internal rotation of the tibial tubercle, which medializes the landmark, decreasing the "Q" angle. (C) Lateralization and external rotation of the tibial component are demonstrated to cause an additive effect of medializing the tibial tubercle, decreasing the "Q" angle and minimizing the risk of lateral maltracking. M = medial, L = lateral. (Adapted from Scott WN. *Insall and Scott's Surgery of the Knee.* 4th ed. Philadelphia, PA: Elsevier; 2006.)

cut surface of the tibia causes a relative internal rotation of the tibial tubercle, medializing the structure and decreasing the "Q" angle. In order to minimize the "Q" angle, the surgeon should aim for slight external rotation of the tibial component. The corresponding preferred rotational position of the tibial component is centered over the medial third of the tibial tubercle.[11]

The medial-lateral positioning of the tibial component also indirectly influences the position of the tibial tubercle in space (see Figure 11-11). Lateral positioning of the tibial component on the cut surface of the tibia leads to a relative medialization of the tibial tubercle and medialization of the component has the opposite effect. In order to minimize the "Q" angle, the surgeon should aim for maximal lateralization of the component on the cut surface of the tibia without creating overhang.

The concave shape of the trochlea of the femoral component, the translational and rotational orientation of the femoral component, and the tensioning of the medial and lateral retinacula all affect patellofemoral tracking (see Figure 11-10). When the surgeon has flexibility in establishing its medial-lateral position, lateralization of the component is preferred in order to decrease the "Q" angle and optimize patellar tracking.

The rotational positioning of the femoral component similarly influences patellar tracking. External rotation of the femoral component, coincidentally used to tension the soft tissues in flexion symmetrically, directs the trochlea laterally and facilitates improved patellar tracking. Conversely, surgical errors that lead to significant medialization and/or internal rotation of the femoral component oppose proper patellar tracking and should be avoided.

## Surgical Principles of Soft Tissue Balancing

Although the tibial and femoral bone cuts play an important role in achieving appropriate component alignment in total knee arthroplasty, it is soft tissue tensioning that determines the ultimate balance and stability of the reconstructed joint. There are 2 general approaches used to achieve both goals of component alignment and soft tissue balancing in total knee arthroplasty. With the measured resection technique, the surgeon uses guides and jigs to achieve appropriate component alignment and subsequently, the soft tissues are balanced to accommodate to the alignment. With the gap balancing technique, the surgeons primarily balances the knee by releasing soft tissues to correct preoperative deformity. Subsequently, the surgeon uses a tensioning device to achieve appropriate alignment by creating bone cuts based on the balanced soft tissues. In practice, surgeons often use concepts from both approaches in achieving alignment and balance. If a stable knee cannot be achieved for any reason, the level of constraint must be increased until the knee is stable. Some varus-valgus laxity can be addressed with a stabilized polyethylene. More severe instabilities in the coronal or sagittal plane may require a hinged knee replacement. Regardless of the technique, it is crucial to leave the operating room with a stable knee.

Soft tissue balancing in the coronal plane is determined by the relative tension of the medial and lateral soft tissues that cross the axis of the joint line, and preoperative varus or valgus deformity may lead to asymmetric soft tissue tensioning. Correction of the deformity without addressing the soft tissue imbalance may lead to instability and poor clinical results. A severe preoperative varus deformity causes contracture of the medial soft tissues and stretching of the lateral soft tissues, whereas a severe preoperative valgus deformity has the opposite effect. The first step in balancing the medial and lateral soft tissues is the removal of the femoral and tibial osteophytes, which cause extrinsic soft tissue tensioning. If asymmetry persists, the soft tissue on the contracted side may be released in a progressive manner until coronal balance is achieved. A detailed description of techniques used to achieve coronal balance with preoperative varus and valgus deformity is reserved for the chapter on complex TKA (see Chapter 21).

In the sagittal plane, the surgeon achieves soft tissue balancing by releasing tight soft tissue structures and by adjusting both the level of bone resection and the thickness of the implanted components in flexion and extension. Because the tibia articulates with the femur in both flexion and extension, the level of the tibia cut and the thickness of the implanted tibial components influence soft tissue tensioning in flexion and extension. Because the distal femur articulates with the tibia in extension but not in flexion, the level of the distal femoral cut and the thickness of the distal aspect of the femoral component influence soft tissue tensioning in extension only. Because the posterior femur articulates with the tibia in flexion but not in extension, the level of the posterior femoral cut and the thickness of the posterior aspect of the femoral component influence soft tissue tensioning in flexion only.

Soft tissue balance in the sagittal plane is influenced by preoperative deformities, which lead to soft tissue contracture or laxity, and by the relative level of bone resections performed during the procedure. After the tibial and femoral resections have been made, the surgeon assesses the flexion and extension gaps, which refer to the empty spaces between the cut surfaces of the tibia and femur in full extension and 90 degrees of flexion (Figure 11-12). When necessary, subsequent adjustments are made to the tension of the soft tissues, as described next, in order to achieve balance in full extension and 90 degrees of flexion.

Laxity in extension, manifested as a recurvatum deformity with the trial components in place, can be corrected by increasing the thickness of the distal aspect of the femoral component or the thickness of the tibial component. Practically, these goals can be achieved by adding metal augments to the distal aspect of the femoral component or by upsizing the tibial polyethylene component. These maneuvers increase the fill of the extension gap and, as a result, further tension the posterior soft tissue structures.

Tightness in extension, manifested as the inability to fully extend the knee with the trial components in place, is caused by tightness of posterior soft tissue structures and can be corrected by several techniques. Tight posterior structures can be directly addressed by releasing the capsule of the knee from the posterior aspect of the distal femur. Loosening of tight posterior structures can also be achieved by decreasing the fill of the extension gap. This goal is met by advancing the level of resection of the distal femoral cut, by advancing the level of the tibial cut, or by decreasing the size of the tibial polyethylene when the option is available. It is important to note that maneuvers that lead to mismatch between the amount of resected bone and the dimensions of the components that replace them may change the level of the joint line. Elevation of the joint line results in a relative patella baja while depression of the joint line results in a relative patella alta.

Laxity in flexion manifests as an abnormal drawer test during trialing of the knee in 90 degrees of flexion. The surgeon addresses this scenario by increasing the fill of the flexion gap with the components. This goal is met either by upsizing the femoral component and adding posterior femoral augments to fill the resulting gap, by flexing the femoral component, or by upsizing the tibial polyethylene component.

Tightness in flexion manifests as a limitation in maximal flexion with the trial components in place. The surgeon addresses this scenario by decreasing the fill of the flexion gap with the components. This goal is met by downsizing the femoral component, by advancing the level of the tibial cut, or by decreasing the size of the tibial polyethylene when the option is available.

In practice, the surgeon's specific approach to addressing sagittal soft tissue imbalance depends on the number and specific combinations of deformities in flexion and extension. Table 11-1 demonstrates each of the 8 possible combinations of soft tissue imbalance in the sagittal plane and reviews the appropriate solutions for each combination.

## Summary

The concepts used to align and implant total knee replacements have remained fairly constant over the last 20 years. The surgeon needs to pay close attention to both the bony alignment and the soft tissue balance issues. Mastering the basic principles in total knee arthroplasty will lead to well-aligned, well-balanced implants.

## References

1. Johnson F, Leitl S, Waugh W. The distribution of load across the knee. *J Bone Joint Surg Br.* 1980;62:346-349.
2. Hsu WW, Himeco S, Coventry MB, et al. Normal axial alignment of the lower extremity and load bearing distribution of the knee. *Clin Orthop.* 1990;225:215-227.
3. Caillouette JT, Anzel AH. Fat embolism syndrome following an intramedullary alignment guide in total knee arthroplasty. *Clin Orthop Relat Res.* 1990;251:198-199.
4. Church JS, Scadden JE, Gupta RR, et al. Embolic phenomena during computer-assisted and conventional total knee replacement. *J Bone Joint Surg Br.* 2007;89:481-485.

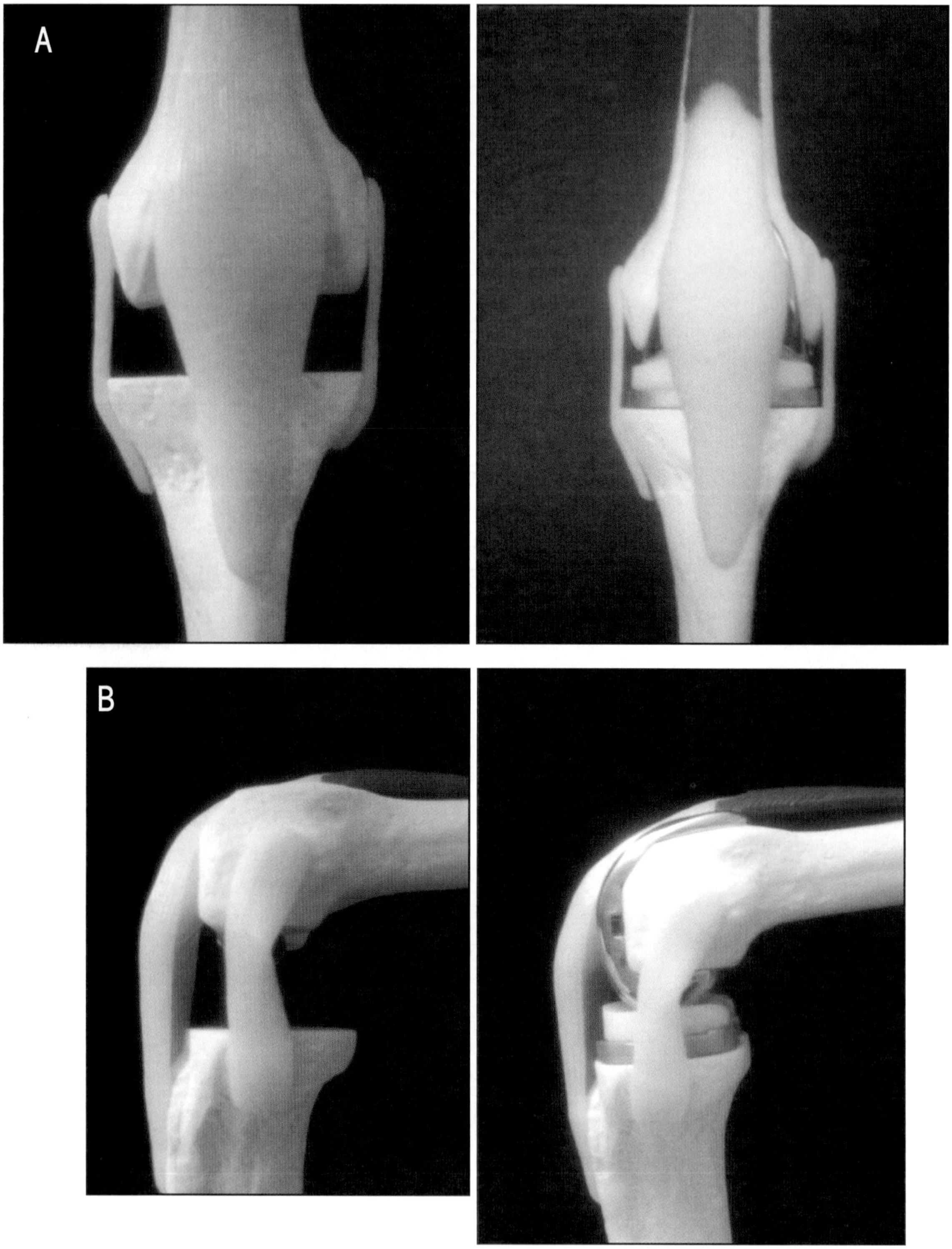

**Figure 11-12.** Flexion and extension gaps. (A) Anteroposterior view of a symmetric extension gap (left) and of the same flexion gap filled with the tibial components and distal aspect of the femoral component (right). (B) Lateral view of a symmetric flexion gap (left) and the same flexion gap filled with the tibial components and posterior aspect of the femoral component (right).

Table 11-1

## Flexion/Extension Balancing in Total Knee Arthroplasty

| Problem | Flexion | Extension | Solutions |
|---|---|---|---|
| 1 | Balanced | Loose | Add a distal femoral augment<br>Downsize the femoral component (converting to problem 4) and upsize the tibial polyethylene<br>Upsize the tibial polyethylene (converting to problem 6) and downsize the femoral component |
| 2 | Balanced | Tight | Release the capsule from the posterior femur and remove posterior femoral osteophytes<br>Resect more distal femoral bone |
| 3 | Loose | Balanced | Upsize the femoral component and fill the gap with cement or a posterior femoral augment |
| 4 | Loose | Loose | Upsize the tibial polyethylene |
| 5 | Loose | Tight | Upsize the femoral component and fill the gap with cement or a posterior femoral augment, resect more distal femoral bone |
| 6 | Tight | Balanced | Check the sagittal slope of the tibia and recut it if it is anteriorly oriented<br>Downsize the femoral component |
| 7 | Tight | Loose | Downsize the femoral component and add a distal femoral augment |
| 8 | Tight | Tight | Downsize the tibial polyethylene<br>Resect more proximal tibial bone |


5. Maestro A, Harwin SF, Sandoval MG, et al. Influence of intramedullary versus extramedullary alignment guides on final total knee arthroplasty component position: a radiographic analysis. *J Arthroplasty.* 1998;13:552-558.
6. Green GV, Berend KR, Berend ME, et al. The effects of varus tibial alignment on proximal tibial surface strain in total knee arthroplasty: the posteromedial hot spot. *J Arthroplasty.* 2002;17:1033-1039.
7. Lotke PA, Ecker ML. Influence of positioning of prosthesis in total knee replacement. *J Bone Joint Surg Am.* 1977;59:77-79.
8. Ritter MA, Faris PM, Keating EM, et al. Postoperative alignment in total knee replacement: its effect on survival. *Clin Orthop.* 1994;299:153-156.
9. Collier MB, Engh CA Jr, McAuley JP, et al. Factors associated with loss of thickness of polyethylene tibial bearings after knee arthroplasty. *J Bone Joint Surg Am.* 2007;89:2306-2314.
10. Culp RW, Schmidt RG, Hanks G, et al. Supracondylar fracture of the femur following prosthetic knee arthroplasty. *Clin Orthop.* 1987;222:212-222.
11. Ritter MA, Thong AE, Keating EM, et al. The effect of femoral notching during total knee arthroplasty on the prevalence of postoperative femoral fractures and on clinical outcome. *J Bone Joint Surg Am.* 2005;87:2411-2414.
12. Grace JN, Rand JA. Patellar instability after total knee arthroplasty. *Clin Orthop Relat Res.* 1988;237:184-189.
13. Berger RA, Crossett LS, Jacobs JJ, et al. Malrotation causing patellofemoral complications after total knee arthroplasty. *Clin Orthop Relat Res.* 1998;256:144-153.

# 12

# Avoiding and Overcoming Your Nightmares

*Michael R. Pagnotto, MD and Brian A. Klatt, MD*

Primary total knee arthroplasty (TKA) is a safe and effective treatment option for end-stage arthritis.[1] The rate of major intraoperative and postoperative complications are low.[2] However, knee arthroplasty is an elective procedure, and some complications may have devastating outcomes. Arterial injury, patella tendon rupture, medial collateral ligament (MCL) rupture, wound complications, postoperative foot drop, and postoperative stiffness can significantly affect patient outcome and satisfaction.

Certainly arterial injury, patellar tendon rupture, and wound dehiscence can be devastating, but not all complications mandate a poor result. When the surgeon reacts properly, he or she can often salvage a very good result even in the face of potential disaster. After the shock of an MCL injury passes, it can—in most cases—be dealt with quite easily and safely. It is not an untold story to hear of an accidental lateral parapatellar approach to the knee, and yet this will likely lead to no adverse outcome.

This chapter reviews the complications of TKA and identifies the patients who are most at risk. Techniques are discussed to keep the surgeon out of trouble. Prompt identification and proper management of perioperative complications is crucial and can be the difference between acceptable outcomes and major morbidity. Other complications such as infection, periprosthetic fracture, loosening, and thromboembolic disease will not be addressed in this chapter because they are each covered in detail throughout the text.

## Arterial Injury

Arterial injury is the nightmare of all nightmares in TKA. Every time the tibia is cut, the surgeon and assistant must think about the popliteal artery and the potential for a devastating complication. The reported incidence of arterial injury in total knee replacement is 0.017% to 0.2%.[3,4] Arterial injury leads to limb loss in 10% to 43% of cases.[5,6] Though residents are always thinking about direct injury with an oscillating saw, injuries occur via a number of mechanisms. The artery can be lacerated by a saw, scalpel, or other sharp instrument, but the artery can also thrombose due to intimal tears, plague disruption, or prolonged low flow. Tourniquets can also lead to plaque disruption or thrombosis.[5,7,8]

An understanding of anatomy and preoperative risk factors is the best defense against arterial injury. Ninomiya et al performed a study in which they examined popliteal artery anatomy and behavior using serial angiography while performing arthroplasty on cadaveric specimens.[9] Their findings were supplemented with magnetic resonance imaging (MRI) data. The authors showed that the popliteal artery is a consistently lateral structure as it crosses the knee. In extension, they found the artery to be within 1 cm of the tibial plateau while in flexion, the distance increased to more than 2 cm. While flexing the knee clearly protected the artery, both hyperflexion and hyperextension led to severe tenting of the artery. They also showed that a single



Parvizi J, Klatt B.
*Essentials in Total Knee Arthroplasty* (pp 91-100).

posterior retractor placed in a position lateral to the posterior cruciate ligament (PCL) or a single retractor placed more than 1 cm into the soft tissue placed the artery at risk. A double pronged retractor placed over the PCL appeared to be a safer alternative. The authors concluded that consistently placing posterior retractors medial to the midline and avoiding extremes in flexion and extension decrease the risk of injury. The risk of popliteal artery injury from retractor placement outweighs the benefit of placing a retractor between the artery and the saw during the tibial cuts. If the surgeon chooses to place a retractor on the lateral side, it is imperative that the retractor be placed with patience. Cautious release of the posterior capsule off the tibia at the lateral, posterior position can allow for safe placement of this retractor on bone.

A history of vascular disease, such as vascular insufficiency, previous vascular surgery, or a popliteal aneurysm, is the biggest risk factor for arterial injury.[4,7,8] One study showed an astonishing 25% incidence of arterial injury in patients with pre-existing vascular disease.[7] In their review of the literature, Smith et al recommended that patients with a history of arterial insufficiency, absence of pedal pulses, a suspected popliteal artery aneurysm, or radiographic evidence of calcification of the superficial femoral artery or popliteal artery should undergo evaluation by a vascular surgeon preoperatively and that those patients may benefit from TKA without the use of a tourniquet (Table 12-1).[8] Preoperative vascular disease can also cloud the postoperative assessment. Incorrectly attributing an abnormal vascular exam postoperatively to preoperative baseline can be devastating. It is essential to have a well-documented preoperative vascular exam.

Prompt identification and appropriate treatment of arterial injury can be limb saving. The first vascular check should be done in the operating room while the patient is still anesthetized. A complete neurovascular exam should be performed as soon as the patient is awake and regional anesthesia wears off. The presence of a "warm" foot is absolutely not sufficient to rule out a vascular injury. Pulses must be confirmed with palpation or Doppler evaluation. Collateral blood flow can lead to a warm foot even in the presence of a vascular injury. In one report, nearly half of all vascular injuries secondary to TKA or total hip arthroplasty were not identified until more than 24 hours postoperatively.[10] The authors identified several factors that contributed to delay in diagnosis, including epidural anesthesia masking neurologic changes, and postoperative dressing and antithrombotic pumps, making assessment difficult. When there is any question about postoperative vascular exam, we recommend prompt vascular surgery consultation. Once arterial injury is identified, aggressive revascularization is critical to avoid amputation.[10]

Table 12-1

**Preoperative Risk Factors for Arterial Injuries**

- Vascular insufficiency
- History of vascular surgery
- Popliteal aneurysm
- Absence of pedal pulses
- Radiographic evidence of arterial calcification

Compartment syndrome is a major concern any time there is an arterial injury. Arterial bleeding into the leg can easily cause an acute compartment syndrome. The hallmark of any compartment syndrome is pain. Unfortunately, in the immediate postoperative setting, pain may not be a reliable indicator because the patient's pain is masked by postoperative pain management. Nerve blocks, epidurals, or patient-controlled analgesics could hide the pain of a compartment syndrome. By the time the epidural or nerve block wears off, irreversible soft tissue injuries may have occurred. Furthermore, even when an acute compartment syndrome is avoided, patients can still develop a delayed compartment syndrome secondary to a reperfusion injury. Anytime an arterial injury occurs, compartments should be monitored with extreme caution and the surgeon should have a very low threshold for compartment release. All of the benefits of limb-sparing revascularization procedures will be negated if a compartment syndrome is missed. Although extremely rare, compartment syndromes may occur outside of vascular injuries. Nadeem et al reported a thigh compartment syndrome that developed 3 days after TKA after the patient was started on heparin for a deep vein thrombosis (DVT).[11]

In summary, arterial injury in TKA is rare, but with reported rates as high as 1 in 500, it is a complication that will be seen in any high-volume joint practice. An awareness of preoperative risk factors and vascular anatomy combined with meticulous surgical technique and thorough postoperative monitoring will help surgeons avoid this complication and minimize the damage if it occurs.

## Medial Collateral Ligament Rupture

MCL injury is an uncommon complication. The incidence is reported to be around 2%, although 1 study reported 8% in morbidly obese patients.[12,13] Injury patterns

Table 12-2

**PREOPERATIVE RISK FACTORS FOR MEDIAL COLLATERAL LIGAMENT INJURY**

- Obesity
- Varus alignment
- Osteopenia

include intrasubstance tears as well as femoral and tibial avulsion injuries. This section reviews MCL anatomy, preoperative risk factors, common injury mechanisms, tips to avoid injury, and treatment options.

In their classic article, Warren and Marshall describe a 3-layer classification system for the medial-sided structures of the knee.[14] As they describe, the MCL is composed of deep and superficial layers. The deep MCL is in layer III. It originates on the medial epicondyle of the femur, attaches to the medial meniscus, and then inserts on the medial tibia just below the articular surface. The deep MCL is a thickening of the joint capsule. The superficial MCL is in layer II. It originates from the medial epicondyle of the femur and inserts onto the tibia deep and distal to the insertion of the gracilis and semitendinosus. The anterior border of the superficial MCL is the primary static stabilizer on the medial side of the knee against valgus and rotational stress.[15] The deep MCL is normally released off the joint line during preparation of the tibia so when an "MCL" injury is referenced, it is the superficial MCL that is injured.

The 3 major risk factors for MCL injury are morbid obesity, osteopenia, and varus alignment. Winiarsky et al reported an 8% MCL avulsion rate in morbidly obese patients compared to no injuries in their nonobese control group.[13] All of their reported injuries were avulsion injuries off the tibia during retraction. The added soft tissue in the obese leg seemed to place the MCL at greater risk. Osteopenic patients are also at increased risk for avulsion injuries. The weakened bone fails more easily when a valgus load is placed on the knee. Patients with pre-existing varus deformity are often tight medially, requiring a more extensive soft tissue release, and the MCL can be injured directly during the release (Table 12-2).

The MCL is most at risk for sharp injury during preparation of the tibial plateau and when making the tibial cuts. As soft tissue is released medially, especially when the medial-sided structures are tight due to varus alignment, care must be taken to protect the superficial MCL. When the medial-sided tibial cut is made, the medial border of

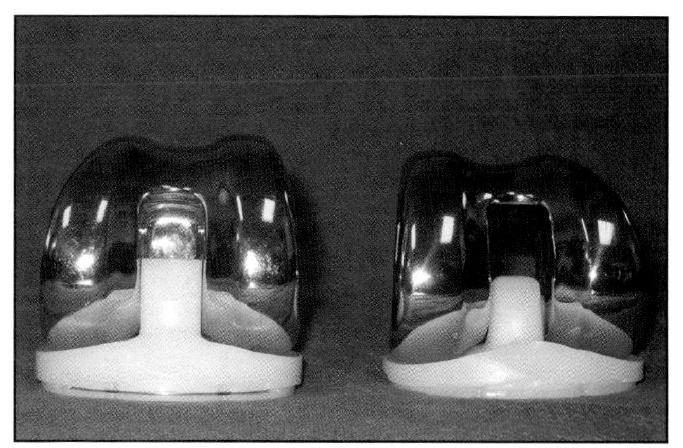

**Figure 12-1.** A constrained condylar implant on the left compared to a standard posterior stabilized implant on the right. Notice the increased height and width of the polyethylene post and the closed box femoral design on the left. These features give the CCK added stability.

the tibial plateau should be well visualized and a retractor should be in place to protect the MCL. Avulsion injuries are usually due to excessive anterior subluxation of the tibia. It is important to adequately release the deep medial soft tissue prior to subluxating the tibia, and the tibia should only be brought forward with gentle traction. If the MCL has been insufficiently released and the tibia is forced forward, this can lead to a traumatic intrasubstance tear.[16] Avulsion injuries are usually obvious when they occur. A pop is heard, and in an instant a difficult exposure becomes easy.[12]

There are 2 accepted treatment options once an MCL injury is recognized. The "standard teaching" is to implant a condylar constrained knee (CCK). These constrained implants provide greater stability by having a large polyethylene post that prevents varus and valgus movement of the knee. The CCK, however, is believed to increase the stress on the implant and lead to higher rates of aseptic loosening. Intramedullary rods should be added to the CCK to provide better fixation of the components, which makes the TKA significantly more invasive. Figure 12-1 highlights the differences between a CCK prosthesis and a standard posterior stabilized knee.

In an attempt to avoid the long-term consequence of higher rates of loosening, one study reported fixing MCL injuries either primarily for midsubstance tears or via suture anchors when the injuries were avulsion injuries followed by up to 6 weeks of postoperative bracing.[12] The authors reported good results on 14 patients treated in this manner at a minimum of 2 years follow-up. An avulsion off the tibia can also be fixed to the tibial bone with a single staple in the tibia.

Table 12-3

**PREOPERATIVE RISK FACTORS FOR PATELLA TENDON INJURY**

- Decreased preoperative range of motion
- Revision surgery
- Difficult exposure

MCL injury should be repaired in all patients. The younger, healthier, higher-demand patients have a higher likelihood of healing the repair and will benefit more from the theoretical lower rates of loosening by avoiding a constrained knee. They should be treated with a hinged brace for 8 weeks. Older, lower-demand, less healthy patients who have a less likely chance of healing the repair can be treated with a CCK implant to supplement the MCL repair. They will benefit less from avoiding a constrained knee. They do not require bracing since the knee is inherently more stable in the valgus direction.

## PATELLA TENDON RUPTURE

Patella tendon rupture is a rare complication. Nearly all of the literature regarding patella tendon rupture in TKA discusses patella tendon rupture in the postoperative period rather then discussing acute intraoperative injuries. The reported incidence after TKA is 0.17%; however, this group ranged in presentation from 0 to 42 months postoperatively.[17] Latent postoperative extensor mechanism disruption will be addressed in other chapters. This section focuses on acute patella injury, preoperative risk factors, operative techniques to protect the tendon, and the appropriate management.

Patella tendon avulsion and direct patella tendon laceration during patella tendon preparation are the 2 mechanisms of patella tendon injury during TKA.[16] Avulsion injuries are far more common. The 3 main risk factors are preoperative limited range of motion, revision knee surgery, and overall difficult exposure (Table 12-3).[17,18] Inverting the patella places significant stress on the insertion of the patella tendon. The insertion site should be consistently visualized to ensure that the tissue is not separating from the tibial tubercle. Furthermore, in a contracted knee that cannot bend to 90 degrees, simply flexing the knee past 90 degrees places the tendon at risk.

Adherence to a few basic principles can decrease the force on the patellar tendon insertion and avoid avulsion injuries. The medial incision should extend down directly on the medial border of the tubercle. Patella femoral ligaments should be released. If the patella is still not easily inverted, check the proximal extent of the exposure. Increasing the split in the quad tendon will make the patella more mobile. Removing extensive patellar or femoral osteophytes can improve the patellar mobility. By this point, the patella is usually easily inverted in the primary knee. Some descriptions of minimally invasive techniques advocate making the patella cut prior to inverting the patella.[16] If the patella is cut prior to inverting the patella, care should be taken not to damage the soft cancellous bone of the remaining patella.[16] When making patella cuts, a retractor should always be in place to protect the tendon. If the patella is fully visualized whenever making patella cuts and the retractors are in place, the risk of cutting the tendon is low.

Often, extensive synovium and fibrous scar tissue must be completely excised before proceeding with TKA. This can be seen in a revision, infection, or a complex primary TKA. It is often surprising how much more knee motion will result, and many times the patella will easily evert after this débridement is complete. Often the fat pad will be scarred to the joint and the surgeon must carefully release this from the joint. When the patella cannot safely be inverted or when the knee is too stiff to adequately flex, a lateral retinacular release can loosen the soft tissues.[18] When a lateral release is not sufficient, a proximal soft tissue release or tibial tubercle osteotomy can also be performed.[19] It is the preference of the authors to use a quad snip. A quad snip can be repaired easily and leads to no delay in the rehabilitation of the knee. Figure 12-2 demonstrates a standard quad snip technique.

When injuries to the tendon are noted intraoperatively, they should be fixed acutely. Partial avulsion injuries may not require any repair; however, a suture anchor can be added to reattach the partially avulsed portion of the tendon. Primary repair with or without augmentation is the standard.[18] We recommend limited range of motion for 4 to 6 weeks postoperatively to allow for tendon healing. Injury to the patella tendon is rare but can have devastating outcomes. Surgeons should be wary of forcefully flexing a stiff knee or forcefully inverting the patella in patients who are at risk.

## THE ACCIDENTAL LATERAL PARAPATELLAR APPROACH

At most institutions, there is a story of a surgeon who accidentally made a lateral parapatellar incision rather than

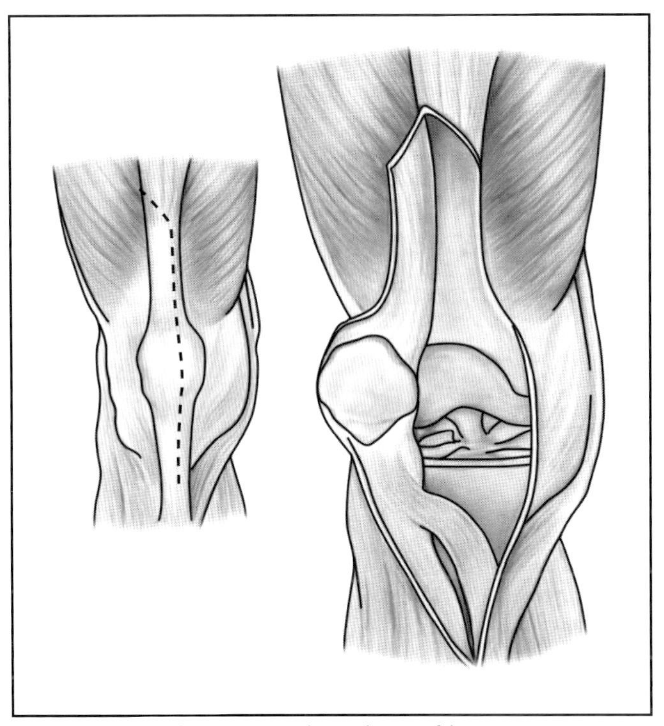

**Figure 12-2.** A quadriceps snip can be used in to safely gain exposure.

a medial parapatellar incision. The mistake is not as frightening as a resident would imagine. The knee can, in fact, be replaced through a lateral parapatellar approach.

Once the capsular incision has been placed laterally, it is better to proceed with the knee from this side. The lateral parapatellar approach is outlined in the chapter on surgical approaches to TKA (see Chapter 9). It is used regularly by surgeons in valgus knees where they believe it makes more sense to release the lateral side. The greatest challenges are everting the patella and setting the rotation of the tibial component. It is best not to close the capsule and make a new incision on the medial side of the joint. This will compromise the circulation to the patella, and for that reason may lead to avascular necrosis and patellar issues.

## Postoperative Foot Drop

Postoperative foot drop or peroneal nerve palsy encompasses a wide spectrum of clinical manifestations from subtle extensor hallucis longus weakness to a complete foot drop. The long-term prognosis and potential disability are equally as varied. Given the spectrum of manifestations, it is difficult to precisely define the incidence of peroneal nerve injury; however, several large studies have identified the incidence between 0.3% to 1.3%.[20] Preoperative valgus deformity and possibly flexion contracture are the most common risk factors.[20,21] Although less clearly linked, epidural analgesia, previous neuropathy (the so-called double crush phenomenon), rheumatoid arthritis, tourniquet, constrictive dressings, and postoperative hematoma have all been proposed as risk factors for peroneal nerve palsy.[20, 22-24]

A thorough physical exam should follow once a nerve palsy is detected. As we discussed, an abnormal neurological exam can be the first sign of a vascular injury or a compartment syndrome. The postoperative dressing should be cut down to relieve any pressure on the peroneal nerve, the knee should be flexed, and the soft tissue around the nerve should be examined for a postoperative hematoma. Most studies report at least 50% of postoperative nerve palsies will resolve with time; anecdotally, however, the number seems even higher.[20,21,23,25] If there is no recovery after 3 months, electromyography (EMG) should be obtained. Also, when there is a complete foot drop, patients should be braced with the foot in neutral to prevent the development of an equinus contracture while the nerve recovers.

## Wound Complications

Postoperative wound complications are rare but potentially devastating. Wound complications include skin necrosis, persistent drainage, hemarthrosis, and superficial wound infection. When wound complications are not the result of deep infection, they can rapidly lead to deep infection and therefore must be addressed in a timely and appropriate manner.[26] Preoperative risk factors for wound complication are similar to the risk factors for infection in general and they include prior surgical scars, immunosuppression, malnutrition, hypokalemia, diverticulosis, concurrent infection, diabetes, obesity, smoking, renal failure, hypothyroidism, alcohol abuse, rheumatoid arthritis, and peripheral vascular disease.[27-29] Clearly, some of these factors such as nutrition or concurrent infection may be optimized preoperatively; however, most of the preoperative risk factors cannot be significantly affected prior to surgery.

Multiple intraoperative and postoperative factors may also increase the risk of wound complications. Skin necrosis is more commonly seen on the lateral skin edge.[26] It is thought that the lateral skin is at a higher risk because the blood supply across the knee flows in a medial to lateral direction. Following that logic, it is usually safest to choose the most lateral incision whenever multiple old incisions are present. As with all surgery, it is important to maintain thick skin flaps and to handle the skin edges with care. Tourniquet time, overall operative time, early knee

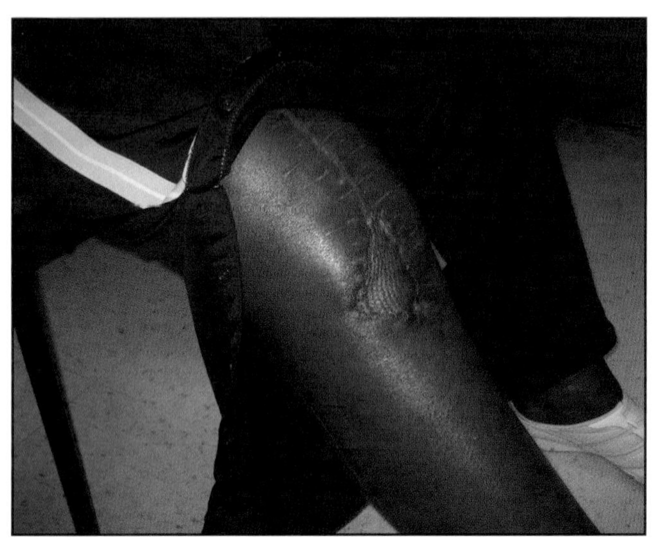

**Figure 12-3.** After wound breakdown following a TKA, local wound care followed by a rotation flap and skin grafting led to an ultimately good outcome with retention of the original implant.

flexion, anticoagulation, and poor postoperative oxygenation have all been associated with increased wound complications.[11,26,30,31] Finally, the use of postoperative drains remains controversial.

When skin necrosis occurs, prompt recognition and treatment can minimize the risk of deep infection. In one review of 9 cases, successful wound healing and implant salvage was achieved in all 9 cases.[27] The authors recommend local wound care and skin grafting for necrosis over the patella with muscle flap coverage for wounds over the patella tendon or tibial tubercle. Figure 12-3 demonstrates a knee that was treated with local wound care, a rotational flap, and skin grafting after skin necrosis over the patella. The authors also noted that immobilization and prophylactic antibiotics serve as a useful adjuvant. A closed but persistently draining wound creates a diagnostic and therapeutic dilemma. Prophylactic antibiotics and skin swabs are not recommended because they usually only cloud the picture.[32,33] When deep infection is not otherwise suspected and there is no evidence of superficial infection, wound drainage can be treated with immobilization and wound care for 5 to 7 days.[26] When wound drainage persists and especially when it does not decease with time, then early irrigation and débridement may be warranted to prevent a deep infection. Similarly, a nondraining hemarthrosis can be followed, but a persistently draining hemarthrosis should be evacuated. Also, a nondraining hemarthrosis that is causing tension on the skin edges, preventing physical therapy, or causing persistent postoperative pain may also be evacuated. Superficial infections usually present with a dry, erythematous, non-purulent wound that does not have significant loculation or induration. Superficial wound infections may be treated with antibiotic; however, it becomes very difficult to diagnose a deep infection once antibiotics are started. Therefore, arthrocentesis should be performed prior to antibiotic initiation.

Table 12-4

**Risk Factors for Postoperative Stiffness**

- Preoperative decreased ROM
- Poor intraoperative ROM
- Pre- or postoperative patella infera
- Increased number of medical comorbidities

## Stiffness

Stiffness after TKA is a relatively common complication with an incidence of 1.3% to 12%.[19,34] Objectively, stiffness is difficult to define because a good outcome in a low-demand elderly patient with limited preoperative range of motion (ROM) is far different than a good outcome in a young, healthy active patient.

Biomechanical studies show that the swing phase of gait requires 67 degrees of flexion, ascending stairs requires 83 degrees, descending stairs 90 to 100 degrees, and rising from a chair 105 degrees.[35,36] In general, patients will be symptomatic with a flexion contracture of 10 to 15 degrees and flexion of less than 90 degrees. Flexion contracture prevents the knee from locking in full extension, making walking more difficult because the quad must continuously fire.

The main predictor of postoperative ROM is preoperative ROM.[37,38] Intraoperative ROM, preoperative or postoperative patella infera, and an increased number of medial comorbidities are all also predictive of decreased postoperative ROM (Table 12-4).[37]

There are a number of intraoperative and postoperative factors that may contribute to stiffness. Improper balancing of flexion and extension gaps may lead to a stiff knee. For example, tightness in flexion could be caused by an oversized polyethylene component that was used to compensate for a loose extension gap. Translating the femoral component posteriorly will narrow the flexion gap, as will oversizing the femoral component or internally or externally rotating the femoral component. A tight PCL in a cruciate-retaining (CR) knee can lead to tightness in flexion and extension. Tight extension gaps are usually caused by oversizing the

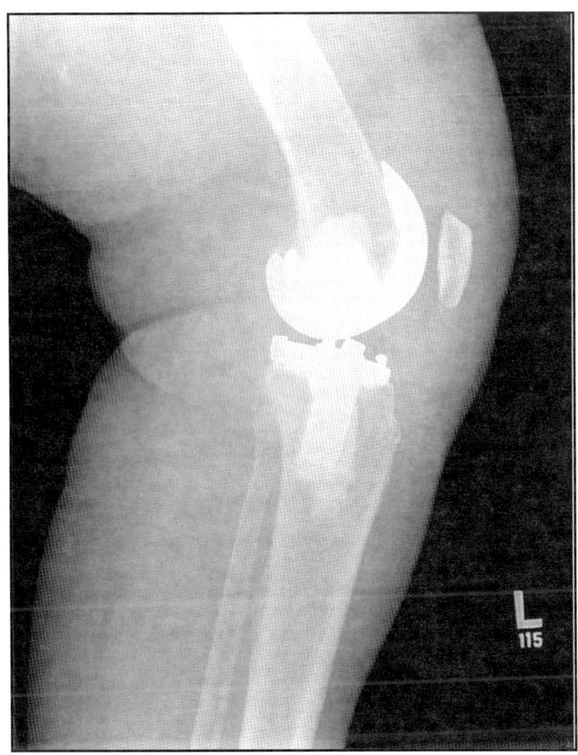


**Figure 12-4.** With an anterior sloping tibial component, this primary TKA required revision due to postoperative stiffness.

polyethylene component. Anything that tightens the extensor mechanism can lead to postoperative stiffness. Elevating the joint line that leads to a relative patella infera and scarring of the patella tendon leading to patella baja postoperatively will both lead to decreased ROM.[39] Overstuffing the patella has been implicated in postoperative stiffness, but recently this has been questioned in the literature.[40] Regardless, a poorly tracking, unstable, or generally painful patellofemoral joint may lead to increased postoperative pain and delayed therapy and thus leads to postoperative stiffness. Cutting the tibia with an anterior slope, especially in a CR knee, can lead to stiffness. Figure 12-4 demonstrates a primary TKA that required revision due to stiffness. Notice the anterior sloping tibial cut. Obviously large posterior osteophytes that are not removed may limit flexion.

Postoperative factors that may lead to stiffness are primarily related to inadequate or delayed rehabilitation. Patient motivation and willingness to work hard postoperatively may be the most important factor. A surgeon can put in a technically perfect knee but if the patient does not do the required rehabilitation, the knee will remain stiff and painful. There are other factors that are outside the patient's control as well. Infection, hemarthrosis, wound complications, medical issues such as myocardial infarct or pneumonia, and periprosthetic fracture can all lead to delayed or inadequate rehabilitation and ultimately a stiff knee. Concurrent orthopedic pathology, specifically hip pain or spinal stenosis, may limit rehabilitation after a total knee. It is always preferable to treat hip pathology prior to a TKA. Reflex sympathetic dystrophy (RSD) and heterotopic ossification (HO) are both uncommon complications, but both can lead to stiffness.[41,42] One study found that HO greater than >5 cm reliably led to postoperative stiffness.[41] Arthrofibrosis is the development of pathologic fibrous scar tissue postoperatively. Arthrofibrosis will certainly lead to stiffness, though it is often difficult to decipher if the arthrofibrosis was the cause or the effect.

When evaluating a stiff knee postoperatively, always start with a thorough history and physical. It is important to establish what the indication for the primary surgery was and what the preoperative ROM was. Always think about infection. Check peripheral blood work for a complete blood count, sedimentation rate, and C-reactive protein. The joint should be aspirated whenever there is any concern. X-rays and possibly CT scan should be obtained to look for technical factors that may cause stiffness as previously described, such as rotation, sizing, tibial slope, posterior osteophytes, joint line elevation, and others. It is critical to try to find an underlying etiology of the stiffness. Whenever an underlying etiology can be established, it should be treated (eg, infection, RSD, posterior osteophytes). Unfortunately, more often than not there is no obvious culprit. When a patient has a well-fixed, well-aligned knee with no evidence of infection or RSD that continues to be stiff, most authors recommend manipulation under anesthesia between 6 and 12 weeks.[36,43] When stiffness persists beyond 3 months, there are several surgical options. Arthroscopic lysis of adhesions, open lysis, and possibly arthroscopic release of the PCL have all been shown to offer some benefit.[44-47] The knee is also manipulated at the time of open or arthroscopic lysis. Open lysis with polyethylene exchange has been shown to be of questionable benefit.[48] Revision arthroplasty offers the best results when there is an identifiable cause of stiffness.[19] Exposure is often difficult in extremely stiff knees and a quadriceps snip, patella turndown procedure, or even tibial tubercle osteotomy may be needed to avoid patella tendon rupture.

## Summary

A successful elective surgery can quickly become complicated by a nightmare. Surgeons should always be cognizant of the potential for arterial injury, MCL rupture, patella tendon rupture, postoperative foot drop, compartment syndromes, wound complications, and postoperative stiffness. The lateral parapatellar approach can be used to do a TKA without any real trouble, but this can be avoided by careful attention to the task at hand. By screening for preoperative risk factors and remembering some basic technical points, the risks of a nightmare occurring can be minimized. Thorough intraoperative and postoperative monitoring is essential to detect and treat complications properly.

## References


1. Mahomed NN, Barrett J, Katz JN, Baron JA, Wright J, Losina E. Epidemiology of total knee replacement in the United States Medicare population. *J Bone Joint Surg Am.* 2005;87(6):1222-1228.
2. Parvizi J, Mui A, Purtill JJ, Sharkey PF, Hozack WJ, Rothman RH. Total joint arthroplasty: when do fatal or near-fatal complications occur? *J Bone Joint Surg Am.* 2007;89(1):27-32.
3. Rand JA. Vascular complications of total knee arthroplasty: report of three cases. *J Arthroplasty.* 1987;2(2):89-93.
4. Calligaro KD, DeLaurentis DA, Booth RE, Rothman RH, Savarese RP, Dougherty MJ. Acute arterial thrombosis associated with total knee arthroplasty. *J Vasc Surg.* 1994;20(6):927-930; discussion 930-922.
5. Da Silva MS, Sobel M. Popliteal vascular injury during total knee arthroplasty. *J Surg Res.* 2003;109(2):170-174.
6. Kumar SN, Chapman JA, Rawlins I. Vascular injuries in total knee arthroplasty: a review of the problem with special reference to the possible effects of the tourniquet. *J Arthroplasty.* 1998;13(2):211-216.
7. DeLaurentis DA, Levitsky KA, Booth RE, et al. Arterial and ischemic aspects of total knee arthroplasty. *Am J Surg.* 1992;164(3):237-240.
8. Smith DE, McGraw RW, Taylor DC, Masri BA. Arterial complications and total knee arthroplasty. *J Am Acad Orthop Surg.* 2001;9(4):253-257.
9. Ninomiya JT, Dean JC, Goldberg VM. Injury to the popliteal artery and its anatomic location in total knee arthroplasty. *J Arthroplasty.* 1999;14(7):803-809.
10. Calligaro KD, Dougherty MJ, Ryan S, Booth RE. Acute arterial complications associated with total hip and knee arthroplasty. *J Vasc Surg.* 2003;38(6):1170-1177.
11. Nadeem RD, Clift BA, Martindale JP, Hadden WA, Ritchie IK. Acute compartment syndrome of the thigh after joint replacement with anticoagulation. *J Bone Joint Surg Br.* 1998;80(5):866-868.
12. Leopold SS, McStay C, Klafeta K, Jacobs JJ, Berger RA, Rosenberg AG. Primary repair of intraoperative disruption of the medical collateral ligament during total knee arthroplasty. *J Bone Joint Surg Am.* 2001;83-A(1):86-91.
13. Winiarsky R, Barth P, Lotke P. Total knee arthroplasty in morbidly obese patients. *J Bone Joint Surg Am.* 1998;80(12):1770-1774.
14. Warren LF, Marshall JL. The supporting structures and layers on the medial side of the knee: an anatomical analysis. *J Bone Joint Surg Am.* 1979;61(1):56-62.
15. Warren LA, Marshall JL, Girgis F. The prime static stabilizer of the medical side of the knee. *J Bone Joint Surg Am.* 1974;56(4):665-674.
16. Berend KR, Lombardi AV Jr. Avoiding the potential pitfalls of minimally invasive total knee surgery. *Orthopedics.* 2005;28(11):1326-1330.
17. Rand JA, Morrey BF, Bryan RS. Patellar tendon rupture after total knee arthroplasty. *Clin Orthop Relat Res.* 1989;(244):233-238.
18. Colwell CW Jr. The extensor mechanism in total knee replacement. *Clin Orthop Relat Res.* 2003;(416):74-75.
19. Kim J, Nelson CL, Lotke PA. Stiffness after total knee arthroplasty: prevalence of the complication and outcomes of revision. *J Bone Joint Surg Am.* 2004;86-A(7):1479-1484.
20. Nercessian OA, Ugwonali OF, Park S. Peroneal nerve palsy after total knee arthroplasty. *J Arthroplasty.* 2005;20(8):1068-1073.
21. Asp JP, Rand JA. Peroneal nerve palsy after total knee arthroplasty. *Clin Orthop Relat Res.* 1990(261):233-237.
22. Horlocker TT, Cabanela ME, Wedel DJ. Does postoperative epidural analgesia increase the risk of peroneal nerve palsy after total knee arthroplasty? *Anesth Analg.* 1994;79(3):495-500.
23. Idusuyi OB, Morrey BF. Peroneal nerve palsy after total knee arthroplasty: assessment of predisposing and prognostic factors. *J Bone Joint Surg Am.* 1996;78(2):177-184.
24. Knutson K, Leden I, Sturfelt G, Rosen I, Lidgren L. Nerve palsy after knee arthroplasty in patients with rheumatoid arthritis. *Scand J Rheumatol.* 1983;12(3):201-205.
25. Schinsky MF, Macaulay W, Parks ML, Kiernan H, Nercessian OA: nerve injury after primary total knee arthroplasty. *J Arthroplasty.* 2001;16(8):1048-1054.
26. Vince K, Chivas D, Droll KP. Wound complications after total knee arthroplasty. *J Arthroplasty.* 2007;22(4 Suppl 1):39-44.
27. Ries MD. Skin necrosis after total knee arthroplasty. *J Arthroplasty.* 2002;17(4 Suppl 1):74-77.
28. Greene KA, Wilde AH, Stulberg BN. Preoperative nutritional status of total joint patients: relationship to postoperative wound complications. *J Arthroplasty.* 1991;6(4):321-325.
29. Peersman G, Laskin R, Davis J, Peterson M. Infection in total knee replacement: a retrospective review of 6489 total knee replacements. *Clin Orthop Relat Res.* 2001;392:15-23.
30. Abdel-Salam A, Eyres KS. Effects of tourniquet during total knee arthroplasty: a prospective randomised study. *J Bone Joint Surg Br.* 1995;77(2):250-253.
31. Johnson DP. The effect of continuous passive motion on wound-healing and joint mobility after knee arthroplasty. *J Bone Joint Surg Am.* 1990;72(3):421-426.
32. Leone JM, Hanssen AD. Management of infection at the site of a total knee arthroplasty. *J Bone Joint Surg Am.* 2005;87(10):2335-2348.
33. Zimmerli W, Trampuz A, Ochsner PE. Prosthetic-joint infections. *N Engl J Med.* 2004;351(16):1645-1654.

34. Mauerhan DR, Mokris JG, Ly A, Kiebzak GM. Relationship between length of stay and manipulation rate after total knee arthroplasty. *J Arthroplasty.* 1998;13(8):896-900.
35. Laubenthal KN, Smidt GL, Kettelkamp DB. A quantitative analysis of knee motion during activities of daily living. *Phys Ther.* 1972;52(1):34-43.
36. Bong MR, Di Cesare PE. Stiffness after total knee arthroplasty. *J Am Acad Orthop Surg.* 2004;12(3):164-171.
37. Gandhi R, de Beer J, Leone J, Petruccelli D, Winemaker M, Adili A. Predictive risk factors for stiff knees in total knee arthroplasty. *J Arthroplasty.* 2006;21(1):46-52.
38. Ritter MA, Stringer EA. Predictive range of motion after total knee replacement. *Clin Orthop Relat Res.* 1979;(143):115-119.
39. Figgie HE III, Goldberg VM, Heiple KG, Moller HS III, Gordon NH. The influence of tibial-patellofemoral location on function of the knee in patients with the posterior stabilized condylar knee prosthesis. *J Bone Joint Surg Am.* 1986;68(7):1035-1040.
40. Pierson JL, Ritter MA, Keating EM, et al. The effect of stuffing the patellofemoral compartment on the outcome of total knee arthroplasty. *J Bone Joint Surg Am.* 2007;89(10):2195-2203.
41. Dalury DF, Jiranek WA. The incidence of heterotopic ossification after total knee arthroplasty. *J Arthroplasty.* 2004;19(4):447-452.
42. Katz MM, Hungerford DS, Krackow KA, Lennox DW. Reflex sympathetic dystrophy as a cause of poor results after total knee arthroplasty. *J Arthroplasty.* 1986;1(2):117-124.
43. Keating EM, Ritter MA, Harty LD, et al. Manipulation after total knee arthroplasty. *J Bone Joint Surg Am.* 2007;89(2):282-286.
44. Williams RJ 3rd, Westrich GH, Siegel J, Windsor RE. Arthroscopic release of the posterior cruciate ligament for stiff total knee arthroplasty. *Clin Orthop Relat Res.* 1996;(331):185-191.
45. Scranton PE Jr. Management of knee pain and stiffness after total knee arthroplasty. *J Arthroplasty.* 2001;16(4):428-435.
46. Campbell ED Jr. Arthroscopy in total knee replacements. *Arthroscopy.* 1987;3(1):31-35.
47. Diduch DR, Scuderi GR, Scott WN, Insall JN, Kelly MA. The efficacy of arthroscopy following total knee replacement. *Arthroscopy.* 1997;13(2):166-171.
48. Babis GC, Trousdale RT, Pagnano MW, Morrey BF. Poor outcomes of isolated tibial insert exchange and arthrolysis for the management of stiffness following total knee arthroplasty. *J Bone Joint Surg Am.* 2001;83-A(10):1534-1536.

# 13

# Postoperative Analgesia Options for the Total Knee Arthroplasty Patient

Eric Schwenk, MD; Kishor Gandhi, MD MPH; and Eugene R. Viscusi, MD

The control of postoperative pain in patients who undergo total knee arthroplasty (TKA) can be a difficult but important task because a large percentage of patients name postoperative pain as one of their primary concerns following surgery.[1] Postoperative pain in TKA patients is severe in over half of all patients and moderate in another third of patients.[2] In addition to creating patient dissatisfaction, postoperative pain can impair patient rehabilitation, a crucial component of regaining muscle strength and functional status back to normal.[1] This is particularly true for recovery from TKA, which can be significantly prolonged by inadequate rehabilitation. Hospitalization time may also increase for patients with poor pain control. Clearly, choosing an effective method of pain control for these patients is paramount to both their physical and mental recovery.

There are several available options for controlling pain after TKA. However, these drugs and techniques do not have to be used in isolation as monotherapy. To the contrary, combinations of drugs and techniques with different mechanisms of action, also known as multimodal analgesia, can be very effective as an analgesia strategy in the perioperative period (Figure 13-1). The available modalities include neuraxial analgesia (injection of local anesthetics, opioids, or other agents into the spinal or epidural space), peripheral nerve blockade, nonopioid (nonsteroidal anti-inflammatory drugs [NSAIDs] and antineuropathic drugs), and opioid drugs. Each analgesic technique has its associated advantages and disadvantages, and all require careful monitoring of the patient for signs of potentially harmful side effects. This chapter will discuss the various analgesia options for these patients and the potential risks and complications, emphasizing the use of a multimodal approach.

## Neuraxial Analgesia

### Spinal Analgesia

The use of local anesthetics in the intrathecal space is a well-established method of analgesia for the surgical procedure in TKA. Spinal anesthesia commonly used for total joint arthroplasty involves the insertion of a spinal needle (Quincke, Sprotte, or Whitacre) into the intrathecal space of a seated or laterally positioned patient. Onset of anesthesia is rapid with this method, and height of the spinal blockade depends on the baricity and volume of the local anesthetic used. Opioids, such as morphine and fentanyl, may be added to the mixture to prolong postoperative pain control. Morphine has a higher degree of patient satisfaction when compared to fentanyl due largely to its prolonged analgesic effect. However, intrathecal morphine does not reduce the need for supplemental IV morphine in the postoperative period for TKA patients, perhaps because of the high degree of postoperative pain associated with these surgeries.[3] Intrathecal opioids are most useful in TKA patients when used as adjuncts to local anesthetics.

Nonopioid drugs can be added to spinal local analgesics as part of a multimodal approach and decrease the amount of intravenous (IV) opioids needed after TKA. Clonidine is an $\alpha 2$-adrenergic agonist that potentiates the analgesia



Parvizi J, Klatt B.
*Essentials in Total Knee Arthroplasty* (pp 101-108).

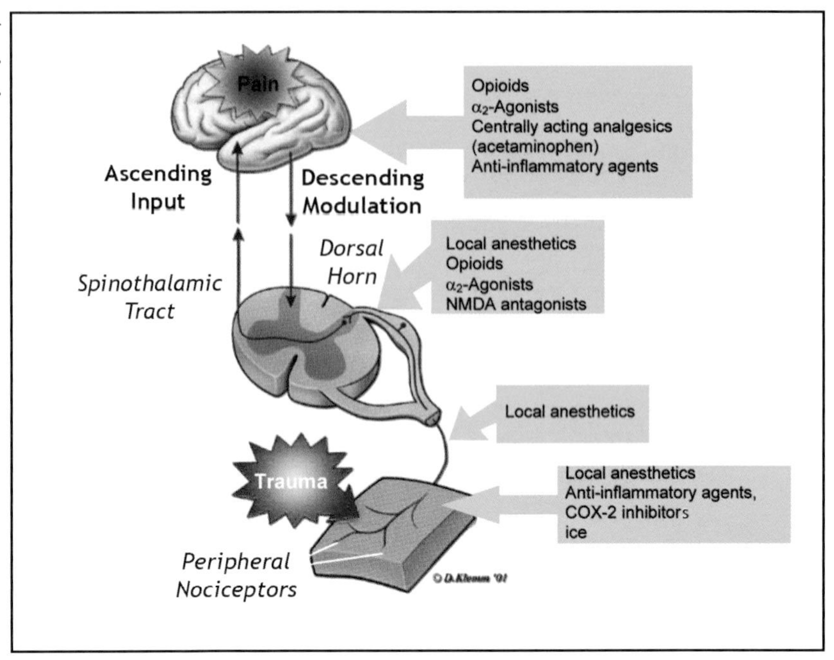


**Figure 13-1.** Pain pathways and multimodal analgesic therapy. (Reprinted with permission from Gottschalk A, Smith DS. New concepts in acute pain therapy: pre-emptive analgesia. *Am Fam Physician*. 2001;63:1979-1985.)

of local anesthetics in the intrathecal space. Together with morphine, clonidine in an intrathecal regimen leads to significant improvements in postoperative pain and decreased IV morphine requirements for 12 hours after TKA.[4] Patients must be monitored for hypotension because this is a possible side effect of clonidine.

Overall, spinal analgesia can be an effective method of pain control for TKA patients. The addition of opioids or clonidine to the intrathecal mix may lead to improved pain control as part of a multimodal strategy. These advantages must be weighed against the lack of ability to titrate analgesic postoperatively. In addition, patients must be monitored for the adverse effects of opioids, which include pruritis, nausea and vomiting, urinary retention, and—perhaps most importantly—respiratory depression. Depression of ventilation is dose dependent and typically manifests itself clinically as a decreased frequency of breathing, often accompanied by a compensatory increase in tidal volume. Clinicians must closely monitor patients for a decreased frequency of breathing, oxygen desaturation seen with pulse oximetry, or depressed level of consciousness. A lower dose of 100 μg of morphine added to the spinal anesthetic may be appropriate for some older patients in whom there is a higher concern for respiratory depression.

## Epidural Analgesia

Epidural analgesia involves the insertion of a special needle (Hustead, Tuohy, or Crawford) into the epidural space, followed by injection of local anesthetic and/or opioid or a catheter may be inserted. Commonly, a combined spinal-epidural (CSE) technique is employed in which a one-time dose of local anesthetic is injected into the intrathecal space through a spinal needle that is inserted through the lumen of an epidural needle. The epidural catheter is inserted following the spinal procedure. The epidural catheter can then provide continuous analgesia following TKA. The obvious advantage of the CSE is that the rate of infusion can be adjusted during the postoperative period according to the pain level of the patient. Epinephrine can be added to intensify the effect by causing vasoconstriction of the vessels in the epidural space and therefore decreasing systemic absorption of the analgesic.[5]

In addition to local anesthetics, opioids can be injected into the epidural space to provide postoperative analgesia. They can be used with or without a local anesthetic. Compared with parenteral opioid use after surgery, continuous infusion of epidural opioid provides superior postoperative pain relief with a similar side effect profile.[6] Another agent that has shown potential benefit when used with other epidural analgesics is ketamine. This drug, a N-methyl-D-aspartate antagonist, exerts its analgesic effects by blocking peripheral afferent pain as well as preventing the central sensitization of nociceptors. There may be an additive effect when ketamine is added to other epidural agents as part of a multimodal approach to postoperative pain control.[7]

Potential limitations of epidural analgesia include failed or dislodged catheters, unilateral blocks, and incompatibility in patients who are anticoagulated (Table 13-1). There is

Table 13-1

**Postoperative Analgesia Options After Total Knee Arthroplasty and Their Compatibility With Anticoagulation**

| *Technique* | *Compatible With Anticoagulation?* |
|---|---|
| Neuraxial analgesia | No* |
| Peripheral nerve block | Depends on the block |
| Nonopioid analgesics | Yes |
| PCA | Yes |
| Oral opioids | Yes |
| Extended-release epidural morphine | Yes |

*The 2010 American Society of Regional Anesthesia and Pain Medicine Guidelines[32] recommend performing neuraxial procedures at least 1 hour before starting intravenous unfractionated heparin and removing catheters after coagulation studies (PTT) become normal. For low molecular weight heparin (LMWH), neuraxial procedures should not be performed until 12 hours after the last LMWH dose. LMWH should not be given until 6 to 8 hours after the procedure and catheters should not be removed until 12 hours after the last dose. For warfarin, the INR should be normal before placement of a neuraxial block, patients on low-dose warfarin postoperatively should have the INR checked daily, and catheters should be removed only once the INR is less than 1.5.

also the risk of epidural hematoma formation, which usually occurs after a traumatic placement of the epidural needle or catheter, although it has been reported to occur spontaneously as well. Some clinicians prefer other postoperative analgesic options due to the fact that TKA patients are typically anticoagulated in the postoperative period and may be at a higher risk of getting an epidural hematoma.

A recent addition to the epidural analgesia drugs is DepoDur, an extended-release epidural morphine (EREM) that has recently been approved by the Food and Drug Administration (FDA) in the United States. DepoDur uses microscopic multivesicular, liposomal spherical particles with internal aqueous chambers containing morphine, resulting in 48 hours of analgesia after a single epidural injection.[8] Patients given EREM may have decreased supplemental opioid requirements in the postoperative period as well as a decreased incidence of hypotension.[8] Problems related to the epidural catheter itself or a patient-controlled analgesia (PCA) pump are theoretically eliminated with EREM.[9] In addition, EREM is compatible with anticoagulation therapy because it does not require an indwelling epidural catheter (see Table 13-1). Like other opioids, the side effects of EREM include nausea and vomiting, pruritis, urinary retention, constipation, and respiratory depression. Almost all instances of respiratory depression after receiving EREM occurred in the first 24 hours of the postoperative period.[9] The incidence of respiratory depression may be higher with EREM than standard PCA, so patients need to be monitored closely, particularly during the first 24 hours.[10] In particular, caution should be exercised in the elderly and patients with pre-existing sleep apnea.

## Peripheral Nerve Blocks

### Lumbar Plexus Block

One peripheral nerve block option for postoperative analgesia after TKA is a lumbar plexus block. The lumbar plexus arises from the first 4 lumbar spinal nerves and gives off the genitofemoral, lateral femoral cutaneous, femoral, and obturator nerves. The femoral nerve innervates the quadriceps muscles, the skin of the anteromedial thigh, and the medial aspect of the leg below the knee and foot. The obturator nerve sends motor branches to the adductors of the hip and a highly variable cutaneous branch to the medial thigh or knee, although the obturator nerve likely does not contribute significantly to postoperative pain after TKA. The lateral femoral cutaneous nerve supplies the lateral thigh. Continuous blockade of the lumbar plexus with local anesthetic via a catheter provides at least equal if not superior analgesia after TKA compared to epidural infusions or PCA with morphine. It is also associated with fewer adverse effects and possibly a more rapid recovery.[11] In addition, it appears that the continuous lumbar plexus block reduces morphine requirements when compared to the single-injection technique.[12] These factors are important to consider when choosing a postoperative analgesia regimen. The lumbar plexus block carries the highest risk of hematoma formation of the 3 blocks discussed, and serious consideration of risks and benefits should be given to anticoagulated patients (see Table 13-1).

### Femoral Nerve Block

As mentioned previously, the femoral nerve supplies motor fibers to the quadriceps muscles, the skin of the anteromedial thigh, and the medial aspect of the leg below the knee and foot. One option for postoperative analgesia is a single-injection femoral nerve block alone. This involves the injection of local anesthetic into the tissue surrounding the femoral nerve, which is located by palpating the femoral artery just below the midpoint of the inguinal ligament and moving 1 to 2 cm laterally. Some clinicians question the efficacy of this technique because the sciatic nerve, not covered in the block, innervates the posterior and lateral aspects of the knee. Studies are not conclusive as to whether femoral nerve blocks alone provide sufficient postoperative analgesia for TKA.[13,14] However, single-injection femoral nerve blocks have been shown to provide significantly improved postoperative analgesia compared to systemic opioids.[13,15] Additionally, they may reduce hospital length of stay after TKA.[15] Potential complications include intravascular injection of local anesthetic, which typically manifests as restlessness, vertigo, tinnitus, metallic taste in the mouth, or slurred speech. Intravascular injection can also lead to seizures or cardiovascular collapse. Despite these limitations, a single-injection femoral nerve block is a good option as part of a multimodal approach.

Another variation of the femoral nerve block is the continuous block afforded by a catheter. Some studies suggest that continuous femoral nerve blocks provide better analgesia than single-injection blocks.[16] However, their effects on hospital stay and functional recovery are not as clear. Continuous catheters introduce their own set of limitations, including the risk of infection of the catheter, nerve injury, and the additional resources needed to maintain and monitor the external infusion pump. The femoral nerve block can, in most cases, be performed in patients receiving anticoagulation. It carries the least risk of hematoma of the 3 peripheral nerve blocks discussed here (see Table 13-1). Nerve injury can include paresthesias, numbness, or weakness. The injury can be temporary or permanent in rare cases.

With the use of femoral nerve blocks, the surgeon must be wary of weakness for early physical therapy because patients can fall from lack of quad strength. Many surgeons use knee immobilizers until femoral nerve blocks are discontinued.

### Sciatic Nerve Block

The sciatic nerve arises from the lumbosacral plexus and innervates the lateral and posterior portions of the knee. On entering the popliteal fossa, it divides into the tibial and common peroneal nerves, which innervate the leg and foot. A sciatic nerve block could, therefore, improve postoperative analgesia. However, the contribution of the sciatic nerve to postoperative pain after TKA remains unclear, with at least one study showing no difference in morphine consumption between patients given a femoral nerve block and those given both femoral and sciatic nerve blocks.[13] As with the femoral nerve block, the sciatic nerve block may be performed with the single-injection technique or with a continuous infusion through a catheter. The sciatic nerve block carries an intermediate risk of hematoma formation compared to the other 2 blocks discussed here, and patients who are anticoagulated should be evaluated individually for risks and benefits of the block (see Table 13-1).

## Multimodal Nonopioid Agents

### Nonsteroidal Anti-Inflammatory Drugs and Cyclooxygenase-2 Inhibitors

Research has shown that the use of nonopioid drugs in the preoperative period may reduce the possible effects of opioid-induced hyperalgesia in the postoperative period.[17] Opioid-induced hyperalgesia is a complex phenomenon that can follow rapid increases in opioids during or after surgery and can paradoxically result in lowering of a patient's pain threshold and lead to greater opioid requirements.[17] Limiting opioids while maximizing the use of nonopioid drugs can minimize opioid-induced hyperalgesia.

NSAIDS and cyclooxygenase-2 (COX-2) inhibitors given in the preoperative period can also create an "opioid-sparing effect" in the postoperative period. As a result, opioid-related side effects may decrease and patient satisfaction may increase as a result of better analgesia. NSAIDs and COX-2 inhibitors act in the peripheral nervous system by inhibiting prostaglandin synthesis and stimulation of nociceptors, whereas opioids exert their effects in the central nervous system. NSAIDs or COX-2 inhibitors can be used preoperatively to reduce the incidence of central and peripheral sensitization syndromes after surgery.[18] If not prevented, these syndromes can lead to increased opioid consumption postoperatively.

Preoperative use of NSAIDs such as ketorolac and ibuprofen can decrease postoperative pain scores and postoperative opioid requirements.[19] However, some surgeons are concerned about NSAID use prior to surgery due to the decrease in platelet aggregation, potentially increased bleeding time, and poor wound and bone healing associated with them. COX-2 inhibitors may eliminate some of these problems. Recently, concerns have been raised about the potential increased risk of cardiovascular side effects with long-term COX-2-inhibitor use, particularly with rofecoxib and valdecoxib, which have both been withdrawn from the market. These effects have not been associated with short-term use, such as during the perioperative period. Patients given short-term regimens of COX-2 inhibitors before and after TKA may have better outcomes, including reduced opioid requirements, faster time to rehabilitation, decreased nausea and vomiting, better sleep patterns, and greater overall satisfaction.[20]

Table 13-2

**NONOPIOID ANALGESICS AND SUGGESTED DOSING FOR TOTAL KNEE ARTHROPLASTY PATIENTS**

| Drug | Dose | Route of Administration | Time Before Surgery | Time After Surgery |
|---|---|---|---|---|
| **NSAIDs** | | | | |
| Ketorolac | 15 to 30 mg | PO/IV | 1 to 2 hours | 15 to 30 mg every 6 hrs |
| Ibuprofen | 800 mg | PO | 1 to 2 hours | 800 mg every 6 hrs |
| **COX-2 Inhibitors** | | | | |
| Celecoxib | 400 mg | PO | 1 hour | 200 mg X 1 (2 hrs after surgery) |
| **Anti-neuropathic** | | | | |
| Gabapentin | 1200 mg | PO | 1 to 2 hours | 1200 mg X 1 (24 hrs after surgery) |
| Pregabalin | 150 mg | PO | 1 hour | 150 mg X 1 (12 hrs after surgery) |
| Acetaminophen | 1 g | PO/IV | 15 minutes | 1 g every 4 hours |

### Gabapentin and Pregabalin

Gabapentin (Neurontin) and pregabalin (Lyrica), originally studied in patients with seizures and neuropathic pain syndromes, are now playing a role in postoperative analgesia. Studies have shown that preoperative administration of gabapentin leads to decreased postoperative pain and opioid consumption.[21,22] Patients undergoing knee surgery experience decreased anxiety preoperatively and better range of knee motion postoperatively after receiving gabapentin in the preoperative period.[23] The results of a meta-analysis suggest that gabapentin reduces postoperative pain scores and opioid consumption and would be a reasonable component of a multimodal treatment plan.[24] The combination of gabapentin and a COX-2 inhibitor may be synergistic.[25]

Pregabalin also plays an important role in postoperative analgesia after TKA. A recent prospective trial found that perioperative pregabalin reduces the incidence of chronic neuropathic pain after TKA, as well as opioid consumption, and improves range of motion during the first 30 days of rehabilitation.[26] Other advantages of adding these and other nonopioid agents to a multimodal analgesia regimen are the decrease of unwanted opioid side effects and ability to continue usage after discharge from the hospital (Table 13-2).

### Ketamine

Ketamine is a phencyclidine derivative and an N-methyl D-aspartate (NMDA) antagonist and can reduce postoperative morphine consumption as well as nausea and vomiting.[27] Postoperative ketamine infusions may be particularly effective in opioid tolerant patients who undergo surgery.[28] In the TKA patient, ketamine may be a useful adjunct in the perioperative period. When combined with a femoral nerve block, ketamine has been shown to reduce opioid consumption and lead to faster rehabilitation after TKA. Despite the potential for psychological side effects, the incidence of hallucinations did not differ between the ketamine and control groups in that study.[29]

## OPIOID ANALGESIA

### Intravenous Patient-Controlled Analgesia

IV patient-controlled analgesia (PCA) is the most widely used method of postoperative analgesia offered to patients after surgery.[30] It involves infusion pumps programmed to deliver patient-activated, fixed, and small doses of opioids with a lockout period, as well as a maximum hourly dose. The most commonly used opioids include morphine, hydromorphone, and fentanyl. PCA provides a good option for patients who are willing to actively participate in their care, and patient satisfaction is generally high with PCA. Opioid-related side effects, such as nausea and vomiting, pruritis, urinary retention, and respiratory depression, occur commonly with PCA. In addition, the elderly are especially vulnerable to confusion and delirium after PCA use.

As the prototype opioid agonist, morphine deserves some special consideration. It is a commonly used opioid in PCA therapy and is the opioid to which all others are compared. IV morphine requires 15 to 30 minutes to take peak effect,

Table 13-3

**ORAL OPIOIDS AND SUGGESTED DOSING FOR TOTAL KNEE ARTHROPLASTY PATIENTS IN THE POSTOPERATIVE PERIOD**

| DRUG | DOSAGE (MG) | FREQUENCY (HOURS) | DURATION (HOURS) |
|---|---|---|---|
| Codeine | 300 | q4 to 6 | 4 to 6 |
| Hydromorphone | 4 | q3 to 4 | 3 to 4 |
| Oxycodone | 15 to 20 | q12 | 3 to 4 |
| Oxymorphone | 10 | q4 to 6 | 3 to 6 |
| Hydrocodone | 20 to 30 | q4 to 6 | 4 to 8 |
| Propoxyphene | 130 to 200 | q4 | 4 to 6 |

which is slower than the highly lipid-soluble fentanyl and its derivatives. An additional important point to consider is the metabolism of morphine. Morphine-3-glucuronide and morphine-6-glucuronide, morphine's 2 major metabolites, are excreted principally by the kidneys. In patients with renal failure, elimination may be impaired and even small amounts of morphine can lead to respiratory depression. Therefore, extreme caution should be exercised before administering morphine to patients with renal failure.

Multimodal analgesic approaches typically involve one or more nonopioid drugs in combination with opioids. These other drugs often can help reduce opioid consumption and their associated side effects, as well as provide better pain control in the postoperative period. For the TKA patient, this may reduce the time to rehabilitation.

## Oral Opioids

Oral opioids are generally an important component of postoperative analgesia for the TKA patient. Opioids commonly used in the postoperative period and during the transition to home include hydromorphone, oxycodone, oxymorphone, hydrocodone, and propoxyphene (Table 13-3). Meperidine used to be commonly given for postoperative analgesia but has fallen out of favor for several reasons, the first of which is the fact that one of its metabolites, normeperidine, causes central nervous system (CNS) excitation and can cause seizures, particularly in renal failure patients.[31(pp103-104)] Another limitation of meperidine involves its depression of myocardial contractility, a unique feature among opioid agonists.[31(pp103-104)] Finally, meperidine is associated with a high incidence of nausea and vomiting.

Hydromorphone is 5 times as potent as morphine with a slightly shorter duration of action. It is effective for moderate to severe pain and must be taken orally every 4 hours to maintain analgesia.[31(p116)] Oxycodone is available as a sustained-release oral medication for treatment of moderate to severe pain. There is considerable abuse potential due to the ability of users to crush tablets and inject or snort the drug.[31(p116)] For appropriate patients, it is a good analgesia option in the weeks following TKA. Oxymorphone is a metabolite of oxycodone that is 10 times more potent than morphine and causes significant nausea and vomiting. Physical dependence is a major concern.[31(p116)] However, it comes in an immediate-release form that provides rapid analgesia, which can be useful for breakthrough pain. It also comes in an extended-release form. Hydrocodone is most commonly paired with either acetaminophen or aspirin. Its peak plasma concentration occurs after 80 minutes. As with several other oral opioids, abuse potential is high.[31] Propoxyphene, a weak synthetic opioid, has some utility in managing mild to moderate pain. It is limited by extensive first-pass hepatic metabolism. It is commonly prescribed with acetaminophen, and its utility as a postoperative analgesic is limited.

## ACKNOWLEDGMENT

The authors would like to thank Madhavi Pradhan, MD for assistance with the chapter.

## REFERENCES

1. Joshi GP, Ogunnaike BO. Consequences of inadequate postoperative pain relief and chronic persistent postoperative pain. *Anesth Clinics N America*. 2005;23:21-36.
2. Apfelbaum JL, Chen C, Mehta SS, Gan TJ. Postoperative pain experience: results from a national survey suggest postoperative pain continues to be undermanaged. *Anesth Analg*. 2003;97:534-540.

3. Rathmell JP, Pino CA, Taylor R, Patrin T, Viani BA. Intrathecal morphine for postoperative analgesia: a randomized, controlled dose-ranging study after hip and knee arthroplasty. *Anesth Analg.* 2003;97:1452-1457.
4. Sites BD, Beach M, Biggs R, et al. Intrathecal clonidine added to a bupivacaine-morphine spinal anesthetic improves postoperative analgesia for a total knee arthroplasty. *Anesth Analg.* 2003;96:1083-1088.
5. Barash PG, Cullen BF, Stoelting RK. *Clinical Anesthesia.* 5th ed. Philadelphia, PA: Lippincott Williams and Wilkins, 2006;459.
6. Singelyn FJ, Deyaert M, Pendeville E, Gouverneur JM. Effects of intravenous patient-controlled analgesia with morphine, continuous epidural analgesia, and continuous three-in-one block on postoperative pain and knee rehabilitation after unilateral total knee arthroplasty. *Anesth Analg.* 1998;87:88-89.
7. Chia Y, Liu K, Liu YC, Chang HC, Wong CS. Adding ketamine in a multimodal patient-controlled epidural regimen reduces postoperative pain and analgesic consumption. *Anesth Analg.* 1998;86:1245-1249.
8. Viscusi ER, Martin G, Hartrick CT, Singla N, Manlevian G. 48 hours of postoperative pain relief following total hip arthroplasty with a novel, extended-release epidural morphine formulation. *Anesthesiology.* 2005;102:937-947.
9. Viscusi ER. Emerging techniques in the management of acute pain: epidural analgesia. *Anesth Analg.* 2005;101:S23-S29.
10. Sumida S, Lesley MR, Hanna MN, Kumar K, Wu CL. Meta-analysis of the effect of extended-release epidural morphine versus intravenous patient-controlled analgesia on respiratory depression. *J Opioid Manag.* 2009;5:301-305.
11. Watson MW, Mitra D, McLintock TC, Grant SA. Continuous versus single-injection lumbar plexus blocks: comparison of the effects on morphine use and early recovery after total knee arthroplasty. *Reg Anesth Pain Med.* 2005;30(6):541-547.
12. Morin AM, Kratz CD, Eberhart LHJ, et al. Postoperative analgesia and functional recovery after total-knee replacement: comparison of a continuous posterior lumbar plexus (psoas compartment) block, a continuous femoral nerve block, and the combination of a continuous femoral and sciatic nerve block. *Reg Anesth Pain Med.* 2005;30(5):434-445.
13. Allen HW, Liu SS, Ware PD, Nairn CS, Ownes BD. Peripheral nerve blocks improve analgesia after total knee replacement surgery. *Anesth Analg.* 1998;87:93-97.
14. Dang CP, Gautheron E, Guilley J, et al. The value of adding sciatic block to continuous femoral block for analgesia after total knee replacement. *Reg Anesth Pain Med.* 2005;30:128-133.
15. Wang H, Boctor B, Verner J. The effect of single-injection femoral nerve block on rehabilitation and length of hospital stay after total knee replacement. *Reg Anesth Pain Med.* 2002;27(2):139-144.
16. Salinas FV, Liu SS, Mulroy MF. The effect of single-injection femoral nerve block versus continuous femoral nerve block after total knee arthroplasty on hospital length of stay and long-term functional recovery within an established clinical pathway. *Anesth Analg.* 2006;102:1234-1239.
17. Mercadante S, Ferrera P, Villari P, Arcuri E. Hyperalgesia: an emerging iatrogenic syndrome. *J Pain Symp Mgmt.* 2003;26:769-775.
18. Samad TA, Moore KA, Sapirstein A, et al. Interleukin-1 β-mediated induction of COX-2 in the cns contributes to inflammatory pain hypersensitivity. *Nature.* 2001;410:471-475.
19. Fischer HBJ, Simanski CJP. A procedure-specific systematic review and consensus recommendations for analgesia after total hip replacement. *Anaesthesia.* 2005;60:1189-1202.
20. Buvanendran A, Kroin JS, Tuman KJ, et al. Effects of perioperative administration of a selective cyclooxygenase 2 inhibitor on pain management and recovery of function after knee replacement: a randomized controlled trial. *JAMA.* 2003;290:2411-2418.
21. Turan A, Karamanlioglu B, Memis D, et al. Analgesic effect of gabapentin after spinal surgery. *Anesthesiology.* 2004;100:935-938.
22. Dierking G, Duedahl TH, Rasmussen ML, et al. Effects of gabapentin on postoperative morphine consumption and pain after abdominal hysterectomy: a randomized, double-blind trial. *Acta Anaesthesiol Scand.* 2004;48:322-327.
23. Menigaux C, Adam F, Guignard B, Sessler DI, Chauvin, M. Preoperative gabapentin decreases anxiety and improves early functional recovery from knee surgery. *Anesth Analg.* 2005;100:1394-1399.
24. Hurley RW, Cohen SP, Williams KA, Rowlingson AJ, Wu CL. The analgesic effects of perioperative gabapentin on postoperative pain: a meta-analysis. *Reg Anesth Pain Med.* 2006;31:237-247.
25. Turan A, White PF, Karamanlioglu B, et al. Gabapentin: an alternative to the cyclooxygenase-2 inhibitors for perioperative pain management. *Pain Med.* 2006;102:175-181.
26. Buvanendran A, Kroin JS, Della Valle CJ, Kari M, Moric M, Tuman KJ. Perioperative oral pregabalin reduces chronic pain after total knee arthroplasty: a prospective, randomized, controlled trial. *Anesth Analg.* 2010;110:199-207.
27. Bell RF, Dahl JB, Moore RA, Kalso EA. Perioperative ketamine for acute postoperative pain (Review). *Acta Anaesthesiol Scand.* 2005;49:1405-1428.
28. Urban MK, Ya Deau JT, Wukovits B, Lipnitsky JY. Ketamine as an adjunct to postoperative pain management in opioid tolerant patients after spinal fusions: a prospective randomized trial. *HSS J.* 2008;4:62-65.
29. Adam F, Chauvin M, Du Manoir B, Langlois M, Sessler DI, Fletcher D. Small-dose ketamine infusion improves postoperative analgesia and rehabilitation after total knee arthroplasty. *Anesth Analg.* 2005;100:475-480.
30. Grass JA. Patient-controlled analgesia. *Anesth Analg.* 2005;101: S44-S61.
31. Stoelting RK, Hillier SC. *Pharmacology and Physiology in Anesthetic Practice.* 4th ed. Philadelphia, PA: Lippincott, Williams, and Wilkins; 2006.
32. Horlocker TT, Wedel DJ, Rowlingson JC, et al. Regional anesthesia in the patient receiving antithrombotic or thrombolytic therapy. American Society of Regional Anesthesia and Pain Medicine Evidence-Based Guidelines (Third Edition). *Reg Anesth Pain Med.* 2010;35:64Y101.

# 14

# Controversies in Total Knee Arthroplasty

*James J. Purtill, MD and Khalid A. Azzam, MD*

## Posterior Cruciate Ligament: Retain, Sacrifice or Substitute?

### Function

The role of the posterior cruciate ligament (PCL) after total knee arthroplasty (TKA) has been stated as two-fold: preventing posterior tibial displacement and preserving normal knee kinematics (primarily femoral roll-back).[1] Femoral roll-back increases the quadriceps lever arm by moving the femorotibial contact location posteriorly with knee flexion.[2] Using anatomical and theoretical models, several authors[2-4] have agreed that roll-back is preserved in PCL-retaining TKA.

Andriacchi and Galante[5] in 1988 argued that retaining the posterior cruciate ligament improves range of motion as well as the mechanical efficiency of the knee. This theoretically improves stair climbing and reduces stress at the cement interfaces. Dorr et al[1] studied the gait of 11 patients with bilateral TKA: PCL-retaining on one side and cruciate-sacrificing on the other. Cruciate-sacrificing TKA was found to be less efficient, with greater medial loading and higher joint reaction forces. However, Knee Society scores, patient satisfaction, and roentgenographic examinations were not found to be different at 5 years.

Range of motion may be better in TKA when the PCL is sacrificed and a posterior stabilized implant is used to maintain femoral roll-back.[3] In kinematic analysis, cruciate-substituting TKA had more consistent and natural function than the cruciate-retaining TKA (Figure 14-1).[6] Fluoroscopic studies demonstrated that anteroposterior translation in posterior-stabilized, cruciate-sacrificing TKA is similar to that of a normal knee during normal gait and deep knee bend.[7]

Mahoney et al[8] compared cruciate-retaining, cruciate-sacrificing, and cruciate-substituting TKA. They found that with cruciate-retaining TKA, femoral roll-back decreased by an average of 36% and there was a 15% loss in extensor efficiency. In PCL-sacrificing TKA, roll-back decreased by 70% and extensor efficiency decreased 19%. However, in cruciate-substituting TKA there was only a 12% loss in roll-back and an 11% decrease in extensor efficiency.

In several clinical trials[6,7,9,10] no significant functional advantage has been observed for PCL-retaining TKA designs. Moreover, it appears that cruciate-substituting TKA has more consistent results.

With a PCL-retaining device and a cruciate-sacrificing device, less bone is removed for the femoral implant. There is more bone removed for the notch in the cruciate-substituting type of knee. It is uncertain how this is beneficial.

Cruciate-substituting knees can have post wear if the knee hyperextends. In most PCL substituting knee systems, the front of the post will not usually impinge on the femoral component until approximately 10 degrees of hyperextension occurs. If the impingement occurs, it is another source of wear debris.

Both types of knees can have flexion instability, but with a PCL substituting device there can be a complete knee



Parvizi J, Klatt B.
*Essentials in Total Knee Arthroplasty* (pp 109-120).

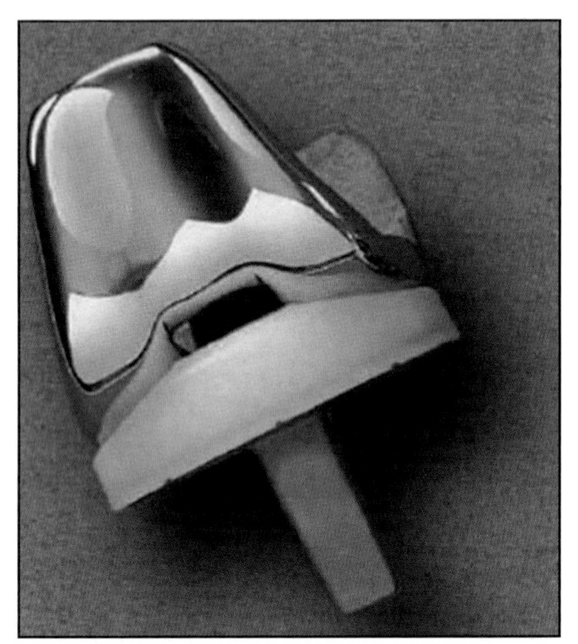

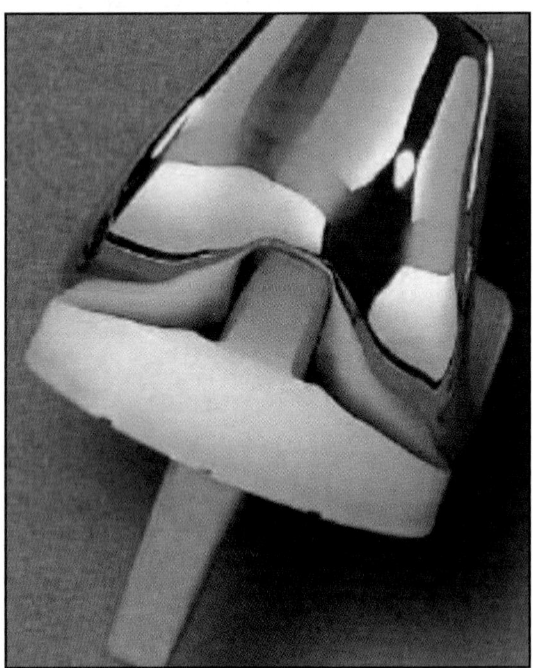

**Figure 14-1.** (A) PCL-retaining implant. (B) Post-stabilized implant.

dislocation if the flexion gap is so loose it allows the implant to jump over the post. This cannot happen in PCL-retaining knees because there are late ruptures of the PCL that can result in a similar behavior. These ruptures are seen more in patients with inflammatory arthritis.

## Proprioception

Another potential advantage of retaining the PCL in TKA is preserving proprioception.[11] However, this theoretical advantage has not been proven in clinical studies.[12-15] Simmons et al[12] measured proprioception following TKA with PCL retained and substituting designs. Passive motion threshold-to-detection was quantified as a measure of proprioception. No difference was found comparing these 2 TKA designs. In patients with severe preoperative arthritis, proprioception with cruciate-substituting TKA was significantly better than cruciate-retaining TKA.

In another study, Lattanzio et al[13] compared proprioception for PCL-retaining and PCL sacrificing TKA using the absolute angular error (defined as the difference between the arc-of-motion angle and the perceived arc of motion). No significant difference was found between PCL-retaining and PCL sacrificing TKA.

## Survivorship

The use of either PCL-retaining or substituting total knee replacement has not been implicated as a significant factor influencing the survival of knee implants. In a recent study, Gioe et al[16] prospectively followed 1047 patients who underwent knee arthroplasty in a community joint registry over a 14-year period. They found that cemented TKAs performed best, with a cumulative revision rate of 15.5%, compared to 32.3% in unicompartmental knee arthroplasty patients and 34.1% in cementless designs. Men had a higher cumulative revision rate than women, 31.9% compared to 20.6%. Adjusting for implant type and gender, there was no difference in cumulative revision rate based on diagnosis (OA versus other) or age group or between cruciate-retaining and cruciate-substituting designs. Cementless designs and unicompartmental knee arthroplasty increased revision risk independently.

## Pre-Existing Deformity

The PCL may be contracted when there is significant deformity associated with a severely arthritic knee. This may affect range of motion with PCL-retaining TKA. Laskin[17] reviewed a series of patients with a preoperative varus deformity greater than 15 degrees who underwent either PCL-retaining or posterior stabilized TKA. In the PCL-retaining group, there was a decreased range of motion, an increased incidence of pain, bone-cement radiolucency, and revision.

## Underlying Cause of Arthritis

Inflammatory arthritis is frequently noted as an indication for PCL substituting TKA. Schai et al[18] reported 97% survivorship at 13 years with PCL-retaining TKA for patients with rheumatoid arthritis. Palmer et al[19] reported an 80% success rate for PCL-retaining TKA in patients with juvenile rheumatoid arthritis at 12 years.

Laskin and O'Flynn,[20] however, reported at 8.2-year follow-up posterior instability and recurvatum deformity, resulting in an increased revision rate in a series of patients with rheumatoid arthritis who underwent PCL-retaining TKA.

## Points to Remember

- No significant differences in clinical or radiographic outcome between PCL-sacrificing and PCL-retaining TKA.
- There is no solid basis from available randomized studies on which one would suggest the superiority of either technique irrespective of the cause of arthritis, although correction of knee deformities and adjusting soft tissue balance is more difficult with PCL retention.
- PCL retention has the theoretical advantage of mimicking the normal knee joint biomechanics by maintaining femoral roll-back and knee joint proprioception, increasing quadriceps efficiency and improving stair-climbing ability. These potential advantages have yet to be proven.

# Alignment Instrumentation: Intramedullary Versus Extramedullary

## Femur

Intramedullary TKA instrumentation is frequently used to establish coronal alignment of the femur. The entry point for the femoral alignment rod is typically placed a few millimeters medial to the midline at a point anterior to the origin of the PCL (Figure 14-2). Preoperative roentgenograms should be carefully scrutinized for a wide canal or excessive femoral bowing, which may result in alignment errors.[21]

Extramedullary femoral alignment is useful with severe bowing, malunion, or stenosis of the femur. Extramedullary instrumentation may also be necessary when an ipsilateral total hip replacement or other hardware fills the femoral canal.[21]

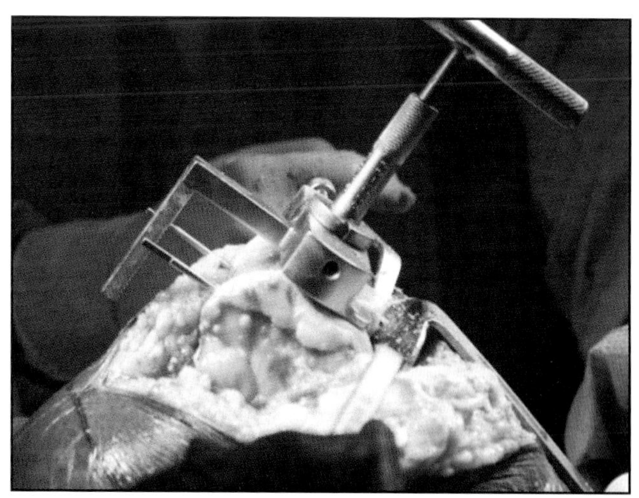

**Figure 14-2.** Intramedullary femur.

## Tibia

### Intramedullary

In a prospective randomized study, Reed et al[22] found that intramedullary guides were superior to extramedullary guides for tibial component alignment (85% versus 65% correct alignment, respectively). In a prospective study of 116 TKA comparing intramedullary and extramedullary tibial resection guides, Maestro et al[23] found no significant difference in sagittal plane positioning (posterior tilt) of the tibial component. However, in the coronal plane, intramedullary guides were found to be superior to extramedullary guides. In addition, using either technique, obese patients and those with wide intramedullary canals were prone to tibial malpositioning.

### Extramedullary

In a study of 116 TKAs comparing the accuracy of intramedullary and extramedullary tibial resection guides, Dennis et al[24] concluded that satisfactory alignment can be obtained with either resection guide, although a wider range of error was encountered with the intramedullary guide use. They emphasized the importance of positioning the extramedullary guide over the center of the talus rather than the midpoint of the ankle to avoid varus tibial resection. Simmons et al[25] studied the accuracy of a tibial

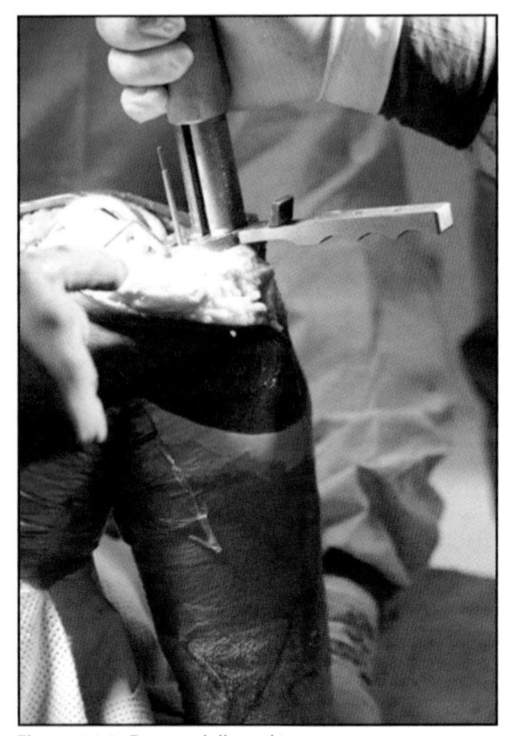

**Figure 14-3.** Extramedullary tibia.

extramedullary alignment guide in TKAs with either varus and valgus preoperative deformity. They found that extramedullary alignment guides are accurate for varus knees; however, up to 5 degrees of malalignment may result when used with valgus knees. Tibial bowing, present in up to 66% of valgus knees, was felt to be the main source of error (Figure 14-3).

### Complications: Intramedullary Versus Extramedullary Instrumentation

Increased intramedullary pressures and subsequent fat embolization are concerns with the use of intramedullary alignment devices. Stern et al[26] studied a series of 26 patients undergoing bilateral cemented TKA who were randomized to either extramedullary tibial/vented intermedullary guides or intramedullary tibial/unvented femoral cutting guides. They found that postoperatively, the intramedullary group had lower cardiac indices and higher pulmonary pressures. This increase in pulmonary vascular resistance with the use of intramedullary instrumentation may represent fat embolism and lung injury in this group.

Fahmy et al[27] found a significant increase in intramedullary pressure after insertion of both solid and fluted 8-mm alignment rods through an 8-mm hole in both vented and unvented femoral canals. In addition, bone marrow contents and fat were retrieved from samples of blood from the right atrium. A reduction in oxygen saturation, arterial oxygen tension ($PaO_2$), and end-tidal carbon-dioxide tension ($PETCO_2$) was also noted during insertion of the alignment rod. These changes were completely eliminated by the use of a 12.7-mm drill hole as the entry site of the 8-mm fluted rod.

### Points to Remember

- Intramedullary alignment instrumentation is useful on the femoral side of a TKA as femoral landmarks are not easily palpable.[21]
- Extramedullary guides may avoid fat embolization and hypoxia, associated with the use of intramedullary guides. A larger femoral entry hole may prevent these problems.[24]

## Fixed-Bearing Versus Mobile-Bearing Knee Replacements

### Theoretical

Mobile-bearing TKA designs may decrease polyethylene wear and mechanical loosening by reducing contact stresses in the polyethylene as well as minimizing bone-prosthesis stress at the tibial surface. In an in vivo kinematic study, Delport et al[28] found that mobile-bearing total knee designs had rotation of the tibial polyethylene during flexion, whereas fixed-bearing posterior-stabilized designs had rotation at the proximal surface of the bearing. Mobile-bearing TKA designs allow the femur to move in the anteroposterior direction on the upper surface and the tibia to rotate on its lower surface. This potentially leads to less wear compared to the multidirectional movement (sliding and rotation) at the proximal surface of the fixed-bearing designs.[28]

In addition, mobile-bearing TKA designs may allow correction of malalignment of the tibial component, which could increase the stresses on the polyethylene insert and lead to early wear.[29] Matsuda et al[30] showed that a mobile meniscal-bearing surface may offer an advantage with regard to contact stresses over a standard fixed tibial component when rotational malalignment of the tibial component occurs. However, severe rotational malalignment caused edge contact increased undersurface stress, which could cause deformity and subluxation.[30]

### Functional

Despite the theoretical advantages, long-term studies of fixed-bearing and mobile-bearing knees have shown no difference in the rate of osteolysis.[31] Aglietti et al[32] compared a fixed-bearing (Legacy Posterior Stabilized [LPS], Zimmer Inc., Warsaw, IN) with a mobile-bearing (Meniscal Bearing Knee [MBK], Zimmer Inc.) knee prosthesis and showed no difference in early results. Callaghan[33] found 95% to 100% survivorship rates at 11- and 12-year follow-up for low contact stress rotating platform knee replacements.

Stiehl et al[34] reviewed a multicenter study of primary mobile bearing and reported that the most common cause of revision was bearing-related problems (chronic instability, bearing subluxation, bearing dislocation, or bearing wear).

Bhan and Malhotra[35] reported on a series of patients with significant preoperative deformity undergoing low-contact stress (LCS) rotating-platform TKA. They reported an unacceptably high reoperation rate of 10% and concluded that rotating platform design is unsuitable for severely deformed knees.

### Points to Remember

- Although a mobile-bearing TKA design allows rotation of the tibial polyethylene, which may reduce contact stress and polyethylene wear and result in less mechanical loosening, there are no long-term studies that show superior functional outcome or improved survivorship.
- Mobile-bearing TKA design is associated with a slightly higher incidence of complications related to subluxation or dislocation of the bearing, especially in cases with severe preoperative deformity or ligamentous pathology.

## Simultaneous Bilateral Versus Staged Bilateral Total Knee Arthroplasty

Controversy still exists as to whether it is safe to perform bilateral TKA simultaneously.

### Simultaneous Bilateral Total Knee Arthroplasty

#### Outcome

Ritter et al[36] showed that patients who had unilateral TKA had significantly lower Knee Society scores than those who had simultaneous bilateral surgery at all follow-up intervals. Ritter et al[37] also demonstrated, in a series of 62,730 patients who had undergone bilateral TKA (either simultaneously or in a staged fashion), that wound infections were nearly twice as common when done in a staged fashion compared to simultaneously. In addition, overall hospital length of stay and cost were much less for the simultaneous procedure group.

#### Risks

Liu and Chen[38] reported on a series of patients undergoing bilateral simultaneous or staged TKA. They found that simultaneous bilateral TKA did not increase the incidence of complications or blood loss. Knee Society score was similar for both groups; however, operative time and duration of hospitalization were significantly shorter in the simultaneous bilateral group.

Bullock et al[39] showed rates of myocardial infarction, postoperative confusion, and the need for intensive monitoring were greater after the bilateral arthroplasties compared to unilateral TKA. However, 30-day and 1-year mortality rates as well as the rate of pulmonary embolism, infection, and deep venous thrombosis were similar for unilateral and bilateral TKA. Lombardi et al[40] reported that patients who underwent simultaneous bilateral TKA had higher blood loss and gastrointestinal complications than patients who had unilateral TKA. However, they found that age had a more significant effect on morbidity than unilateral or bilateral TKA.

#### Costs

Reuben et al[41] found that bilateral simultaneous TKA was 36% less costly than staged bilateral TKA.

### Staged Bilateral Total Knee Arthroplasty

Lane et al[42] found that postoperative confusion was approximately 4 times greater, cardiopulmonary complications were approximately 3 times greater, and there was a 17 times greater need for banked blood in simultaneous bilateral total knee arthroplasties compared to unilateral TKA. Although hospital length of stay was similar, 89% of the patients with simultaneous bilateral TKA required a rehabilitation stay compared with 45% of the patients with unilateral TKA.

Ritter et al[36] showed that patients who had simultaneous bilateral TKA had a significantly higher incidence of thrombophlebitis (0.9%) than those who underwent unilateral TKA (0.3%). In addition, Ritter et al[37] found that patients who underwent simultaneous bilateral TKA experienced

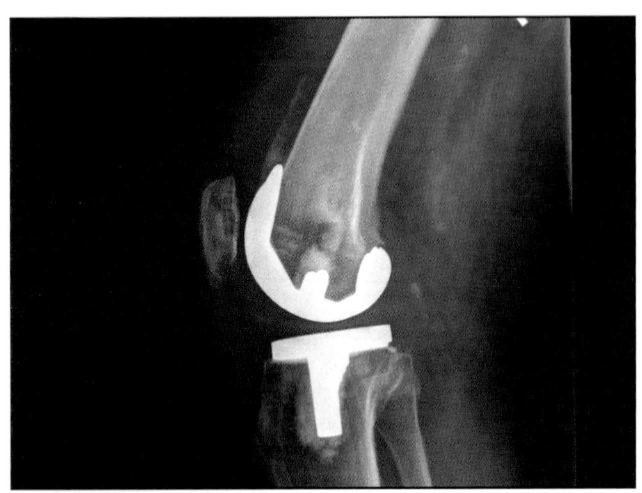

**Figure 14-4.** Lateral radiograph of a knee showing resurfaced patella.

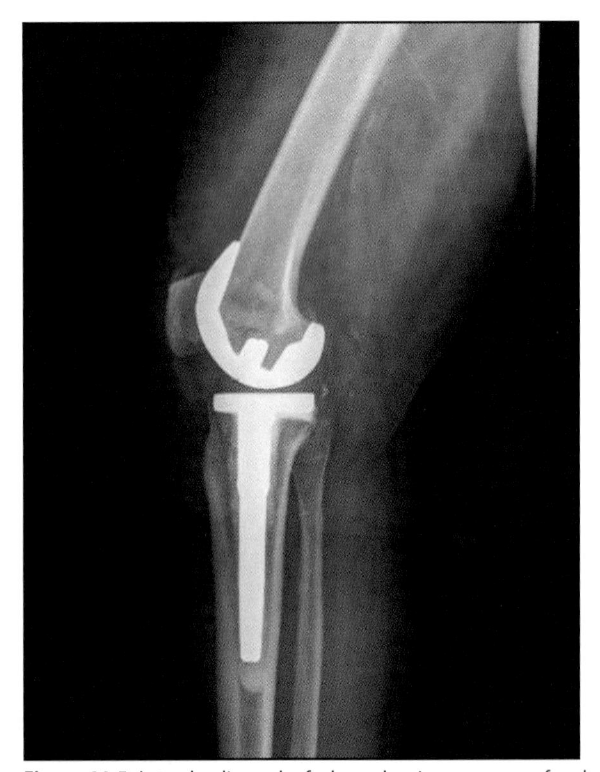

**Figure 14-5.** Lateral radiograph of a knee showing a non-resurfaced patella.

twice the number of intensive care days than those choosing staged procedures. Staging bilateral TKA 3 to 6 months apart offered the fewest disadvantages, was only slightly more expensive, and had the lowest mortality rate.

Mangaleshkar et al[43] found that age was the only significant risk factor associated with mortality following simultaneous bilateral total knee replacement. Staged bilateral TKA was found to be safer for patients who are 75 years or older.

### Costs Are Equivalent

Although simultaneous bilateral TKA offers a clear economic advantage during the acute hospitalization over staged bilateral TKA, the cost savings are partially offset by the approximately 2 times greater need for rehabilitation.[42]

## *Points to Remember*

- There is concern with bilateral simultaneous TKA that there is a higher incidence of perioperative complications (blood loss, cardiac, neurologic, gastrointestinal, genitourinary, and pulmonary) than with staged bilateral TKA.
- The increased stress on the cardiopulmonary system with simultaneous bilateral total knee arthroplasties may make this procedure contraindicated in certain patients with pre-existing disease and advanced age.[42]
- Despite the lack of prospective randomized studies, orthopedic literature suggests limiting bilateral simultaneous total knee replacements to younger patients (< 70 years of age) without pre-existing cardiopulmonary disease.[44]
- With appropriate patient selection and operative technique, patients who present with bilateral symptomatic knee arthritis can enjoy the benefits of simultaneous sequential bilateral total knee replacement without increasing their risks of complications.[45]

# Patella: Unresurfaced Versus Resurfaced

Whether to resurface the patella during a primary TKA performed for the treatment of degenerative osteoarthritis remains a controversial issue (Figures 14-4 and 14-5).

## *Resurfacing*

In a prospective randomized study, Schroeder-Boersch et al[46] found that patients undergoing TKA with a resurfaced patella had better Knee Society score, better stair climbing, and better overall function. Wood et al[47] in a prospective, randomized study of 220 osteoarthritic knees, found a higher incidence of anterior pain in the knees that had not had patellar resurfacing (anterior knee pain, however, did still occur in some patients with patellar resurfacing).

Finally, Pakos et al,[48] in a meta-analysis of randomized controlled trials comparing TKA with- and without patellar resurfacing, found that patellar resurfacing reduced the risk of postoperative anterior knee pain by 13.8%.

Kajino et al,[49] in a randomized trial of bilateral TKA in patients with rheumatoid arthritis, found that Knee Society score (as well as individual scores for pain, function, range of motion), muscle strength, flexion contracture, and instability were not significantly different between the knees that had a patellar replacement and those that had not. However, pain on standing and on ascending or descending stairs as well as tenderness of the patellofemoral joint were only noted in knees that had not had a patellar replacement. Replacement of the patella during TKA is preferable for patients who have rheumatoid arthritis.

### Nonresurfacing

Feller et al[50] found that stair-climbing ability was significantly better in a group of patients who underwent primary TKA without patella resurfacing for osteoarthritis in whom the patella was not severely deformed preoperatively (regardless of the state of the patellar articular cartilage). Burnett et al[51] found in a randomized trial of resurfaced versus nonresurfaced patellae in patients undergoing bilateral TKA that results were equivalent at 10 years.

In a kinematic study, Smith et al[52] found that there were no significant differences in gait between TKA performed with or without patellar resurfacing. In addition, Pollo et al[53] found that there were no significant differences in the biomechanics of walking, stair climbing, or chair rising after TKA with or without patella resurfacing.

### Selective Patellar Resurfacing

Patella resurfacing has been recommended in patients with obvious patellofemoral disease, maltracking patella, age greater than 60 years, and patients with inflammatory arthritis.[54] Other parameters that may guide the decision to resurface the patella include height and weight[55] and the presence of anterior knee pain preoperatively.[56]

### Points to Remember

- Whether there is any advantage to resurfacing the patella in patients with osteoarthritic knees in the absence of severe patellofemoral arthritis is still unclear from available prospective randomized clinical trials.[57]
- The concern about resurfacing the patella with every total knee replacement is patellofemoral complications, which include wear, loosening, avascular necrosis, and fracture. However, over the past decade, patellofemoral complications have become less frequent due to improvement in prosthetic design and improvement in surgical techniques.[57]
- Not resurfacing the patella in TKA may result in a higher incidence of anterior knee pain[58] and reoperation and less patient satisfaction.

## Computer Navigation Versus Conventional Guides

### Theoretical

Computer-assisted systems were developed to improve the alignment of total knee components. Proper axial and coronal alignment is of paramount importance for proper function and patellar tracking and to avoid early wear and loosening of the implant. With computer navigation, the cuts can be theoretically made more accurately. The coronal alignment and slope of the tibia can be accurately measured and corrected intraoperatively. With computer navigation, the distal femur cut can be calculated to match the mechanical alignment of the limb by intraoperatively finding the center of rotation of the femoral head.

Although improved alignment after navigated TKA has been reported, only a few studies meet the criteria of a level-1 evidence.[59]

### Functional

Several prospective randomized clinical trials[59-63] have shown significant improvement in alignment with computer navigation for TKA. However, no functional improvement or survivorship advantage has been demonstrated.

Kim et al[64] studied computer navigation versus convention methods for TKA and found that operating and tourniquet times were significantly longer in the navigation group. There were no significant pre- or postoperative differences in Knee Society scores. Computer navigation did not result in more accurate orientation or alignment of the components.

Novak et al[65] has shown that computer-assisted surgery is potentially a cost-effective technique for TKA. This depends on the cost of the use of navigation and whether a true reduction in revisions is realized with the improved alignment.

### Points to Remember

- Improved alignment after navigated knee surgery has been reported.
- Whether the added cost, learning curve, and operative time that result from the use of computer-navigation in TKA have a real influence on knee function and implant survivorship is still controversial.

## Medial Parapatellar Versus Vastus-Splitting Approach

A vastus-splitting approach for TKA has been advocated to preserve function of the extensor mechanism and to decrease the prevalence of lateral release. Critics have claimed that there is greater blood loss and compromised exposure in obese patients who are managed with this approach.[66]

### Midvastus Better

Engh et al[67] compared the rate of lateral retinacular release in 2 groups of patients undergoing TKA: medial parapatellar and midvastus. Lateral retinacular release was necessary in 50% of the medial parapatellar group but only 3% of the midvastus group. White et al[68] compared midvastus and medial parapatellar approach for primary TKA and found that the midvastus approach had fewer lateral retinacular releases, less pain at 8 days and 6 weeks, and better straight leg raise at 8 days. However, pain relief, range of motion, and straight leg raise were no different at 6 months.

### Midvastus Not Better

In a prospective randomized study of bilateral TKA, Keating et al[69] found no differences in range of motion, straight leg raise, terminal knee extension, extensor lag, lateral release, or rehabilitation comparing the side with midvastus TKA and the side with the medial parapatellar TKA.

### Point to Remember

- The vastus-splitting approach to TKA may result in a lower incidence of lateral retinacular release. There is little evidence that there is any functional advantage in the long-term. The exposure may be more difficult using the midvastus approach.

## Minimally Invasive, Quadriceps-Sparing Total Knee Arthroplasty

The minimally invasive, quadriceps-sparing approach was described by Tria and Coon.[70] The principles touted by surgeons using the technique include no eversion of the patella, the tibiofemoral joint is not dislocated, and a shorter anteromedial incision (2x the patella length), rather than a longer direct anterior incision, is used.[71]

### Benefits of Minimally Invasive Total Knee Arthroplasty

Berger et al[72] reported a series of 50 patients who underwent minimally invasive TKA. Ninety-six percent of these patients were discharged the day of surgery and there were no intraoperative complications and only 3 readmissions. They concluded that in selected patients, minimally invasive outpatient TKA was safe. In a recent study by King et al,[71] minimally invasive TKA technique compared with traditional medial parapatellar approach resulted in shorter length of stay, less need for inpatient rehabilitation, less narcotic usage at 2 and 6 weeks, and less need for assistive devices. No significant differences were noted in implant alignment between the minimally invasive group and the medial parapatellar approach.

### No Benefit From Minimally Invasive Total Knee Arthroplasty

Dalury and Dennis[73] compared mini-incision TKA to TKA with a standard length incision. The small-incision group used less pain medication and had earlier improvement in range of motion, but these advantages dissipated by 3 months. Importantly, 4 of the 30 patients with small incisions had varus tibial malalignment (< 87 degrees), while no patients with the standard length incision had malalignment.

### Points to Remember

- From the data available, it appears that a minimally invasive quadriceps-sparing approach could result in faster recovery and accelerated rehabilitation, but risk of malposition of the components is higher.
- Clinical outcome may initially be better with minimally invasive surgical techniques, but these advantages may not persist in the long term.

## Gender-Specific Knee

A new controversy began with the recent introduction of the Zimmer Gender Solutions knee implant (Zimmer, Inc, Warsaw, IN) that is being promoted for use in a woman's knee due to its narrower and thinner shape and a special design to accommodate the higher average Q angle in women. In addition to a modified ML/AP aspect ratio, the Zimmer Gender Solutions knee system also decreases the thickness of the anterior flange and increases the trochlear groove angle in comparison to the original NexGen knee (Zimmer, Inc).[74]

Intraoperative measurements suggest that for any given anteroposterior femoral dimension, women tend to have a narrower mediolateral dimension than men.[75,76] Subsequently, for women, there is a significant association between the component size and the amount of medial-lateral overhang, with larger sizes having more overhang.[77] Regarding the rotatory measurements, a significant difference between the genders was found for the trochlear groove, which is angled somewhat externally relative to the epicondylar line in females.[76] The anterior extent of the trochlea seems to be smaller in females, but according to Poilvache et al,[76] this difference can be explained by the smaller size of their femurs.

Despite these differences, there is no evidence in the literature that the outcome of TKA is influenced by gender. Furthermore, there is a paucity of literature as to how much overhang is acceptable and to what degree it affects total knee results.[78]

The implant has been in use less than 1 year,[74] and studies will show if there is any added benefit from its use.

## References


1. Dorr LD, Ochsner JL, Gronley J, Perry J. Functional comparison of posterior cruciate-retained versus cruciate-sacrificed total knee arthroplasty. *Clin Orthop Relat Res.* 1988;236:36-43.
2. Sorger JI, Federle D, Kirk PG, Grood E, Cochran J, Levy M. The posterior cruciate ligament in total knee arthroplasty. *J Arthroplasty.* 1997;12:869-879.
3. Stiehl JB, Komistek RD, Dennis DA, Paxson RD, Hoff WA. Fluoroscopic analysis of kinematics after posterior-cruciate-retaining knee arthroplasty. *J Bone Joint Surg Br.* 1995;77:884-889.
4. Li G, Zayontz S, Most E, Otterberg E, Sabbag K, Rubash HE. Cruciate-retaining and cruciate-substituting total knee arthroplasty: an in vitro comparison of the kinematics under muscle loads. *J Arthroplasty.* 2001;16:150-156.
5. Andriacchi TP, Galante JO. Retention of the posterior cruciate in total knee arthroplasty. *J Arthroplasty.* 1988;3 Suppl:S13-S19.
6. Victor J, Banks S, Bellemans J. Kinematics of posterior cruciate ligament-retaining and -substituting total knee arthroplasty: a prospective randomised outcome study. *J Bone Joint Surg Br.* 2005;87:646-655.
7. Udomkiat P, Meng BJ, Dorr LD, Wan Z. Functional comparison of posterior cruciate retention and substitution knee replacement. *Clin Orthop Relat Res.* 2000;378:192-201.
8. Mahoney OM, Noble PC, Rhoads DD, Alexander JW, Tullos HS. Posterior cruciate function following total knee arthroplasty: a biomechanical study. *J Arthroplasty.* 1994;9:569-578.
9. Straw R, Kulkarni S, Attfield S, Wilton TJ. Posterior cruciate ligament at total knee replacement: essential, beneficial or a hindrance? *J Bone Joint Surg Br.* 2003;85:671-674.
10. Clark CR, Rorabeck CH, MacDonald S, MacDonald D, Swafford J, Cleland D. Posterior-stabilized and cruciate-retaining total knee replacement: a randomized study. *Clin Orthop Relat Res.* 2001;392:208-212.
11. Warren PJ, Olanlokun TK, Cobb AG, Bentley G. Proprioception after knee arthroplasty: the influence of prosthetic design. *Clin Orthop Relat Res.* 1993;297:182-187.
12. Simmons S, Lephart S, Rubash H, Borsa P, Barrack RL. Proprioception following total knee arthroplasty with and without the posterior cruciate ligament. *J Arthroplasty.* 1996;11:763-768.
13. Lattanzio PJ, Chess DG, MacDermid JC. Effect of the posterior cruciate ligament in knee-joint proprioception in total knee arthroplasty. *J Arthroplasty.* 1998;13:580-585.
14. Cash RM, Gonzalez MH, Garst J, Barmada R, Stern SH. Proprioception after arthroplasty: role of the posterior cruciate ligament. *Clin Orthop Relat Res.* 1996;331:172-178.
15. Swanik CB, Lephart SM, Rubash HE. Proprioception, kinesthesia, and balance after total knee arthroplasty with cruciate-retaining and posterior stabilized prostheses. *J Bone Joint Surg Am.* 2004;86-A:328-334.
16. Gioe TJ, Novak C, Sinner P, Ma W, Mehle S. Knee arthroplasty in the young patient: survival in a community registry. *Clin Orthop Relat Res.* 2007;464:83-87.
17. Laskin RS. The Insall Award. Total knee replacement with posterior cruciate ligament retention in patients with a fixed varus deformity. *Clin Orthop Relat Res.* 1996;331:29-34.
18. Schai PA, Scott RD, Thornhill TS. Total knee arthroplasty with posterior cruciate retention in patients with rheumatoid arthritis. *Clin Orthop Relat Res.* 1999;367:96-106.
19. Palmer DH, Mulhall KJ, Thompson CA, Severson EP, Santos ER, Saleh KJ. Total knee arthroplasty in juvenile rheumatoid arthritis. *J Bone Joint Surg Am.* 2005;87:1510-1514.
20. Laskin RS, O'Flynn HM. The Insall Award. Total knee replacement with posterior cruciate ligament retention in rheumatoid arthritis: problems and complications. *Clin Orthop Relat Res.* 1997;345:24-28.
21. Crockarell JR Jr, Guyton JL. Arthroplasty of ankle and knee. In: Canale ST, ed. *Campbell's Operative Orthopaedics.* 10th ed. St. Louis, MO: Mosby; 2003.
22. Reed MR, Bliss W, Sher JL, Emmerson KP, Jones SM, Partington PF. Extramedullary or intramedullary tibial alignment guides: a randomised, prospective trial of radiological alignment. *J Bone Joint Surg Br.* 2002;84:858-860.

23. Maestro A, Harwin SF, Sandoval MG, Vaquero DH, Murcia A. Influence of intramedullary versus extramedullary alignment guides on final total knee arthroplasty component position: a radiographic analysis. *J Arthroplasty.* 1998;13:552-558.
24. Dennis DA, Channer M, Susman MH, Stringer EA. Intramedullary versus extramedullary tibial alignment systems in total knee arthroplasty. *J Arthroplasty.* 1993;8:43-47.
25. Simmons ED Jr, Sullivan JA, Rackemann S, Scott RD. The accuracy of tibial intramedullary alignment devices in total knee arthroplasty. *J Arthroplasty.* 1991;6:45-50.
26. Stern SH, Sharrock N, Kahn R, Insall JN. Hematologic and circulatory changes associated with total knee arthroplasty surgical instrumentation. *Clin Orthop Relat Res.* 1994;299:179-189.
27. Fahmy NR, Chandler HP, Danylchuk K, Matta EB, Sunder N, Siliski JM. Blood-gas and circulatory changes during total knee replacement: role of the intramedullary alignment rod. *J Bone Joint Surg Am.* 1990;72:19-26.
28. Delport HP, Banks SA, De SJ, Bellemans J. A kinematic comparison of fixed- and mobile-bearing knee replacements. *J Bone Joint Surg Br.* 2006;88:1016-1021.
29. Kaper BP, Smith PN, Bourne RB, Rorabeck CH, Robertson D. Medium-term results of a mobile bearing total knee replacement. *Clin Orthop Relat Res.* 1999;367:201-209.
30. Matsuda S, White SE, Williams VG, McCarthy DS, Whiteside LA. Contact stress analysis in meniscal bearing total knee arthroplasty. *J Arthroplasty.* 1998;13:699-706.
31. Kim YH, Kook HK, Kim JS. Comparison of fixed-bearing and mobile-bearing total knee arthroplasties. *Clin Orthop Relat Res.* 2001;392:101-115.
32. Aglietti P, Baldini A, Buzzi R, Lup D, De LL. Comparison of mobile-bearing and fixed-bearing total knee arthroplasty: a prospective randomized study. *J Arthroplasty.* 2005;20:145-153.
33. Callaghan JJ. Mobile-bearing knee replacement: clinical results: a review of the literature. *Clin Orthop Relat Res.* 2001;392:221-225.
34. Stiehl JB, Hamelynck KJ, Voorhorst PE. International multicenter survivorship analysis of mobile bearing total knee arthroplasty. *Int Orthop.* 2006;30:190-199.
35. Bhan S, Malhotra R. Results of rotating-platform, low-contact-stress knee prosthesis. *J Arthroplasty.* 2003;18:1016-1022.
36. Ritter MA, Harty LD, Davis KE, Meding JB, Berend M. Simultaneous bilateral, staged bilateral, and unilateral total knee arthroplasty: a survival analysis. *J Bone Joint Surg Am.* 2003;85-A:1532-1537.
37. Ritter M, Mamlin LA, Melfi CA, Katz BP, Freund DA, Arthur DS. Outcome implications for the timing of bilateral total knee arthroplasties. *Clin Orthop Relat Res.* 1997;345:99-105.
38. Liu TK, Chen SH. Simultaneous bilateral total knee arthroplasty in a single procedure. *Int Orthop.* 1998;22:390-393.
39. Bullock DP, Sporer SM, Shirreffs TG Jr. Comparison of simultaneous bilateral with unilateral total knee arthroplasty in terms of perioperative complications. *J Bone Joint Surg Am.* 2003;85-A:1981-1986.
40. Lombardi AV, Mallory TH, Fada RA, et al. Simultaneous bilateral total knee arthroplasties: who decides? *Clin Orthop Relat Res.* 2001;392:319-329.
41. Reuben JD, Meyers SJ, Cox DD, Elliott M, Watson M, Shim SD. Cost comparison between bilateral simultaneous, staged, and unilateral total joint arthroplasty. *J Arthroplasty.* 1998;13:172-179.
42. Lane GJ, Hozack WJ, Shah S, et al. Simultaneous bilateral versus unilateral total knee arthroplasty: outcomes analysis. *Clin Orthop Relat Res.* 1997;(345):106-112.
43. Mangaleshkar SR, Prasad PS, Chugh S, Thomas AP. Staged bilateral total knee replacement: a safer approach in older patients. *Knee.* 2001;8:207-211.
44. Dennis DA. Debate: bilateral simultaneous total knee arthroplasty. *Clin Orthop Relat Res.* 2004;428:82-83.
45. Alemparte J, Johnson GV, Worland RL, Jessup DE, Keenan J. Results of simultaneous bilateral total knee replacement: a study of 1208 knees in 604 patients. *J South Orthop Assoc.* 2002;11:153-156.
46. Schroeder-Boersch H, Scheller G, Fischer J, Jani L. Advantages of patellar resurfacing in total knee arthroplasty: two-year results of a prospective randomized study. *Arch Orthop Trauma Surg.* 1998;117:73-78.
47. Wood DJ, Smith AJ, Collopy D, White B, Brankov B, Bulsara MK. Patellar resurfacing in total knee arthroplasty: a prospective, randomized trial. *J Bone Joint Surg Am.* 2002;84-A:187-193.
48. Pakos EE, Ntzani EE, Trikalinos TA. Patellar resurfacing in total knee arthroplasty: a meta-analysis. *J Bone Joint Surg Am.* 2005;87:1438-1445.
49. Kajino A, Yoshino S, Kameyama S, Kohda M, Nagashima S. Comparison of the results of bilateral total knee arthroplasty with and without patellar replacement for rheumatoid arthritis: a follow-up note. *J Bone Joint Surg Am.* 1997;79:570-574.
50. Feller JA, Bartlett RJ, Lang DM. Patellar resurfacing versus retention in total knee arthroplasty. *J Bone Joint Surg Br.* 1996;78:226-228.
51. Burnett RS, Boone JL, McCarthy KP, Rosenzweig S, Barrack RL. A prospective randomized clinical trial of patellar resurfacing and nonresurfacing in bilateral TKA. *Clin Orthop Relat Res.* 2007;464:65-72.
52. Smith AJ, Lloyd DG, Wood DJ. A kinematic and kinetic analysis of walking after total knee arthroplasty with and without patellar resurfacing. *Clin Biomech (Bristol, Avon).* 2006;21:379-386.
53. Pollo FE, Jackson RW, Koeter S, Ansari S, Motley GS, Rathjen KW. Walking, chair rising, and stair climbing after total knee arthroplasty: patellar resurfacing versus nonresurfacing. *Am J Knee Surg.* 2000;13:103-108.
54. Bourne RB, Burnett RS. The consequences of not resurfacing the patella. *Clin Orthop Relat Res.* 2004;428:166-169.
55. Picetti GD 3rd, McGann WA, Welch RB. The patellofemoral joint after total knee arthroplasty without patellar resurfacing. *J Bone Joint Surg Am.* 1990;72:1379-1382.
56. Barrack RL, Bertot AJ, Wolfe MW, Waldman DA, Milicic M, Myers L. Patellar resurfacing in total knee arthroplasty: a prospective, randomized, double-blind study with five to seven years of follow-up. *J Bone Joint Surg Am.* 2001;83-A:1376-1381.

57. Hanssen AD. Orthopaedic crossfire: all patellae should be resurfaced during primary total knee arthroplasty: in the affirmative. *J Arthroplasty.* 2003;18:31-34.
58. Boyd AD Jr, Ewald FC, Thomas WH, Poss R, Sledge CB. Long-term complications after total knee arthroplasty with or without resurfacing of the patella. *J Bone Joint Surg Am.* 1993;75:674-681.
59. Bertsch C, Holz U, Konrad G, Vakili A, Oberst M. [Early clinical outcome after navigated total knee arthroplasty: comparison with conventional implantation in TKA: a controlled and prospective analysis]. *Orthopade.* 2007;36:739-745.
60. Sparmann M, Wolke B, Czupalla H, Banzer D, Zink A. Positioning of total knee arthroplasty with and without navigation support: a prospective, randomised study. *J Bone Joint Surg Br.* 2003;85:830-835.
61. Spencer JM, Chauhan SK, Sloan K, Taylor A, Beaver RJ. Computer navigation versus conventional total knee replacement: no difference in functional results at two years. *J Bone Joint Surg Br.* 2007;89:477-480.
62. Perlick L, Bathis H, Perlick C, Luring C, Tingart M, Grifka J. Revision total knee arthroplasty: a comparison of postoperative leg alignment after computer-assisted implantation versus the conventional technique. *Knee Surg Sports Traumatol Arthrosc.* 2005;13:167-173.
63. Ensini A, Catani F, Leardini A, Romagnoli M, Giannini S. Alignments and clinical results in conventional and navigated total knee arthroplasty. *Clin Orthop Relat Res.* 2007;457:156-162.
64. Kim YH, Kim JS, Yoon SH. Alignment and orientation of the components in total knee replacement with and without navigation support: a prospective, randomised study. *J Bone Joint Surg Br.* 2007;89:471-476.
65. Novak EJ, Silverstein MD, Bozic KJ. The cost-effectiveness of computer-assisted navigation in total knee arthroplasty. *J Bone Joint Surg Am.* 2007;89:2389-2397.
66. Kelly MJ, Rumi MN, Kothari M, et al. Comparison of the vastus-splitting and median parapatellar approaches for primary total knee arthroplasty: a prospective, randomized study. Surgical technique. *J Bone Joint Surg Am.* 2007;89(Suppl 2 Pt.1):80-92.
67. Engh GA, Parks NL, Ammeen DJ. Influence of surgical approach on lateral retinacular releases in total knee arthroplasty. *Clin Orthop Relat Res.* 1996;331:56-63.
68. White RE Jr, Allman JK, Trauger JA, Dales BH. Clinical comparison of the midvastus and medial parapatellar surgical approaches. *Clin Orthop Relat Res.* 1999;367:117-122.
69. Keating EM, Faris PM, Meding JB, Ritter MA. Comparison of the midvastus muscle-splitting approach with the median parapatellar approach in total knee arthroplasty. *J Arthroplasty.* 1999;14:29-32.
70. Tria AJ Jr, Coon TM. Minimal incision total knee arthroplasty: early experience. *Clin Orthop Relat Res.* 2003;440:185-190.
71. King J, Stamper DL, Schaad DC, Leopold SS. Minimally invasive total knee arthroplasty compared with traditional total knee arthroplasty: assessment of the learning curve and the postoperative recuperative period. *J Bone Joint Surg Am.* 2007;89:1497-1503.
72. Berger RA, Sanders S, Gerlinger T, Della VC, Jacobs JJ, Rosenberg AG. Outpatient total knee arthroplasty with a minimally invasive technique. *J Arthroplasty.* 2005;20:33-38.
73. Dalury DF, Dennis DA. Mini-incision total knee arthroplasty can increase risk of component malalignment. *Clin Orthop Relat Res.* 2005;440:77-81.
74. Greene KA. Gender-specific design in total knee arthroplasty. *J Arthroplasty.* 2007;22:27-31.
75. Chin KR, Dalury DF, Zurakowski D, Scott RD. Intraoperative measurements of male and female distal femurs during primary total knee arthroplasty. *J Knee Surg.* 2002;15:213-217.
76. Poilvache PL, Insall JN, Scuderi GR, Font-Rodriguez DE. Rotational landmarks and sizing of the distal femur in total knee arthroplasty. *Clin Orthop Relat Res.* 1996;331:35-46.
77. Hitt K, Shurman JR, Greene K, et al. Anthropometric measurements of the human knee: correlation to the sizing of current knee arthroplasty systems. *J Bone Joint Surg Am.* 2003;85-A (Suppl 4):115-22.
78. Lo CS, Wang SJ, Wu SS. Knee stiffness on extension caused by an oversized femoral component after total knee arthroplasty: a report of two cases and a review of the literature. *J Arthroplasty.* 2003;18:804-808.

# 15

# Early Failure in Primary Total Knee Arthroplasty

*William V. Arnold, MD, PhD*

Total knee arthroplasty (TKA) is an overwhelmingly successful surgery. Excellent long-term survivorship on the order of 95% over 15 years has been reported.[1] In addition, significant improvement in patient quality of life has been found after TKA. Partly because of this success, it is disappointing for both the patient and the surgeon when knee arthroplasty fails. Failure in knee arthroplasty also creates a practical problem. One estimate projects an increase from 37,544 revision knee arthroplasties in 2005 to 56,918 in 2030 with projected hospital costs in excess of $2 billion by 2030.[2] Therefore, knee arthroplasty surgeons and the patients they serve have a vested interest in minimizing the need for revision arthroplasty.

While long-term follow-up studies of knee arthroplasty have routinely reported on revision rates, the mechanisms of failure have often been less well studied. However, a few recent studies of knee revision attempted to clarify these mechanisms of failure. Fehring et al[3] studied 440 patients who required revision knee arthroplasty between 1986 and 1999. They reported that 279 (63%) of the patients required revision within 5 years of their original surgery. Sharkey et al[4] reported on 212 revision arthroplasty cases from 1997 to 2000. Greater than half (55.6%) of these revisions were performed within 2 years of the primary surgery. In a more recent study, Mulhall et al[5] studied 318 revision patients and found that 99 (31%) required revision within 2 years of their primary surgery. While Mulhall et al did not present their data in the same breakdown (early versus late) as the 2 previous reports, the modes of failure were similar: infection, instability, loosening, polyethylene wear, and patellar complications.

It has become clear from these studies that there seems to be 2 types of failure: early and late.

Late failure from polyethylene wear with subsequent bone osteolysis or from late hematogenous infection is, to some degree, beyond the surgeon's control. Early failure, however, seems to be dependent on surgical technique and therefore is more amenable to immediate improvement. The mechanisms of early failure found by Fehring et al[3] and by Sharkey et al[4] are summarized in Table 15-1. It should be noted that the most common mechanism of early failure, infection, is somewhat beyond surgeon control. However, the surgeon can have a key role in lowering early infection rates, and this will be discussed next. Most of the remaining modes of failure are specifically related to surgical technique and decision making. Each mechanism of failure is discussed in turn next.

## Infection

Infection is a particularly dreaded complication in knee arthroplasty because of the significant morbidity associated with it. Patients must often undergo 2-stage surgical procedures with the associated investment of time, pain, and recovery. Reported rates of infection vary. In a retrospective analysis of 6489 knee replacement surgeries, Peersman et al reported an infection rate of 0.39% for primary knee replacement and 0.97% for revision knee replacement.[6] Infection rates of 1% have also been reported for primary TKA,[7] and the ideal rate probably approximates these values.



Parvizi J, Klatt B.
*Essentials in Total Knee Arthroplasty* (pp 121-128).

Table 15-1

## Early Mechanisms of Failure in Total Knee Arthroplasty

| | Fehring et al (N = 279)* | Sharkey et al (N = 118)** |
|---|---|---|
| Infection | 38% | 25.4% |
| Instability | 27% | 21.2% |
| Loosening | 13% | 16.9% |
| Patellofemoral problems | 8% | See note |
| Wear/osteolysis | 7% | 11.8%[a] |
| Arthrofibrosis | | 16.9% |
| Malalignment | | 11.9% |

*Revision within 5 years of index procedure
**Revision within 2 years of index procedure. N is calculated from the reported 55.6% of 212 cases requiring revision within 2 years of the index procedure.
[a] Reported in this percentage of early failures, although it was not the primary reason for failure
Note: Sharkey et al reported failures in categories of extensor mechanism deficiency, avascular necrosis of the patella, and revision of an unresurfaced patella. These failures accounted for 11.7% of the revisions in the early and late groups combined. Patellar resurfacing (0.9% of failures) was reported in only the early failure group.

Surgeons must take the practical steps necessary to minimize the rate of perioperative infection. Some of these are quite simple to implement, such as the use of body exhaust suits and laminar flow operative suites, but require hospital investment. Personnel flow in and out of the operating room during surgery should be minimized. The value of using prophylactic antibiotics prior to surgery has been well established.[8] Specifically, cefazolin or cefuroxime should be given within 60 minutes of the incision time. In the case of a β-lactam allergy, clindamycin or vancomycin should be given. Clindamycin should be given within 60 minutes of the incision time; vancomycin should be given within 120 minutes of the incision time. Patients with methicillin-resistant Staphylococcus aureus (MRSA) colonization should be treated with vancomycin. Antibiotic prophylaxis should be discontinued within 24 hours of the end of surgery. The importance of antibiotic prophylaxis cannot be overemphasized. Unfortunately, timely administration of prophylactic antibiotics preoperatively has been a challenge. In a review of 8137 major surgical procedures, Hawn et al found a 23.8% failure rate in meeting the time demand for preoperative antibiotic administration.[9] Bratzler et al found a failure rate of 44.3%.[10] A recently published recommendation[11] to improve the appropriate timing of preoperative antibiotic administration required that the prophylactic antibiotic as well as its time of administration be identified during the surgical "time-out" protocol, which many hospitals have instituted as a preventive measure against wrong-side surgery. This simple measure improved compliance for proper preoperative antibiotic administration from 65% to 97% when a prestudy patient group was compared with a poststudy patient group. In addition to better attention to detail with regard to prophylactic antibiotic administration, surgeons should also regularly consult with their infectious disease colleagues to optimize antibiotic choices. For example, if a significant percentage of local community staphylococcus or streptococcus strains are resistant to clindamycin, then this may be a poor choice for antibiotic prophylaxis.

Other ways to minimize infection risk involve surgical technique and experience.

Low surgeon volume has been associated with an increased infection risk[12] as has prolonged surgical times.[6] Attention to detail with surgical closure is a simple but important measure in infection control. Patel et al[13] reported that each day of prolonged wound drainage increases the risk of wound infection in knee arthroplasty by 29%. Surgical incisions should be carefully planned. When multiple incisions are present, the most recently healed or the most lateral incision should be used.[14] The use of surgical drains in joint arthroplasty has been debated between those who think that they help prevent wound problems and those who believe that they increase the risk of infection. A meta-analysis involving 3495 hip and knee arthroplasty patients suggests that closed suction drainage has no major benefits and does not alter the risk of wound infection.[15] Allogeneic transfusions have been shown to cause immune modulation and increased rates of infection in orthopedic procedures. Employing methods to reduce transfusion may be of benefit. Certainly, it is best to maximize preoperative hemoglobin because low preoperative hemoglobin is a strong predictor for the need to transfuse.

Another factor related to infection is patient selection. Certain patient groups have been shown to have a higher risk of infection including diabetics,[16] obese patients,[17] patients with rheumatoid arthritis,[18] patients with liver cirrhosis,[19] and hemophiliacs.[20] Although some of these patient-related factors are beyond the surgeon's control, a knowledge of their infection-predisposing characteristics can be nonetheless useful. Surgery should be held from brittle diabetics until their blood glucose levels are appropriately controlled. Doctors can enter into agreements with their obese patients to encourage weight loss prior to surgery. The dosing of immunosuppressive medications can be optimized preoperatively to minimize their effects.

Although infection will always be a part of knee arthroplasty surgery, proactive steps can be taken to keep the rate of infection at 1% or less.

## Instability

Instability in knee arthroplasty can manifest as pain as well as mechanical problems, such as knee buckling. Although malalignment of prosthetic components can certainly contribute to joint instability, joint instability can still occur in the setting of well-positioned components. Joint instability basically results from poor ligament balance as well as poor balancing of flexion and extension gaps.[21,22] Surgeons should be knowledgeable about the appropriate soft tissue releases needed to achieve a balanced knee arthroplasty. As a first step, all osteophytes should be removed. Sometimes this alone is enough to balance a knee. Bone cuts should generally not be altered to substitute for varus-valgus soft tissue balancing. Fixed varus and valgus deformities usually manifest during the course of the surgery. The surgeon can often get a sense of a disparity in the tension and functional length of the collateral ligaments when a laminar spreader is placed to separate the cut tibial and femoral surfaces. This disparity is often also noted when placing trial spacer blocks. A fixed varus deformity should be addressed with a release of the medial collateral ligament. Downsizing the polyethylene insert to accommodate the contracted medial structures can leave the knee with a lateral thrust. Upsizing the polyethylene insert to make up for lateral laxity can lead to bony avulsion of the medial collateral ligament. A fixed valgus deformity can be evaluated similarly with laminar spreaders and spacer blocks. In a valgus knee, the usual medial release done for exposure is limited and releases of the lateral structures proceed in a step-wise manner. Ranawat et al[23] recently reviewed this "inside-out technique," which involves a release of the posterolateral capsule, pie-crusting of the iliotibial band, and bony resections of the tibia and femur.

A flexion-extension mismatch in an otherwise balanced knee arthroplasty can be corrected with appropriate additional femoral cuts. Often a flexion contracture can be corrected with the removal of posterior femoral osteophytes and a posterior release. A knee that flexes poorly due to a larger extension gap than flexion gap can be treated in 2 ways. One technique would augment the distal femur and downsize the polyethylene insert. This would decrease the extension gap and make it equal to the flexion gap. The second technique involves downsizing the femoral component to increase the flexion gap. Downsizing the femoral component decreases the anteroposterior diameter of the implant without changing the distal size.

## Malalignment

Improper alignment of knee arthroplasty components can cause increased wear, joint instability, and joint pain.[24] Multiple studies have reaffirmed these problems.[25-27] Essentially there are 3 planes to consider for alignment: the coronal plane, the sagittal plane, and the rotational plane.

The normal anatomic axis (the intersection of the axes of the tibial and femoral shafts) of the knee is 5 to 7 degrees of valgus.[28] Although the normal native tibial surface is in approximately 3 degrees of varus in the coronal plane, most surgeons will try to place their tibial resection perpendicular to the mechanical axis of the tibia. The distal femoral resection is performed in valgus to achieve an overall tibiofemoral angle that approximates the normal angle of 5 to 7 degrees of valgus. A consequence of the perpendicular tibial resection is that an asymmetric flexion gap can result unless the posterior condylar resections compensate for this. This usually requires a larger resection of the medial posterior condyle compared with the lateral posterior condyle. Poor alignment in the coronal plane results in varus and valgus instability. This can result from a poor tibial or distal femoral resection. Poor alignment in the sagittal plane can result in a flexed femoral component that can affect knee extension. Too steep of a posterior tibial slope can contribute to instability in knee flexion.

Proper rotational alignment of the femoral component is essential to achieve balanced flexion and extension gaps as well as proper patellar tracking. Rotational alignment is determined by appropriate bone cuts of the distal femur. Usually this entails proper placement of a 4-in-1 cutting guide on the distal femur. There are 3 axes to consider in placing this guide: the posterior femoral condylar axis, the epicondylar axis, and the anteroposterior axis. The posterior femoral condylar axis is usually internally rotated by approximately 3 degrees. This axis can be somewhat unreliable because of unequal wear of the posterior condyles. The epicondylar axis connects the medial and lateral epicondyles of the femur, which are usually palpable structures. The cutting guide should be placed so that the anterior and posterior femoral bone resections will parallel this axis. These resections will usually be perpendicular to the anteroposterior axis,[29] which extends from the base of the trochlear groove to the apex of the intercondylar notch. This usually results in a larger cut medially of the posterior condyles and a larger cut laterally of the anterior flange of the femur. When done properly, the anterior femoral cut is said to resemble a grand piano. Olcott and Scott[30] compared rotational alignment in 100 total knee arthroplasties using 1 of the 3 axes as the sole reference point during surgery. A symmetric flexion gap occurred in 90%, 83%, and 70% of cases in which the reference axis was the epicondylar axis, the anteroposterior axis, and the posterior femoral transcondylar axis, respectively. It was recommended that more than one reference axis be used, and most surgeons seem to use the epicondylar and the anteroposterior axes for rotational alignment. Rotational alignment on the tibial side usually places the anterior midpoint of the tibial tray at the junction of the medial one third and lateral two-thirds of the tibial tubercle. Another method is to allow the tibial tray to "find" its own alignment by placing a nonkeeled tibial trial and then putting the knee through repeated flexion and extension trials, allowing the tray to rotate to its proper alignment on the cut proximal tibial surface. This method assumes that there is already proper soft tissue balance in the knee.

The instrumentation involved in current knee arthroplasty is reliable and usually involves the use of an extramedullary or intramedullary bone-cutting guide for the proximal tibial resection and an intramedullary bone-cutting guide for the distal femur. These guides can give reliable results but must be used properly.[31] The entrance point for the femoral intramedullary guide is often not the midline of the femur but approximately 5 mm medial to the center of the intercondylar notch. This entry point can change depending on the bow of the femur. The extramedullary tibial guide should be aligned at its distal tip with the center of the ankle joint, not the midmalleolar point as this results in a varus tibial cut. The center of the ankle is medial to the midmalleolar point by approximately 1 cm. Positioning of the extramedullary tibial guide can be challenging in obese patients. Also, a rotational mismatch between the proximal tibia and the ankle has been shown to result in varus tibial cuts. Intramedullary tibial cutting guides should not use the midpoint of the tibial plateau as an entry point as this can result in a valgus tibial cut. Usually the proper entry point is just medial to the midline and at the anterior one-third of the anterior-posterior axis of the tibial plateau.

It has been postulated that computer navigation should improve the overall alignment of arthroplasty components and thereby improve surgical outcomes. Results in this regard have been somewhat mixed. Kim et al[32] compared knee arthroplasty done with a computed tomography (CT)-free computer-assisted navigation system with knee arthroplasty done with conventional techniques in 100 patients undergoing bilateral knee arthroplasties in which one surgery was done with navigation and the other was done without navigation. They found no difference in terms of the accuracy of the orientation and alignment of the prosthetic components between the 2 types. A recent meta-analysis including 33 studies involving 3423 patients showed no difference in the alignment of the mechanical axes between the navigated and non navigated surgical groups, although the navigation results did show a lower risk of malalignment at critical thresholds of more than 2 degrees and more than 3 degrees of malalignment.[33]

It should be emphasized that the quality of a computer-navigated knee arthroplasty, especially in terms of alignment accuracy, is only as good as the data input into the navigation system. For imageless navigation, the anatomic landmarks input into the system by the surgeon are mostly the same as those the surgeon would use routinely for non-navigated arthroplasty. Therefore, the same error can occur under both systems. This may explain why some studies have not found a significant difference between navigated and traditional knee arthroplasties. In the end, computer navigation is just another tool at the surgeon's disposal to facilitate the knee arthroplasty operation. It is no substitute for good surgical technique and judgment.

## Loosening

Loosening as a cause of early failure in both the Fehring et al[3] and Sharkey et al[4] studies refers specifically to loosening of cementless prosthetic components. This is distinct from the late loosening and osteolysis usually attributed to prosthetic wear. While there are supporters of cementless fixation in knee arthroplasty, the conclusion of the Fehring et al[3] and Sharkey et al[4] studies was to consider abandoning this technique altogether. The proposed benefit of cementless fixation is that it provides a more durable implant, which avoids cement-specific problems such as cement wear and debonding. A recent report of a prospective randomized series of 501 primary posterior cruciate-retaining knee replacements, 277 cemented versus 224 cementless, showed a 15-year survival rate of 80.7% and 75.3% for cemented and cementless knees, respectively.[34] This difference was found not to be statistically significant. Another review[35] of 1000 consecutive cementless knee replacements found an impressive survival of 99.14% at 10 years with revision as a measure of failure. Although cementless knee arthroplasty will continue to have its supporters, surgeons performing these surgeries must be rigorous in their fixation techniques because it is ultimately the failure of ingrowth that leads to the early loosening of these prostheses.

## Patellofemoral Problems

Patellofemoral problems can result in knee pain and joint instability and have long been a source of concern in knee arthroplasty. Complication rates as high as 10% have been reported in the older literature.[36] With improvements in technique and component design, the complication rate remains about 4%.[37] An ongoing debate has involved the question of whether to resurface the patella at all during knee arthroplasty. Some of the patellar problems reported by Sharkey et al[4] involved specifically the need to resurface a patella that was left alone at the original knee arthroplasty. Patellar resurfacing as a revision procedure seems to have inferior results when compared with patellar resurfacing done as part of the primary procedure.[38,39] A meta-analysis of the literature from 1966 to 2003 supported patella resurfacing at the time of primary knee arthroplasty.[40] Another meta-analysis involving 1223 cases came to the same conclusion.[41]

Patellofemoral instability usually results from patellar maltracking. Lateral patellar tracking can result from tight lateral structures such as encountered in a valgus degenerative knee. A lateral release can often remedy this problem. In episodes of significant patellar maltracking, the surgeon may need to consider repositioning of the extensor mechanism with a tibial tubercle transfer. It is extremely rare to need to resort to such a measure. When such significant maltracking occurs, it is often due to malrotation of the tibial and femoral prosthetic components, and this is what needs to be corrected.

Periprosthetic fracture of the patella can severely compromise knee arthroplasty results. Studies have documented the treatment of this problem with modest surgical outcomes and often surgical complications.[42,43] Generally, the best strategy is to avoid this problem altogether. Careful attention during patellar resection is needed to avoid over-resection with subsequent weakening of the patella. A cadaver study has noted the fracture risk of patellar resection to 11 mm.[44] Such aggressive bone resection is generally not needed in primary arthroplasty. Care is also needed to avoid oblique patellar cuts that leave the medial and lateral patellar facets either under-resected or over-resected with respect to one another. Under-resection of the patella or oversizing of the femoral component is also a problem because it can cause overstuffing of the patellofemoral joint with subsequent decreased knee flexion, although the overall flexion loss has not been that dramatic in recently reported studies[45,46] (on the order of 2 to 3 degrees of flexion loss for 2 mm of build-up on either the patellar or the anterior femoral side).

Prosthetic component positioning has been discussed with respect to rotational malalignment; however, components also need to be appropriately placed in the coronal plane. Medialization of the femoral or tibial component increases the Q-angle and thereby the lateral pull on the patella. The same occurs if the patellar component is lateralized. Proper surgical exposure should avoid these pitfalls. Attention should also be paid to achieving a proper position of the joint line. Patella infera after TKA has been correlated with decreased functional scores.[47]

## Arthrofibrosis

Arthrofibrosis or knee stiffness in TKA has been long studied but is still not very well understood. Nelson et al[48] reported a prevalence of arthrofibrosis of 1.3% in their series of 1000 consecutive primary total knee arthroplasties. Fisher et al[49] reported on patient factors and poor results from knee pain or stiffness at 1 year after TKA and found significant associations with female gender, obesity, previous knee surgery, diabetes mellitus, pulmonary disease, depression, and employment disability. Not surprisingly, postoperative flexion has been correlated with preoperative flexion.[50]

The results of revision arthroplasty for knee stiffness are not impressive. Simple tibial insert exchange with lysis of adhesions has shown poor outcomes with minimal change in the mean Knee Society pain and function scores.[51] More aggressive revision arthroplasty can improve motion, but the reported gains are modest.[48,52,53] Nelson et al[48] reported the results of 56 revisions of primary knee arthroplasties with arthrofibrosis. The arc of motion increased in 93% of the cases, but the mean arc of motion only improved from 54.6 degrees to 82.2 degrees. Haidukewych et al[52] reported on the revision of 16 well-fixed primary total knee arthroplasties. The mean arc of motion only improved from 40 degrees to 73 degrees. Ries and Badalamente[53] reported an increase in the mean arc of motion from 36 degrees to 86 degrees in 6 knee arthroplasty revisions. Perhaps these less-than-satisfying results simply reflect our ignorance of the true source of this problem. Obviously, attention to an aggressive therapy regimen with adequate treatment of pain is warranted for the less motivated patient. Attention to surgical detail is needed to avoid any expected impediments to motion. However, in the end, more research is needed to better clarify the causative factors of this frustrating problem.

## Summary

Various causes of poor outcome and early failure in TKA have been reviewed. Most of these causes are amenable to improvement with improved surgical technique. As in the past, continued advances in knee replacement components as well as improved understanding into the various modes of arthroplasty failure should lead to improved outcomes in the future. It is incumbent on joint arthroplasty surgeons to incorporate these improvements into their practice with the goal of achieving the best and most durable functional results for their patients.

## References

1. Vessely MB, Whaley AL, Harmsen WS, Schleck CD, Berry DJ. The Chitranjan Ranawat Award: long-term survivorship and failure modes of 1000 cemented condylar total knee arthroplasties. *Clin Orthop Relat Res.* 2006;452:28-34.
2. Lavernia C, Lee DJ, Hernandez VH. The increasing financial burden of knee revision surgery in the United States. *Clin Orthop Relat Res.* 2006;446:221-226.
3. Fehring TK, Odum S, Griffen WL, Mason JB, Nadaud M. Early failures in total knee arthroplasty. *Clin Orthop Relat Res.* 2001;392:316-318.
4. Sharkey PF, Hozack WJ, Rothman RH, Shastri S, Jacoby SM. Insall Award Paper: why are total knee arthroplasties failing today? *Clin Orthop Relat Res.* 2002;404:7-13.
5. Mulhall KJ, Ghomrawi HM, Scully S, Callaghan JJ, Saleh KJ. Current etiologies and modes of failure in total knee arthroplasty revision. *Clin Orthop Relat Res.* 2006;446:45-50.
6. Peersman G, Laskin R, Davis J, Peterson M. Insall Award Paper: infection in total knee replacement. *Clin Orthop Relat Res.* 2001;392:15-23.
7. Blom AW, Brown J, Taylor AH, Pattison G, Whitehouse S, Bannister GC. Infection after total knee arthroplasty. *J Bone Joint Surg Br.* 2004;86:688-691.
8. Bratler DW, Houck PM, for the Surgical Infection Prevention Guideline Writers Workgroup. Antimicrobial prophylaxis for surgery: an advisory statement from the National Surgical Infection Prevention Project. *Am J Surg.* 2005;189:395-404.
9. Hawn MT, Gray SH, Vick CC, et al. Timely administration of prophylactic antibiotics for major surgical procedures. *J Am Coll Surg.* 2006;203:803-811.
10. Bratzler DW, Houck PM, Richards C, et al. Use of antimicrobial prophylaxis for major surgery: baseline results from the National Surgical Infection Project. *Arch Surg.* 2005;140:174-182.
11. Rosenberg AD, Wanbold D, Kraemer L, et al. Ensuring appropriate timing of antimicrobial prophylaxis. *J Bone Joint Surg Am.* 2008;90:226-232.
12. Muilwijk J, van den Hof S, Wille JC. Associations between surgical site infection risk and hospital operation volume and surgeon operation volume among hospitals in the Dutch nosocomial infection surveillance network. *Infection Control and Hospital Epidemiology.* 2007;28:557-563.
13. Patel VP, Walsh M, Sehgal B, Preston C, DeWal H, Di Cesare PE. Factors associated with prolonged wound drainage after primary total hip and knee arthroplasty. *J Bone Joint Surg Am.* 2007;89:33-38.
14. Vince KG, Abdeen A. Wound problems in total knee arthroplasty. *Clin Orthop Relat Res.* 2006;452:88-90.
15. Parker MJ, Roberts CP, Hay D. Closed suction drainage for hip and knee arthroplasty: a meta-analysis. *J Bone Joint Surg Am.* 2004;86:1146-1152.
16. Namba RS, Paxton L, Fithian DC, Stone ML. Obesity and perioperative morbidity in total hip and total knee arthroplasty patients. *J Arthroplasty.* 2005;20:46-50.
17. Medling JB, Reddleman K, Keating ME, et al. Total knee arthroplasty in patients with diabetes mellitus. *Clin Orthop Relat Res.* 2003;416:208-216.
18. Meding JB, Keating EM, Ritter MA, Faris PM, Berend ME. Long-term followup of posterior-cruciate-retaining TKR in patients with rheumatoid arthritis. *Clin Orthop Relat Res.* 2004;428:146-152.
19. Shih LY, Cheng CY, Chang CH, Hsu KY, Hsu RW, Shih HN. Total knee arthroplasty in patients with liver cirrhosis. *J Bone Joint Surg Am.* 2004;86:335-341.
20. Silva M, Luck JV. Long-term results of primary total knee replacement in patients with hemophilia. *J Bone Joint Surg Am.* 2005;87:85-91.
21. Robbins GM, Bassam AM, Garbuz DS, Duncan CP. Preoperative planning to prevent instability in total knee arthroplasty. *Orthopedic Clinics of North America.* 2001;32:611-626.
22. Clarke HD, Scott WN. Knee: axial instability. *Orthop Clin North Am.* 2001;32:627-637.
23. Ranawat AS, Ranawat CS, Elkus M, Rasquinha VJ, Rossi R, Babhulkar S. Total knee arthroplasty for severe valgus deformity. *J Bone Joint Surg Am.* 2005;87(Suppl 1 [Pt 2]):271-284.
24. Berger RA, Rubash HE. Rotational instability and malrotation after total knee arthroplasty. *Orthop Clin North Am.* 2001;32:639-647.
25. Collier MB, Engh CA, McAuley JP, Engh GA. Factors associated with the loss of thickness of polyethylene tibial bearings after knee arthroplasty. *J Bone Joint Surg Am.* 2007;89:1306-1314.
26. Berend ME, Ritter MA, Meding JB, et al. The Chitranjan Ranawat Award: tibial component failure mechanisms in total knee arthroplasty. *Clin Orthop Relat Res.* 2004;428:26-34.
27. Ritter MA, Faris PM, Keating EM, Meding JB. Postoperative alignment of total knee replacement: its effect on survival. *Clin Orthop Relat Res.* 1994;299:153-156.
28. Pollice P, Lotke PA, Lonner J. Principles of instrumentation and component alignment. In: Callaghan JJ, Rosenberg AG, Rubash HE, Simonian PT, Wickiewicz TL, eds. *The Adult Knee.*

Philadelphia, PA: Lippincott Williams and Wilkins; 2003:1085-1093.

29. Whiteside LA, Arima J. The anteroposterior axis for femoral rotational alignment in valgus total knee arthroplasty. *Clin Orthop Relat Res.* 1995;321:168-172.
30. Olcott CW, Scott RD. A comparison of four intraoperative methods to determine femoral component rotation during total knee arthroplasty. *J Arthroplasty.* 2000;15:22-26.
31. Laskin RS. Instrumentation pitfalls: you just can't go on autopilot. *J Arthroplasty.* 2003;18 (Suppl 1):18-22.
32. Kim YH, Kim JS, Yoon SH. Alignment and orientation of the components in total knee replacement with and without navigation support: a prospective, randomized study. *J Bone Joint Surg Br.* 2007;89:471-476.
33. Bauwens K, Matthes G, Wich M, et al. Navigated total knee replacement: a meta-analysis. *J Bone Joint Surg Am.* 2007;89:261-269.
34. Baker PN, Khaw FM, Kirk LMG, Esler CAN, Greg PJ. A randomized controlled trial of cemented versus cementless press-fit condylar total knee replacement: 15-year survival analysis. *J Bone Joint Surg Br.* 2007;89:1608-1614.
35. Cross MJ, Parish EN. A hydroxyapatite-coated total knee replacement: prospective analysis of 1000 patients. *J Bone Joint Surg Br.* 2005;87:1073-1076.
36. Lynch AF, Rorabeck CH, Bourne RB. Extensor mechanism complications following total knee arthroplasty. *J Arthroplasty.* 1987;2:135-140.
37. Rand JA. Extensor mechanism complications after total knee arthroplasty. *Instr Course Lect.* 2005;54:241-250.
38. Karnezis IA, Vossinakis IC, Rex C, Fragkiadakis EG, Newman JH. Secondary patellar resurfacing in total knee arthroplasty: results of multivariate analysis in two case-matched groups. *J Arthroplasty.* 2003;18:993-998.
39. Muoneke HE, Khan AM, Giannikas KA, Hagglund E, Dunningham TH. Secondary resurfacing of the patella for persistent anterior knee pain after primary knee arthroplasty. *J Bone Joint Surg Br.* 2003;85:675-678.
40. Parvizi J, Rapuri VR, Saleh KJ, Koskowski MA, Sharkey PF, Mont MA. Failure to resurface the patella during total knee arthroplasty may result in more knee pain and secondary surgery. *Clin Orthop Relat Res.* 2005;438:191-196.
41. Pakos EE, Ntzani EE, Trikalinos TA. Patellar resurfacing in total knee arthroplasty: a meta-analysis. *J Bone Joint Surg Am.* 2005;87:1438-1445.
42. Parvizi J, Kim KI, Oliashirazi A, Ong A, Sharkey PF. Periprosthetic patellar fractures. *Clin Orthop Relat Res.* 2006;446:161-166.
43. Ortiguera CJ, Berry DJ. Patellar fracture after total knee arthroplasty. *J Bone Joint Surg Am.* 2002;84:532-540.
44. Lie DT, Gloria N, Amis AA, Lee BP, Yeo SJ, Chou SM. Patellar resection during total knee arthroplasty: effect on bone strain and fracture risk. *Knee Surg Sports Traumatol Arthrosc.* 2005;13:203-208.
45. Mihalko W, Fishkin Z, Krackow K. Patellofemoral overstuff and its relationship to flexion after total knee arthroplasty. *Clin Orthop Relat Res.* 2006;449:283-287.
46. Bengs BC, Scott RD. The effect of patellar thickness on intraoperative knee flexion and patellar tracking in total knee arthroplasty. *J Arthroplasty.* 2006;21:650-655.
47. Meneghini RM, Ritter MA, Pierson JL, Meding JB, Berend ME, Faris PM. The effect of the Insall-Salvati ratio on outcome after total knee arthroplasty. *J Arthroplasty.* 2006;21(6 Suppl 2):116-120.
48. Nelson CL, Kim J, Lotke PA. Stiffness after total knee arthroplasty. *J Bone Joint Surg Am.* 2005;87 (Suppl 1[Pt 2]):264-270.
49. Fisher DA, Dierckman B, Watts MR, Davis K. Looks good but feels bad: factors that contribute to poor results after total knee arthroplasty. *J Arthroplasty.* 2007;22(6 Suppl 2):39-42.
50. Ghandi R, de Beer J, Leone J, Petruccelli D, Winemaker M, Adili A. Predictive risk factors for stiff knees in total knee arthroplasty. *J Arthroplasty.* 2006;21:46-52.
51. Babis GC, Trousdale RT, Pagnano MW, Morrey BF. Poor outcomes of isolated tibial exchange and arthrolysis for the management of stiffness following total knee arthroplasty. *J Bone Joint Surg Am.* 2001;83:1534-1536.
52. Haidukewych GJ, Jacofsky DJ, Pagnano MW, Trousdale RT. Functional results after revision of well-fixed components for stiffness after primary total knee arthroplasty. *J Arthroplasty.* 2005;20:133-138.
53. Ries MD, Badalamente M. Arthrofibrosis after total knee arthroplasty. *Clin Orthop Relat Res.* 2000;380:177-183.

# 16

# Mechanisms of Failure in Total Knee Arthroplasty

*Peter F. Sharkey, MD and Omar Abdul-Hadi, MD*

Total knee arthroplasty (TKA) has been shown to be successful in achieving pain relief and functional improvement.[1] In addition, the long-term survival of these implants is well documented in the literature with greater than 90% survivorship at 10 to 15 years.[2-4] The revision rate as reported by Heck et al[5] was found to be less than 3% in the first 2 years after index TKA. In 1999, 22,000 knee revision operations were done in the United States at an estimated expense of $262 million.[6] Between 1990 and 2002, the rate of primary total knee arthroplasties per 100,000 persons almost tripled. The rate of revision total knee arthroplasties increased by 5.4 procedures per 100,000 persons per decade.[7]

It is currently estimated that about 8.2% of total knee arthroplasties will eventually require a revision.[7] Considering the increasing numbers of primary knee arthroplasties performed each year, one can expect a greater number of revisions in the future. In addition, one must take into account the emotional distress that the operation imparts on the patient as well as the morbidity of the procedure itself.

## Evaluation of the Patient With a Failed Total Knee Arthroplasty

When the results of TKA fall well below the patient's expectations, the operation should be considered a failure. This lack of satisfaction can be attributed to pain, inadequate function, or inconsistent patient expectations. Evaluation of the failed total knee should follow a logical algorithm in order to determine the cause of failure. Initial evaluation always starts with the patient's history and physical examination. The nature of the complaint after arthroplasty can help determine the etiology of failure. Pain is a common symptom associated with failure of the arthroplasty. The nature of the pain should be carefully analyzed, including its character, location, radiation, and aggravating and relieving factors.

Activity-related pain is an indication of a mechanical component to the failure and can signify loosening, component failure, or patellofemoral dysfunction. Continuous pain can be associated with infection or complex regional pain syndrome. Instability should be defined by its nature and inciting activities.

The physical examination is an equally important adjunct in the evaluation of a failed TKA. Gait patterns should be observed. Referred pain from other joints should be considered and examined in conjunction with the knee. The presence of effusion, erythema, warmth, and persistent drainage are findings associated with infection. Other causes of effusion include soft-tissue impingement, ligamentous imbalance, and synovitis.

Passive and active range of motion should be assessed. A discrepancy can be related to muscle or extensor tendon dysfunction. Anteroposterior (AP) and medial-lateral stability are evaluated with the knee in 0, 30, and 90 degrees of flexion. Patellar tracking should be assessed throughout the range of motion to elicit any maltracking, grinding, or the presence of a patellar clunk.[8]

A stiff painful knee with shiny skin and diffuse tenderness suggests complex regional pain syndrome.



Parvizi J, Klatt B.
*Essentials in Total Knee Arthroplasty* (pp 129-140).

## Radiographic Evaluation

Radiographic evaluation starts with AP, lateral, and sunrise view radiographs of the knee. Full-length standing lower extremity radiographs help assess component alignment.

Weight-bearing radiographs of the knee help demonstrate asymmetric wear, failure of the tibial insert, and instability. A sunrise view of the patella helps assess patellar position in the femoral groove. Tilt and medial-lateral position of the patella should be assessed. Lateral radiographs help determine position of the joint and presence of patella baja, which is determined by a distance of less than 10 mm between the lower pole of the patella and the joint line. Osteolysis can be observed and is usually noted at the bone–cement interface. Oblique radiographs are useful when attempting to detect osteolysis. Signs of component loosening should be noted and include the following:

- Change in component position as noted on serial radiographs
- Presence of radiolucent lines, especially when they extend under the entire prosthesis
- Progressive widening of the cement-bone or bone-prosthesis interface
- Cement cracking or fragmentation

Computed tomography (CT) plays a role in quantifying the degree of juxta-articular bone defects, and also in determining both femoral and tibial component rotation.

## Laboratory Evaluation

The white blood cell count (WBC), erythrocyte sedimentation rate (ESR), and the C-reactive protein (CRP) are helpful in ruling out an infectious etiology for the TKA failure. ESR is a nonspecific indicator for infection; however, it can be elevated up to 1 year after surgery.[9] An elevated ESR can signify either an infectious or an inflammatory etiology. The level of CRP, an acute-phase reactant, is elevated after surgery but normalizes in 2 to 4 weeks.[9]

A cell count and culture of the joint aspiration is helpful in ruling out an infectious etiology.

A synovial fluid leukocyte differential of greater than 65% neutrophils or a leukocyte count more than 1.7 X 103/μL is a sensitive and specific test for the diagnosis of deep periprosthetic infection in patients without underlying inflammatory disease.[10]

## Mechanisms of Failure After Primary Total Knee Arthroplasty

There are a number of factors that influence the longevity of total knee arthroplasties. Several studies have attempted to evaluate the causes of failure after TKA. Fehring et al[11] reported on 440 revision arthroplasties done between 1986 and 1999. Failure of total knee arthroplasties frequently occurred in the first 5 years after the index procedure and often was related to infection or surgical error. Sharkey et al[12] evaluated all patients who had revision TKA during a 3-year period (September 1997 to October 2000). They found the most common reasons for failure included polyethylene wear, aseptic loosening, instability, infection, arthrofibrosis, malalignment or malposition, deficient extensor mechanism, avascular necrosis of the patella, periprosthetic fracture, and isolated patellar resurfacing. In many patients, more than one failure mechanism was seen.

## Polyethylene Wear and Aseptic Loosening

Component loosening results in pain as a result of micromotion between the implant and bone. Progressive loosening can result in change in the component position, resulting in mechanical dysfunction. The resulting pain is activity related and occurs with weight bearing.

Loosening of the tibial component in a posterior cruciate ligament (PCL)-substituting TKA is more common in patients with varus tibial femoral alignment, a varus tibial component, and excessive tibial resection.[13] Femoral component loosening has been found to be associated with inaccurate bony cuts, poor cementation technique, and deficient bone.[14]

Several factors have been found to result in patellar component failure. Those include incorrect resection of the patella, lateralization of the patellar component, patellar maltracking, and malposition of the femoral and tibial components.[15] Other factors include increased flexion of the knee, increased weight, increased activity, and male gender.[16]

Polyethylene wear results in the generation of particles that can instigate an osteolytic reaction. This can result in eventual loosening of the component. Polyethylene wear particles can be generated by the motion between the articulation of the femoral component on the polyethylene liner or by motion between the insert and the tibial base plate, which is referred to as backside wear.[17] Post wear can also occur in a PCL-substituting TKA if hyperextension occurs. Factors that may increase the wear and failure rate of a tibial insert include lack of congruency, presence of third-body debris, and methods of production or sterilization. Gamma ray sterilization in air has been shown to alter polyethylene via oxidation, making the components more susceptible to wear.[18]

Metal-backed patellar components have a high rate of failure as a result of wear and fracture of the polyethylene on the edge of the metal backing, dissociation of the polyethylene from the base plate, and fracture of the fixation pegs.

## Extensor Mechanism Rupture

Rupture of the extensor mechanism may occur in conjunction with a patellar fracture. It may also occur with rupture of either the patellar or quadriceps tendon. Quadriceps tendon rupture is less frequent than patellar tendon rupture. The prevalence of patellar tendon rupture has been reported to be 0.22% of 8288 total knee arthroplasties observed over a 12-year period.[19]

Risk factors associated with patellar tendon ruptures include a difficult exposure in a stiff knee, extensive release of the patellar tendon at the time of surgical exposure, manipulation for the treatment of limited motion, revision TKA, and distal realignment of the extensor mechanism to treat patellar maltracking.[19]

Surgical options include direct repair with augmentation with an autogenous semitendinosus tendon graft, an Achilles or whole patellar tendon allograft, or a synthetic ligament. The use of a medial gastrocnemius flap for reconstruction has the advantage of providing viable autogenous tissue to cover the anterior-inferior aspect of the knee; however, this procedure results in a poor cosmetic appearance and weakness of ankle plantar flexion.[20]

The results of allograft reconstruction have been variable. In one study, 3 of 9 knees treated with an Achilles tendon allograft had residual extensor lags ranging from 5 to 20 degrees.[21]

Complications in that series consisted of 2 graft failures requiring repeat repair and one infection treated with débridement.

## Infection

Infection is uncommon after primary TKAs. The prevalence of deep infection is about 1% to 2%.[22,23] The most common organisms are *Staphylococcus aureus* (50% to 65%) and *S. epidermidis* (25% to 30%). Risk factors include inflammatory arthritis, prior surgeries, psoriasis, diabetes, and chronic steroid use.

Antibiotic prophylaxis is the single most effective method of reducing infection in TKA.[24,25] The optimal time for administration of the antibiotics should be within 30 to 60 minutes before incision.[26] The routine use of antibiotic-impregnated cement in primary TKAs remains controversial. In one randomized study, cefuroxime-impregnated cement was shown to be effective in the prevention of early to intermediate deep infection after primary TKA.[27] The current recommendation is for the use of antibiotic-impregnated cement in primary TKA in patients at higher risk for periprosthetic infection.

Appropriate identification and diagnosis of infection after TKA requires a thorough history, physical examination, plain radiographs, arthrocentesis, and hematological studies. The timing of the clinical infection is important in determining the appropriate management strategy.

The onset of the infection could occur intraoperatively, in the early postoperative period, or late (chronic), or it could be a result of an acute hematogenous infection.

Pain is the most common initial symptom and usually occurs at rest. Persistent drainage in the early postoperative period is highly suggestive of infection and should be managed with irrigation and débridement. An acute hematogenous infection presents with a sudden onset of pain, swelling, and stiffness in an otherwise previously well-functioning arthroplasty. Usually, this is a result of a recent invasive procedure resulting in significant bacteremia.[28]

Most cases of infected TKAs are diagnosed in the subacute or chronic setting. Indicators for deep infection include persistent pain since the arthroplasty and knee stiffness despite extensive rehabilitation efforts.

Useful screening tools that aid in the diagnosis of infection in the painful TKA are the combination of ESR and CRP.[29] CRP levels usually peak on postoperative day 2 and decrease to preoperative baseline levels generally 14 to 21 days postoperatively.[30]

Joint arthrocentesis is essential to confirming the diagnosis. A complete discussion of aspiration results is presented in the chapter on infection (see Chapter 19). Evaluation includes Gram stain, quantitative leukocyte count, cultures, aerobic, anaerobic, mycobacterium, and fungus.

The use of the combination of indium 111 leukocyte scanning and technetium 99 sulfur colloid marrow scintigraphy can yield an accuracy of 95% in diagnosing deep prosthetic infections.[31]

A negative indium scan may be helpful in suggesting the absence of infection in cases in which the diagnosis is not otherwise evident. An indium scan will detect acute and chronic white cells, and this can be positive with wear debris. Some suggest the addition of a sulfa colloid scan to the nuclear medicine regimen. The sulfa colloid scan identifies the white cells in the marrow, so that marrow pooling is not confused with infection. All of the nuclear studies are used infrequently. There is a large variability in the accuracy of the nuclear studies, and much of this has to do with the interpretation.

## Treatment

Once the diagnosis of infection is established, there are several variables that dictate the management strategy. Those include location of the infection (superficial versus deep), elapsed time between the index arthroplasty and the diagnosis of infection, host comorbidities, integrity and condition of the soft tissues and extensor mechanism, status of the implant (loose versus well fixed), responsible pathogen, and the patient's functional status.

Treatment options include the following:

- Antibiotic suppression: Usually reserved for cases when removal of the implant is not feasible (medical condition that precludes an operative intervention), the microorganism has low virulence, is susceptible to an oral antibiotic agent, and the implant is not loose. The success rate of antibiotic suppression is about 24%.[32]
- Débridement with retention of the prosthesis: Typically reserved for an acute infection in the early postoperative period or for an acute hematogenous infection. For this procedure to work, the infection generally needs to be less than 2 weeks in duration, with a susceptible gram-positive organism and no evidence of implant loosening. The success rate has been reported at 32.6%.[33] The timing of the débridement is of paramount importance in determining the success of treating the infection. In one study, successful treatment was demonstrated in 100% of the early postoperative infection group and 71% of the acute hematogenous infection group.[34] The virulence of the organism is an important predictor of success of open débridement. *S. aureus* prosthetic joint infection is associated with the lowest success rate after débridement.[35] In contrast, open débridement of prosthetic infections with penicillin-susceptible streptococcal species yields a higher success rate (89.5%) if performed within 10 days of the onset of symptoms.[36]
- Arthrodesis: Once considered the gold standard treatment for infected TKAs. However, the functional limitations incurred by a knee arthrodesis are poorly tolerated by most patients. The elimination of knee motion causes sitting and other activities to be cumbersome. Current indications for arthrodesis include the following:
  - Patients with high functional demands
  - Disruption of the extensor mechanism
  - Poor soft-tissue envelope necessitating extensive reconstruction
  - Systemic immunocompromise
  - Organism resistant to conventional antibiotics

  Arthrodesis surgical fixation options include external and internal fixation either with an intramedullary nail or plate fixation. The union rates associated with intramedullary nails range from 67% to 100% of cases.[32]
- Two-stage reimplantation: This has become the principal method of treatment for patients with chronic TKA infection. A 6-week course of intravenous antibiotics is usually administered prior to reimplantation. This has resulted in excellent success rates and is the most commonly accepted clinical standard for treating persistent infection.[37,38]
- Insall originally described this procedure, which includes soft-tissue débridement, removal of the infected prosthesis, and cement followed by 6 weeks of intravenous antibiotics and subsequent reimplantation.[39] The adjunctive use of antibiotic delivery systems (cement spacers) has gradually led to decreased antibiotic duration and shorter time to reimplantation.[32] The overall success of 2-stage reimplantation ranges from 88% when antibiotic-loaded cement is not used at the time of reimplantation to 92% with antibiotic-loaded cement.[32]

## Arthrofibrosis

Arthrofibrosis creates a functional problem following TKA that can be incapacitating as a result of the limited range of motion. It has been shown recently that there is a direct correlation between a decreased range of motion following surgery and a lower perceived quality of life as evaluated with use of the Short Form-36 health survey questionnaire.[40]

There remains controversy regarding the management of patients for whom initial rehabilitation efforts are unsuccessful following TKA. Nonoperative treatment modalities for restoring range of motion include intensive rehabilitation protocols and static or dynamic splinting.

Manipulation with the patient under anesthesia and invasive procedures, including arthroscopic débridement, open débridement with or without polyethylene exchange, and complete component revision, have been used when initial nonoperative rehabilitation efforts have failed.[41]

Manipulation under anesthesia is usually performed in the first 3 months following arthroplasty. Keating et al selected patients for manipulation as early as 2 months following TKA, and the procedure was used as late as 44 weeks postoperatively.[42] Various protocols can be used for manipulation, and there is no gold standard in this regard. One good protocol is to manipulate the knee with a spinal anesthesia with Duramorph added to the spinal. The patient remains in the hospital for 23 hours. This allows for physical therapy to provide several sessions for range of motion only. After discharge, the physical therapy continues for aggressive range of motion 3 times per week for 6 weeks.

Manipulation is most often done for patients with postoperative flexion of less than 90 degrees after adequate rehabilitation. Keating et al[42] demonstrated an average improvement in flexion of 35 degrees after manipulation. He also reported no significant difference in the improvement in flexion between patients who had been treated within 12 weeks following surgery and those who had the manipulation at more than 12 weeks.

This is in contrast to other studies that showed better results with manipulation when performed less than 3 weeks postoperatively.[43] Other studies revealed no difference in the ultimate range of motion at 1 year between the patients who had received manipulations and those who had not.[44]

Arthroscopy with manipulation has a role in the management of arthrofibrosis after arthroplasty. Arthroscopy is performed with multiple portals to débride scar tissue and to release tissues as needed. Jerosch and Aldawoudy[45] evaluated the efficacy of arthroscopic management of knee stiffness after TKA. In their series of 32 knees, 25 demonstrated improvements in both the range of motion and the Knee Society scores. Williams et al[46] reported on successful arthroscopic release of the PCL in 10 stiff painful knees that had undergone PCL-sparing TKA.

Arthrotomy with débridement is a reasonable option to address arthrofibrosis in patients presenting with severe stiffness of the knee. This is usually accompanied with synovectomy, removal of scar tissue, lateral retinacular release, posterior capsular release, PCL release, and/or exchange of a single component.[47] Generally, at least the modular polyethylene must be removed if a flexion contracture exists and access to the posterior aspect of the knee is needed.

## Malalignment

Implant malalignment is a common cause of failure following TKA.[48,49] Multiple studies have demonstrated that malalignment may affect implant function and lead to decreased survival in TKA.[49,50] This is a result of off-axis loading that ultimately leads to polyethylene wear and implant loosening. Contemporary manual alignment systems may produce significant errors of alignment (mechanical axis alignment of greater than 3 degrees) in 10% of TKAs.[51]

Computer-assisted surgical navigation systems have been developed in order to attain better alignment in the frontal plain and to decrease the number of unsatisfactory alignment outliers. Most studies examining computer-assisted surgery have shown more consistent restoration of neutral mechanical alignment, with improved precision of component placement in one or more of the measured anatomic planes, as compared with mechanical guides. Specifically, computer-assisted surgery results in better alignment in the coronal plane, with significantly fewer outliers.[52,53]

The key determinant of clinical outcomes and cost effectiveness is the effect of computer-assisted surgery on implant survival and revision rates. Long-term outcome studies ultimately will determine the usefulness of this technology, and additional studies examining the long-term outcomes of TKA with regard to implant alignment are needed before reaching any final recommendations regarding the routine use of computer-assisted surgical navigation in TKAs.

## Patellofemoral Complications

The patellofemoral joint is an important source of pain and complications following TKA. The prevalence of complications related to the extensor mechanism is around 4%.[54] Anterior knee pain, fracture, rupture of the extensor mechanism, and patellar instability can adversely affect the TKA outcome.

Lateral subluxation of the patella may occur in midflexion and can cause medial retinacular pain.[55] Patellar maltracking is frequently observed after TKA. In one retrospective review, patellar tilting was noted in 31.2% of cases and displaced patellae were noted in an additional 14.5% of the cases.[56] Multiple factors contribute to patellar maltracking, including femoral or tibial component medialization, excessive internal rotation of the femoral or tibial components, anterior placement of the femoral component, asymmetric patellar resection, and lateral positioning of the patellar component. Assessment of rotational alignment is important in patients who present with complications related to the extensor mechanism after TKA. Rotational malalignment can affect patellar tracking, resulting in anterior knee pain. In one review, combined internal rotation of 1 to 4 degrees resulted in lateral tracking and tilting of the patella, 3 to 8 degrees was associated with patellar subluxation, and 7 to 17 degrees was associated with patellar dislocation or failure.[57]

The geometry of the femoral component plays an important role in patellar tracking. An asymmetric trochlear groove produces 5% less shear and 7% less compressive force on the patella than does a symmetric design, and a deeper trochlear groove results in less shear forces on the patella than does a shallow trochlear groove.[58] The combination of a deepened trochlear groove and a medial position of the patellar implant provides patellar tracking similar to that in the normal knee.[59]

Controversy exists regarding patellar resurfacing during TKAs. Advocates of resurfacing have found it to provide better pain relief, improved patient satisfaction, and fewer complications than nonresurfacing.[60] In one randomized series, 10% of knees with an unresurfaced patella required revision for pain and subsequent patellar resurfacing.[61] Indications for patellar resurfacing include preoperative anterior knee pain, inflammatory arthritis, advanced chondromalacia of Outerbridge grade III or IV, and patellar malalignment.

Patellar baja is another reason for failure of the TKA and can be observed in patients who have had a prior procedure (high tibial osteotomy).[62] Patellar baja can cause impingement of the inferior portion of the patellar component on the anterior aspect of the tibial component, resulting in pain and/or instability.

Patellar clunk syndrome is another cause of pain after posterior stabilized TKA. A palpable suprapatellar fibrous nodule on the posterior surface of the extensor mechanism catches on the anterior aspect of the femur in the intercondylar notch.[63] Original designs for posterior stabilized knees suffered this complication more frequently. Designs with a short femoral flange have been implicated. The occurrence of patellar clunk has been virtually eliminated by redesigning posterior stabilized femoral implants with deep femoral grooves and smooth transitions into the intercondylar notch. If clunk occurs, the clunk can be resolved with open or arthroscopic débridement of the soft tissue mass that is catching in the notch.

The positioning of the femoral and tibial components affects patellar alignment and the rate of complications. The AP and medial-lateral position of the implant and alteration of the joint line affect the patellofemoral joint. The position of the implant and the height of the joint line affect the rate of anterior knee pain.[64] Placement of the femoral component outside of the ideal neutral sagittal alignment results in a higher rate of anterior knee pain.

Also, anterior placement of the tibial component and elevation of the joint line can result in increased strain and abnormal forces on the patellofemoral articulation.[65] Furthermore, medial displacement and internal rotation of the femoral component on the femur can have a similar result.[66]

Rotational alignment of the femoral and tibial components plays an important role in patellofemoral tracking. In vitro, rotation of the femoral component parallel to the epicondylar axis results in the most normal patellar tracking and decreases shear forces early in flexion.[67] The rotational position of the tibial component plays a similarly important role in maintaining proper patellofemoral tracking. The best alignment of the tibial component appears to be symmetric with the femoral component in extension, with the femoral component aligned on the epicondylar axis.[68]

Patellar fractures are another complication and cause of failure after TKA. The prevalence of patellar fracture ranges from <1% to 11%.[69,70] Risk factors associated with patellar fracture include trauma, vascular compromise, implant malalignment, obesity, excessive patellar bone resection, high activity level, a large central fixation lug, and osteoporosis. Vascular compromise of the patella following a medial arthrotomy combined with a lateral retinacular release has been suggested as an etiology for fracture.

Osteonecrosis of the patella with subsequent fragmentation and resorption has been reported after TKA with a lateral retinacular release.[71]

However, an in vitro study assessing a medial parapatellar approach with lateral retinacular release at least 1 cm lateral to the patella did not reveal any impairment of the patellar blood supply.[72]

There are several classification systems for patellar fractures. A commonly used one is the Mayo Clinic Classification System.[70] In this system, there are 3 types of patellar fractures:

1. Type-I fracture is associated with a stable implant and an intact extensor mechanism. These fractures can be treated nonoperatively.
2. Type-II fracture is associated with a disruption of the extensor mechanism. These fractures are less common. Their treatment is controversial but is probably best accomplished with open reduction and fixation.

3. Type-III fracture is associated with a loose patellar implant and an intact extensor mechanism. They are divided into 2 subtypes:
   a. IIIa, which is associated with good bone stock
   b. IIIb, which is associated with poor bone stock (< 10 mm in thickness or marked comminution).

Treatment of most patellar fractures should be nonoperative, with an initial period of immobilization until the pain resolves. Primary operative treatment should be used for fractures associated with disruption of the extensor mechanism.

## Periprosthetic Fracture

Periprosthetic fractures after TKA are a potentially disastrous complication. Various treatment modalities have been developed to manage these fractures. The complication rates from treating these fractures can approach 30% with both nonoperative and operative methods.[73]

Risk factors for supracondylar fractures include osteopenia, rheumatoid arthritis, corticosteroid usage, advanced age, and female gender. Anterior notching of the distal femoral cortex may increase the risk of fracture, with 40% to 52% of reported fractures associated with an anterior notch.[74]

Analysis of cadaveric femora revealed a mean reduction of 18% in bending strength and a mean decrease of 42% in torsional strength when a full-thickness anterior notch is present.[75]

The goals of treatment are to obtain and maintain good postfracture alignment and stability to allow early range of motion. Nonoperative options include skeletal traction, application of a cast, pins and plaster, and cast bracing. The operative options include use of a condylar plate, intramedullary fixation, revision TKA, external fixation, cerclage wiring with strut allograft fixation, and arthrodesis.

Fracture displacement, the degree of osteopenia, and the status of the prosthetic components are the primary determinants of the management method.

Nonoperative treatment is recommended as the initial management technique for nondisplaced fractures that do not exhibit intercondylar extension. Chen et al[73] found an 83% rate of successful results in a literature review.

Culp et al[76] reported the results of 30 patients treated nonoperatively. Fifteen patients (50%) had increased pain or decreased ambulatory status following nonoperative care, whereas this was true of only 13% of patients treated operatively.

Open reduction and fixation with a condylar plate provides the potential advantages of anatomical reconstruction, rigid fixation, and an early range of motion. Rigid supracondylar interlocking rod fixation offers the advantage of being less invasive while providing good axial, angular, and rotational stability. Revision TKA provides the advantage of stable fixation with a diaphysis-engaging intramedullary femoral stem, allowing early range of motion and weight bearing. This is reserved for cases with loose, unstable, substantially malaligned total knee components or in cases when rigid internal fixation is not achievable.

Figgie et al[77] reviewed 10 cases of supracondylar periprosthetic fractures treated with open reduction and internal fixation. Fracture alignment was lost in 8 cases. Zehntner and Ganz[78] reported 100% success rate without malunion in the 6 cases treated with the adjunctive use of polymethylmethacrylate to enhance fixation.

The advent of locking condylar plates has resulted in its expanded use to treat these difficult fractures.

In conclusion, obtaining and maintaining fracture alignment is critical for the success of any treatment method. Rigid fixation allows an early range of motion, resulting in a superior functional result.

## Instability After Total Knee Arthroplasty

Tibio-femoral instability is widely recognized as a common mode of failure after TKA and often requires revision surgery. One study found instability to be responsible for 22% of TKA revisions.[6] Fehring et al reported instability to be the second leading cause of early failure.[11]

Restoration of stability is critically important for a functional and durable knee arthroplasty revision. Surgeons have choices of component design and level of constraint, and it is vital to select the optimum implant for a given patient.

Instability after TKA can be divided into 2 major types:

1. Collateral ligament imbalance (ie, gap asymmetry)
2. Flexion-extension mismatch (ie, gap inequality)

Instability may result from inherent soft-tissue laxity, inadequate flexion/extension gap balancing, improper component positioning or alignment, ligamentous insufficiency, failure to balance the collateral ligaments, or choosing the wrong level of constraint.

Instability can occur in different planes of motion and they can be divided into several categories:

- Varus-valgus (coronal plane) instability

- Recurvatum (hyperextension, sagittal plane) instability
- Anteroposterior (or flexion) instability
- Rotational (cross sectional) instability
- Global

## Varus-Valgus Instability

Medial-lateral instability is the most common type of instability and may result from incompetent collateral ligaments, incomplete correction of a preoperative deformity, or incorrect bone cuts with malalignment.[79]

Clinically, the patient usually presents with complaints of instability, occasional giving way, recurrent knee effusions, and instability in flexion, making stair climbing difficult.[80]

## Recurvatum Instability

Recurvatum deformity may result from a weak quadriceps muscle or an incompetent extensor mechanism. This creates the necessity of walking with compensatory hyperextension. In this situation, the hamstrings substitute for a deficient extensor mechanism. Recurvatum can also be caused by an extension gap that either is or has become larger than the flexion gap, as seen with subsidence of a loose femoral component. Revision arthroplasties for recurvatum often fail. These patients should consider permanent postoperative bracing. A linked constrained prosthesis with a hyperextension stop is a clever but only temporarily successful maneuver. If the hyperextension is a compensatory mechanism for a weak extensor mechanism, over time the patient will hyperextend again to keep the knee from buckling during ambulation.

## Anteroposterior (Flexion Instability)

Flexion instability results in excessive AP translation of the tibia in flexion and usually is associated with a mismatch of the flexion and extension spaces. Flexion instability has been recognized as a source of postoperative pain. On examination, the medial tibial metaphysis or soft tissue envelope may be tender, particularly in the pes anserine region. The patient may also describe a sense of instability and recurrent knee joint effusions.[81]

Similarly, if the flexion gap is larger than the extension gap, the flexed tibia may dislocate posteriorly. This situation may occur after revision surgery if an undersized femoral component was selected because it fit the residual bone and posterior augments were not used. Flexion instability can also be caused by over resection of the posterior femoral condyles, undersizing of the femoral component, and excessive tibial slope.

Frank dislocation of a posterior stabilized prosthesis can occur when there is a relatively tight extension space and a loose flexion space. Most posterior stabilized designs do not require a posterior tibial slope since the slope is usually inherent in the design. Excessive posterior tibial slope can produce a loose flexion space, and laxity in flexion can allow the femoral component to jump the tibial spine.[82]

## Rotational Instability

Malrotation of the tibial and femoral components affects kinematics of the patellofemoral joint and the flexion gap. Isolated internal malrotation of the femoral component results in an asymmetric flexion gap. Clinically, the patient suffers from either lateral instability or medial tightness in flexion. Lateral flexion instability leads to medial tibial pain, difficulties standing up from a chair, or instability during descending stairs or walking downhill. The balanced flexion gap technique seeks to achieve a perfectly balanced extension gap first, and then aligns the femoral component parallel to the tibial resection plane when the knee is under symmetric distraction in 90 degrees of flexion. If the medial collateral ligament is not first properly balanced, the femoral component may be internally rotated. Rotational positioning of the tibial component referenced on the tibial tuberosity is a reliable method, but placing the tibial component according to the femoral component using a floating trial technique may lead to internal malrotation of the tibia.

## Global

Global instability is defined as combined laxity of both the flexion and extension gaps. It can occur when the flexion-extension spaces are balanced but a polyethylene insert of insufficient thickness is used. Global instability can also result from use of an underconstrained implant in the presence of gross ligamentous insufficiency.

# Evaluation and Management of Instability

Initial evaluation of the patient with instability after TKA should include a comprehensive history and physical examination of the knee. Overall ligamentous quality should be assessed. Radiographic evaluation should include long-standing views and appropriate stress radiographs. It is important to assess the overall axial alignment as well as the sagittal alignment of the knee components. Also, evaluation of the rotational alignment of the components is useful. This can be done by obtaining a CT scan to evaluate the position of the femoral component relative to the epicondylar axis.

Correlating the complaints and physical findings is imperative. When the principal complaints are specifically mechanical, such as a sensation of slipping, subluxation, or giving way, there very well may be an instability problem. However, if instability cannot be determined on physical exam, then revision surgery is unlikely to be successful. Buckling has many causes: pain, fixed flexion contracture of the knee, quadriceps weakness, and patellar pathology.

A key principle of TKA is to always choose an implant with as little constraint as needed. Excessive constraint transfers stress to the implant and bone-cement interface and can result in an increased incidence of aseptic loosening. Conversely, failure to use an adequately constrained implant results in instability. The pathology in an arthritic knee relates not only to abnormalities of the cartilage but also of the surrounding soft tissue envelope. Alteration of the cruciate and collateral ligaments in addition to the posterior capsule occurs and must be dealt with properly.

A contracted anterior cruciate ligament/PCL will result in poor range of motion of the knee. Contracted collateral ligaments result in deformity in the frontal plane. Tightness of the posterior capsule will lead to a flexion contracture. This ligamentous pathology must be addressed prior to choosing an implant.

Revision surgery for instability requires the following:

- Achieving a neutral mechanical axis of the limb
- Equalization of the flexion and extension gaps
- Assessment of ligament integrity
- Choosing the proper level of implant constraint

The principles involved in achieving the above goals during reconstruction of a failed TKA include reestablishment of neutral alignment, restoration of joint line position, restoration of functional femoral and tibial component rotation, and flexion and extension gap balancing. It is prudent for the surgeon to have multiple constraint options available during revision knee arthroplasty performed for instability.

## Summary

Failure after TKA must be carefully evaluated. It is imperative to determine the underlying pathology to establish a treatment algorithm.

Revision surgery should be tailored to address the etiology of failure. Simply implanting revision components will not correct the problem. Therefore, a thorough understanding of the mechanism of failure and the development of a structured surgical plan to correct the problem is of paramount importance.

## References


1. Ranawat CS, Luessenhop CP, Rodriquez JA. The press-fit condylar modular total knee system: four to six year results with a posterior-cruciate-substituting design. *J Bone Joint Surg.* 1997;79A:342-348.
2. Weir DJ, Moran CG, Pinder IM. Kinematic condylar total knee arthroplasty: 14-year survivorship analysis of 208 consecutive cases. *J Bone Joint Surg.* 1996;78B:907-911.
3. Rodricks DJ, Patil S, Pulido P, Colwell CW Jr. Press-Fit condylar design total knee arthroplasty: fourteen to seventeen-year follow-up. *J Bone Joint Surg Am.* 2007;89:89-95.
4. Ito J, Koshino T, Okamoto R, Saito T. 15-year follow-up study of total knee arthroplasty in patients with rheumatoid arthritis. *J Arthroplasty.* 2003;18(8):984-992.
5. Heck DA, Melfi CA, Mamlin LA, et al. Revision rates after knee replacement in the United States. *Med Care.* 1998;36:661-669.
6. Ingenix: Data Analyst Group. Columbus, OH, Ingenix 1999.
7. Kurtz S, Mowat F, Ong K, Chan N, Lau E, Halpern M. Prevalence of primary and revision total hip and knee arthroplasty in the United States from 1990 through 2002. *J Bone Joint Surg Am.* 2005;87(7):1487-1497.
8. Beight JL, Yao B, Hozack WJ, Hearn SL, Booth RE Jr. The patellar "clunk" syndrome after posterior stabilized total knee arthroplasty. *Clin Orthop.* 1994;299:139-142.
9. Niskanen RO, Korkala O, Pammo H. Serum C-reactive protein levels after total hip and knee arthroplasty. *J Bone Joint Surg Br.* 1996;78:431-433.
10. Trampuz A, Hanssen AD, Osmon DR, Mandrekar J, Steckelberg JM, Patel R. Synovial fluid leukocyte count and differential for the diagnosis of prosthetic knee infection. *Am J Med.* 2004;117(8):556-562.
11. Fehring TK, Odum S, Griffin WL, Mason JB, Naduad M. Early failures in total knee arthroplasty. *Clin Orthop.* 2001;392:315-318.
12. Sharkey PF, Hozack WJ, Rothman RH, Shastri S, Jacoby SM. Insall Award paper: why are total knee arthroplasties failing today? *Clin Orthop.* 2002;404:7-13.
13. Windsor RE, Scuderi GR, Moran MC, Insall JN. Mechanisms of failure of the femoral and tibial components in total knee arthroplasty. *Clin Orthop.* 1989;248:15-20.
14. King TV, Scott RD. Femoral component loosening in total knee arthroplasty. *Clin Orthop.* 1985;194:285-290.
15. Malkani AL, Rand JA, Bryan RS, Wallrichs SL. Total knee arthroplasty with the kinematic condylar prosthesis: a ten-year follow-up study. *J Bone Joint Surg Am.* 1995;77:423-431.

16. Brick GW, Scott RD. The patellofemoral component of total knee arthroplasty. *Clin Orthop.* 1988;231:163-178.
17. Wasielewski RC, Parks N, Williams I, Surprenant H, Collier JP, Engh G. Tibial insert undersurface as a contributing source of polyethylene wear debris. *Clin Orthop.* 1997;345:53-59.
18. Williams IR, Mayor MB, Collier JP. The impact of sterilization method on wear in knee arthroplasty. *Clin Orthop.* 1998;356:170-180.
19. Rand JA, Morrey BF, Bryan RS. Patellar tendon rupture after total knee arthroplasty. *Clin Orthop.* 1989;244:233-238.
20. Pagnano MW. Patellar tendon and quadriceps tendon tears after total knee arthroplasty. *J Knee Surg.* 2003;16:242-247.
21. Crossett LS, Sinha RK, Sechriest VF, Rubash HE. Reconstruction of a ruptured patellar tendon with achilles tendon allograft following total knee arthroplasty. *J Bone Joint Surg Am.* 2002;84:1354-1361.
22. Wilson MG, Kelley K, Thornhill TS. Infection as a complication of total knee replacement arthroplasty: risk factors and treatment in sixty-seven cases. *J Bone Joint Surg Am.* 1990;72:878-883.
23. Blom AW, Brown J, Taylor AH, Pattison G, Whitehouse S, Bannister GC. Infection after total knee arthroplasty. *J Bone Joint Surg Br.* 2004;86(5):688-691.
24. Oishi CS, Carrion WV, Hoaglund FT. Use of parenteral prophylactic antibiotics in clean orthopedic surgery: a review of the literature. *Clin Orthop Relat Res.* 1993;296:249-255.
25. Hanssen AD, Osmon DR. The use of prophylactic antimicrobial agents during and after hip arthroplasty. *Clin Orthop Relat Res.* 1999;369:124-138.
26. Leigh DA, Griggs J, Tighe CM, et al. Pharmacokinetic study of ceftazidime in bone and serum of patients undergoing hip and knee arthroplasty. *J Antimicrob Chemother.* 1985;16(5):637-642.
27. Chiu FY, Chen CM, Lin CF, Lo WH. Cefuroxime-impregnated cement in primary total knee arthroplasty: a prospective, randomized study of three hundred and forty knees. *J Bone Joint Surg Am.* 2002;84-A(5):759-762.
28. Maniloff G, Greenwald R, Laskin R, Singer C. Delayed postbacteremic prosthetic joint infection. *Clin Orthop Relat Res.* 1987;(223):194-197.
29. Austin MS, Ghanem E, Joshi A, Lindsay A, Parvizi J. A simple, cost-effective screening protocol to rule out periprosthetic infection. *J Arthroplasty.* 2008;23(1):65-68.
30. Niskanen RO, Korkala O, Pammo H. Serum C-reactive protein levels after total hip and knee arthroplasty. *J Bone Joint Surg Br.* 1998;80(5):909-911.
31. Scher DM, Pak K, Lonner JH, Finkel JE, Zuckerman JD, Di Cesare PE. The predictive value of indium-111 leukocyte scans in the diagnosis of infected total hip, knee, or resection arthroplasties. *J Arthroplasty.* 2000;15(3):295-300.
32. Hanssen AD, Rand JA. Evaluation and treatment of infection at the site of a total hip or knee arthroplasty. *Instr Course Lect.* 1999;48:111-122.
33. Silva M, Tharani R, Schmalzried TP. Results of direct exchange or débridement of the infected total knee arthroplasty. *Clin Orthop Relat Res.* 2002;(404):125-131.
34. Mont MA, Waldman B, Banerjee C, Pacheco IH, Hungerford DS. Multiple irrigation, débridement, and retention of components in infected total knee arthroplasty. *J Arthroplasty.* 1997;12(4):426-433.
35. Deirmengian C, Greenbaum J, Lotke PA, Booth RE Jr, Lonner JH. Limited success with open débridement and retention of components in the treatment of acute Staphylococcus aureus infections after total knee arthroplasty. *J Arthroplasty.* 2003;18(7 Suppl 1):22-26.
36. Meehan AM, Osmon DR, Duffy MC, Hanssen AD, Keating MR. Outcome of penicillin-susceptible streptococcal prosthetic joint infection treated with débridement and retention of the prosthesis. *Clin Infect Dis.* 2003;36(7):845-849.
37. Goldman RT, Scuderi GR, Insall JN. 2-stage reimplantation for infected total knee replacement. *Clin Orthop Relat Res.* 1996;(331):118-124.
38. Windsor RE, Insall JN, Urs WK, Miller DV, Brause BD. Management of total knee arthroplasty infection. *Orthop Clin North Am.* 1991;22(3):531-538. Review.
39. Insall JN, Thompson FM, Brause BD. Two-stage reimplantation for the salvage of infected total knee arthroplasty. *J Bone Joint Surg Am.* 1983;65(8):1087-1098.
40. Padua R, Ceccarelli E, Bondi R, Campi A, Padua L. Range of motion correlates with patient perception of TKA outcome. *Clin Orthop Relat Res.* 2007;460:174-177.
41. Mont MA, Seyler TM, Marulanda GA, Delanois RE, Bhave A. Surgical treatment and customized rehabilitation for stiff knee arthroplasties. *Clin Orthop Relat Res.* 2006;446:193-200.
42. Keating EM, Ritter MA, Harty LD, et al. Manipulation after total knee arthroplasty. *J Bone Joint Surg Am.* 2007;89:282-286.
43. Yercan HS, Sugun TS, Bussiere C, Ait Si Selmi T, Davies A, Neyret P. Stiffness after total knee arthroplasty: prevalence, management and outcomes. *Knee.* 2006;13:111-117.
44. Fox JL, Poss R. The role of manipulation following total knee replacement. *J Bone Joint Surg Am.* 1981;63:357-362.
45. Jerosch J, Aldawoudy AM. Arthroscopic treatment of patients with moderate arthrofibrosis after total knee replacement. *Knee Surg Sports Traumatol Arthrosc.* 2007;15:71-77.
46. Williams RJ 3rd, Westrich GH, Siegel J, Windsor RE. Arthroscopic release of the posterior cruciate ligament for stiff total knee arthroplasty. *Clin Orthop Relat Res.* 1996;331:185-191.
47. Maloney WJ. The stiff total knee arthroplasty: evaluation and management. *J Arthroplasty.* 2002;17(4 Suppl 1):71-73.
48. Tew M, Waugh W. Tibiofemoral alignment and the results of knee replacement. *J Bone Joint Surg Br.* 1985;67:551-556.
49. Ritter MA, Faris PM, Keating EM, Meding JB. Postoperative alignment of total knee replacement. its effect on survival. *Clin Orthop Relat Res.* 1994;299:153-156.

50. Wasielewski RC, Galante JO, Leighty R, et al. Wear patterns on retrieved polyethylene inserts and their relationship to technical considerations during total knee arthroplasty. *Clin Orthop Relat Res.* 1994;299:31.
51. Stulberg SD, Loan P, Sarin V. Computer-assisted navigation in total knee replacement: results of an initial experience in thirty-five patients. *J Bone Joint Surg Am.* 2002;84(A Suppl 2):90.
52. Chauhan SK, Scott RG, Breidahl W, Beaver RJ. Computer-assisted knee arthroplasty versus a conventional jig-based technique: a randomised, prospective trial. *J Bone Joint Surg Br.* 2004;86:372-377.
53. Haaker RG, Stockheim M, Kamp M, Proff G, Breitenfelder J, Ottersbach A. Computer-assisted navigation increases precision of component placement in total knee arthroplasty. *Clin Orthop Relat Res.* 2005;433:152-159.
54. Larson CM, Lachiewicz PF. Patellofemoral complications with the Insall-Burstein II posterior-stabilized total knee arthroplasty. *J Arthroplasty.* 1999;14(3):288-292.
55. Scuderi GR, Insall JN, Scott NW. Patellofemoral pain after total knee arthroplasty. *J Am Acad Orthop Surg.* 1994;2:239-246.
56. Bindelglass DF, Cohen JL, Dorr LD. Patellar tilt and subluxation in total knee arthroplasty: relationship to pain, fixation, and design. *Clin Orthop.* 1993;286:103-109.
57. Berger RA, Rubash HE, Seel MJ, Thompson WH, Crossett LS. Determining the rotational alignment of the femoral component in total knee arthroplasty using the epicondylar axis. *Clin Orthop.* 1993;286:40-47.
58. Petersilge WJ, Oishi CS, Kaufman KR, Irby SE, Colwell CW Jr. The effect of trochlear design on patellofemoral shear and compressive forces in total knee arthroplasty. *Clin Orthop.* 1994;309:124-130.
59. Yoshii I, Whiteside LA, Anouchi YS. The effect of patellar button placement and femoral component design on patellar tracking in total knee arthroplasty. *Clin Orthop.* 1992;275:211-219.
60. Kajino A, Yoshino S, Kameyama S, Kohda M, Nagashima S. Comparison of the results of bilateral total knee arthroplasty with and without patellar replacement for rheumatoid arthritis: a follow-up note. *J Bone Joint Surg Am.* 1997;79:570-574.
61. Barrack RL, Wolfe MW, Waldman DA, Milicic M, Bertot AJ, Myers L. Resurfacing of the patella in total knee arthroplasty: a prospective, randomized, double-blind study. *J Bone Joint Surg Am.* 1997;79:1121-1131.
62. Scuderi GR, Windsor RE, Insall JN. Observations on patellar height after proximal tibial osteotomy. *J Bone Joint Surg Am.* 1989;71:245-248.
63. Beight JL, Yao B, Hozack WJ, Hearn SL, Booth RE Jr. The patellar "clunk" syndrome after posterior stabilized total knee arthroplasty. *Clin Orthop.* 1994;299:139-142.
64. Figgie HE 3rd, Goldberg VM, Heiple KG, Moller HS 3rd, Gordon NH. The influence of tibial patellofemoral location on function of the knee in patients with the posterior stabilized condylar knee prosthesis. *J Bone Joint Surg Am.* 1986;68:1035-1040.
65. Singerman R, Heiple KG, Davy DT, Goldberg VM. Effect of tibial component position on patellar strain following total knee arthroplasty. *J Arthroplasty.* 1995;10:651-656.
66. Rhoads DD, Noble PC, Reuben JD, Tullos HS. The effect of femoral component position on the kinematics of total knee arthroplasty. *Clin Orthop.* 1993;286:122-129.
67. Miller MC, Berger RA, Petrella AJ, Karmas A, Rubash HE. Optimizing femoral component rotation in total knee arthroplasty. *Clin Orthop.* 2001;382:38-45.
68. Eckhoff DG, Metzger RG, Vandewalle MV. Malrotation associated with implant alignment technique in total knee arthroplasty. *Clin Orthop.* 1995;321:28-31.
69. Brick GW, Scott RD. The patellofemoral component of total knee arthroplasty. *Clin Orthop.* 1988;231:163-178.
70. Ortiguera CJ, Berry DJ. Patellar fracture after total knee arthroplasty. *J Bone Joint Surg Am.* 2002;84:532-540.
71. Holtby RM, Grosso P. Osteonecrosis and resorption of the patella after total knee replacement: a case report. *Clin Orthop.* 1996;328:155-158.
72. Kayler DE, Lyttle D. Surgical interruption of patellar blood supply by total knee arthroplasty. *Clin Orthop.* 1988;229:221-227.
73. Chen F, Mont MA, Bachner RS. Management of ipsilateral supracondylar femur fractures following total knee arthroplasty. *J Arthroplasty.* 1994;9:521-526.
74. Scott RD. Anterior femoral notching and ipsilateral supracondylar femur fracture in total knee arthroplasty. *J Arthroplasty.* 1988;3:381.
75. Lesh ML, Schneider DJ, Pellegrini VD. Biomechanical evaluation of the effects of anterior cortical notching of the femur in total knee arthroplasty. *Orthop Trans.* 1998;22:122.
76. Culp RW, Schmidt RG, Hanks G, Mak A, Esterhai JL Jr, Heppenstall RB. Supracondylar fracture of the femur following prosthetic knee arthroplasty. *Clin Orthop.* 1987;222:212-222.
77. Figgie MP, Goldberg VM, Figgie HE 3d, Sobel M. The results of treatment of supracondylar fracture above total knee arthroplasty. *J Arthroplasty.* 1990;5:267-276.
78. Zehntner MK, Ganz R. Internal fixation of supracondylar fractures after condylar total knee arthroplasty. *Clin Orthop.* 1993;293:219-224.
79. Fehring TK, Valadie AL. Knee instability after total knee arthroplasty. *Clin Orthop.* 1994;299:157-162.
80. Waslewski GL, Marson BM, Benjamin JB. Early, incapacitating instability of posterior cruciate ligament-retaining total knee arthroplasty. *J Arthroplasty.* 1998;13:763-767.
81. Pagnano MW, Hanssen AD, Lewallen DG, et al. Flexion instability after primary posterior cruciate retaining total knee arthroplasty. *Clin Orthop.* 1998;356:39.
82. Lombardi AV Jr, Mallory TH, Vaughn BK, et al. Dislocation following primary posterior-stabilized total knee arthroplasty. *J Arthroplasty.* 1993;8:633-639.

# 17

# Patella Fracture Following Total Knee Arthroplasty

*Alvin Ong, MD*

Patella fractures following TKA occur infrequently. The reported prevalence has ranged from 0.2% to 21%.[1] Patella fractures can occur without resurfacing the patella but are more common if resurfacing has been performed.[2] Most are asymptomatic and cause little functional limitation. The causes of patella fracture include trauma, implant malalignment, obesity, over- or under-resection, high activity level, and increased range of motion, all of which place excessive stress on the patella, leading to fatigue, failure, and fracture. The blood supply to the patella can be compromised during lateral retinacular release, resection of the fat pad, aggressive stripping of soft tissue around the patella bone, and use of a dull saw blade leading to heat necrosis of the patella bone. This can lead to avascular necrosis and subsequent fracture and disintegration of the patella. Fractures occur more frequently in resurfaced patella and in revision surgery. In addition, there is a higher frequency in males than in females. Most patella fractures can be treated nonoperatively. Surgical management is reserved for symptomatic patients with functional impairment.

## Classification

Classification of patella fractures help guide the surgeon to the optimal treatment. The Mayo Clinic classification[1] is the most popular and is well accepted. In this classification system, patella fractures are grouped by the stability of the patella implant and the integrity of the extensor mechanism. Fractures are divided into 3 types with the third type further divided into 2 subtypes. Type I patella fractures consist of a stable patella implant and an intact extensor mechanism. Type II patella fractures have associated disruption of the extensor mechanism. The patella implant remains well fixed. Type III patella fractures consist of a loose patella component with an intact extensor mechanism. Type IIIa is associated with good bone stock and Type IIIb is associated with poor bone stock (<10 mm in thickness or marked comminution).

## Clinical Findings

Fractures of the patella can present with pain and swelling. If the extensor mechanism is intact, the patient may exhibit active extension with little or no lag. There may be reported weakness that may be subclinical or manifest as occasional giving way or difficulty with stair climbing. The presentation is often of effusion with anterior knee pain, although some patients may be asymptomatic and diagnosis is made only on reviewing routine radiographs. Most will complain of discomfort or difficulty with rising from a seated position or ascending or descending stairs. There is often a history of injury, such as a fall or impaction injury, but on occasion, no injury is reported. Physical examination often reveals tenderness over the patella. If there is fracture displacement, a palpable defect may be appreciated. There is typically a positive grind and compression test. Range of motion should be evaluated both passively and actively. In Type II fractures, appreciable extensor weakness or extensor lag is often noted. Flexion is usually not affected except when there is history of acute injury with associated tense



Parvizi J, Klatt B.
*Essentials in Total Knee Arthroplasty* (pp 141-150).

effusion or hemarthrosis. Aspiration is rarely needed and is done in patients with tense effusion or hemarthrosis to relieve pressure and alleviate pain.

## Radiographic Findings

Standard radiographs should be part of the evaluation process. The lateral and sunrise or merchant views are especially helpful in diagnosis and assessment of fractured patellae. The anterior-posterior (AP) view is less helpful because the femoral implant typically obscures the patella. However, fractures with significant displacement can often be seen in this view. The sunrise or merchant view is helpful in determining patella instability, such as patella tilt or frank subluxation and dislocation. Computed tomography (CT) scans can be helpful in diagnosing malrotation of the femoral and tibial implant but are of little value in determining the management of the patella fracture.

## Treatment

### Type I

Type I fractures are defined as patella fractures associated with stable patella implant and intact extensor mechanism. This type of fracture is best treated nonoperatively. They are frequently asymptomatic, and patients present with no functional limitations. Most are diagnosed on routine follow-up radiographs. Asymptomatic patients can be treated with observation. Patients who have swelling and pain can be treated with 4 to 6 weeks of immobilization followed by resumption of activities as tolerated. According to Ortiguera and Berry,[1] the majority of Type I fractures were asymptomatic at last follow-up with only one patient requiring surgical intervention. In their series, they reported no pain, patella or extensor mechanism instability, or weakness in 82% of patients. However, a small number of patients did have extensor lag and pain. One patient became sufficiently symptomatic to warrant surgical intervention. If surgery becomes necessary in a Type I fracture, treatment involves excision of a marginal fragment/nonunion with soft tissue repair of the extensor mechanism to the remaining patella. This is rarely needed.

### Type II

Type II fractures are defined as patella fractures associated with disruption of the extensor mechanism. The patella implant remains well fixed. The patient usually reports a fall or injury. There is full or partial loss of active extension with associated swelling and pain. Radiographs typically reveal polar fractures of the patella (ie, fractures at the superior or inferior periphery of the patella). The majority of the patella mass is usually preserved. Type II fractures are uncommon. Rand[3] reported on 12 Type II fractures representing only 15% of all patella fractures in his series. Most will require open reduction and internal fixation or suture repair. Fixation can consist of screw or wire fixation if the polar fragment is significant in size. In those fractures where the polar fracture fragment is too small to receive fixation hardware, excision of the fragment (partial patellectomy) can be performed with advancement of the tendon onto bone. The latter can be treated as isolated patella tendon avulsion or patella tendon ruptures after the polar fragment has been excised. According to Ortiguera and Berry,[1] 6 of 12 Type II fractures were treated with open reduction and internal fixation and 5 of 12 fractures were treated with partial patellectomy and tendon advancement. No standard regimen for postoperative rehabilitation is defined for these injuries. Many treat them as patellar tendon tears, but clearly they have a poorer outcome. Ortiguera and Berry reported a 50% complication rate.[1] Five of 12 had a reoperation, and 7 of 12 had pain or patella/extensor mechanism instability or weakness. Resolution of pain and the return to full functional capacity was seen in only a few of the patients. Most complain of some pain and functional limitation at last follow-up.

To increase the success rate of primary repair, the contemporary technique often requires supplemental reconstruction using allograft tendon in addition to primary repair and advancement of the tendon rupture. Crossett et al[4] reported on the use of fresh frozen Achilles tendon allograft in the reconstruction of patella tendon rupture. They had a series of 9 patients. There were 5 patients who ruptured their patella tendon following primary total knee replacement and 4 patients who ruptured their patella tendon following revision knee replacement. The technique they used is similar to the one described next (see Selected Surgical Technique on p. 143). The average extensor lag after reconstruction was 3 degrees, while the average flexion was 107 degrees. There were 2 graft failures that were successfully repaired. Although the patella migrated proximally an average of 18 mm, the authors reported on affect on extensor function. They concluded that the use of Achilles tendon allograft is reliable in the reconstruction of patella tendon ruptures following total knee replacement. Burnett et al[5] recommended proper tensioning of the allograft tendon to prevent extensor lag postoperatively. They recommend that the graft be initially tensioned tight in extension.

## Type III

Type III fractures are defined as patella fractures associated with a loose patella implant. Type III fractures are subdivided into those with good bone stock (Type IIIa) and those with poor bone stock (Type IIIb). Poor bone stock was defined as patella bone thickness less than 10 mm or severe comminution, making it unacceptable for internal fixation or another resurfacing procedure. Rand[3] reported on 38 Type III fractures in which 32 fractures were treated surgically. He reported complications in 18 knees and reoperation in 16 knees. He concluded that Type III fractures should be treated nonoperatively. Ortiguera and Berry reported on 28 Type III patella fractures.[1] Twelve of the 28 had reasonable bone stock (Type IIIa); 4 were treated with observation and the other 8 were treated operatively. Five of 8 were treated with patella component resection and internal fixation of the fracture. There were an unacceptable number of complications and reoperations in the surgically managed group. Of those patients that were the treated with observation, 2 remained symptomatic at latest follow-up.

Sixteen of the 28 Type III fractures had poor bone stock (Type IIIb). Four were treated with observation and 12 were treated surgically. Only 1 of the 4 knees treated nonoperatively had pain at latest follow-up. Seven of the 12 surgically managed knees had pain and patella instability or weakness at latest follow-up. The authors recommend that Type IIIa patella fractures should be managed with revision of the patella component or resection of the patella component with patelloplasty. For Type IIIb fractures, removal of the patella implant with partial or complete patellectomy was recommended.

A porous Tantalum metal patella component (Zimmer, Warsaw, IN) has recently been developed for the treatment of substantial patella bone loss.[6] Although this component has been developed for use with marked patella bone loss and not necessarily for patella fractures, it offers a viable option for the Type IIIb patella fractures where bone stock prevents the use of a standard patella component. We have successfully treated 11 Type IIIb fractures with the use of a porous Tantalum metal patella component. The majority of the patients treated with this technique reported pain relief, resolution of effusion, and improved functional ability. Two failures were seen at latest follow-up. The first failure was due to superior pole fracture of the remnant patella shell. Nelson et al have reported similar complications.[6] They surmise that polar fractures occur because of fatigue failure due to weakness of the thin cortical shell seen in these patients, as well as the stress riser created by the edge of the metal shell on the comprised bone. The second failure was due to nonhealing, as the Tantalum metal implant failed to grow into the bone. This technique requires adequate blood supply to be present for healing to occur and, therefore, is highly patient dependent. We recommend this treatment as an alternative to partial or complete patellectomy in the treatment of the Type IIIb patella fracture.

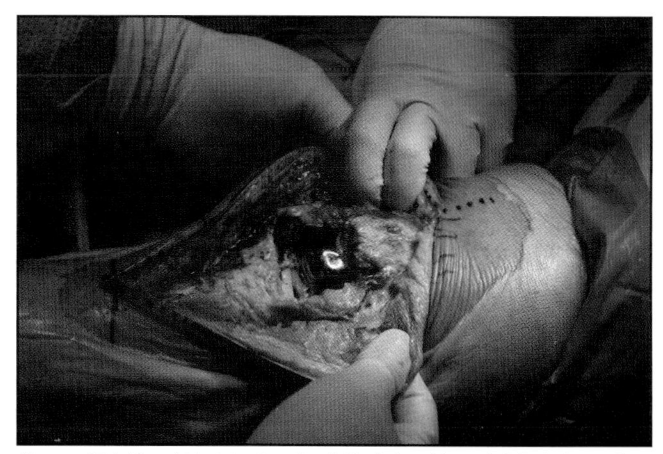

**Figure 17-1.** The old incision is utilized. Medial and lateral, full-thickness flaps are elevated for exposure.

# Selected Surgical Technique

## Type II

The use of Achilles tendon allograft in the reconstruction of Type II patella fracture is a reliable treatment option for this devastating problem. It serves as an excellent adjunct to primary advancement of the native tendon into the patella bone after resection of the polar boney fragment.

The old incision is always used if possible. Medial and lateral full-thickness flaps are elevated for exposure (Figure 17-1). Primary repair of the extensor mechanism is attempted first after excision of the polar fragment, with the creation of 2 parallel tunnels through the patellar bone (Figure 17-2). This can be achieved with a 2- or 3-mm drill bit. A heavy #5 nonabsorbable suture (FiberWire) is passed through the tunnels and sutured to the patella tendon stump (Figure 17-3). If possible, the suture is weaved through native tendon using a Krawkow technique. The suture is tensioned in full extension as tight as possible and tied over a bone bridge at the superior patella pole (Figure 17- 4). The repair is augmented with the use of #1 Vicryl in an interrupted figure-of-eight technique (Figure 17-5). The proximal part of the tibia is prepared for insertion of the calcaneal bone block. A small saw is used to make a rectangular/trapezoidal cavity 2.5-cm long by 1.5-cm wide by

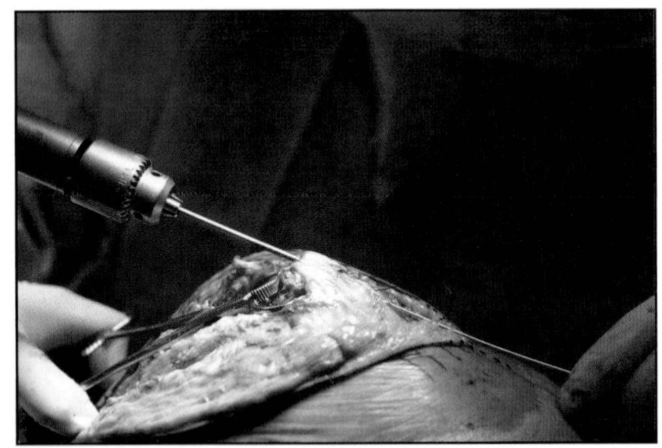

**Figure 17-2.** Primary tendor repair and advancement is attempted after excision of polar fragment. Parallel drill holes are recreated into the patella for suture passage.

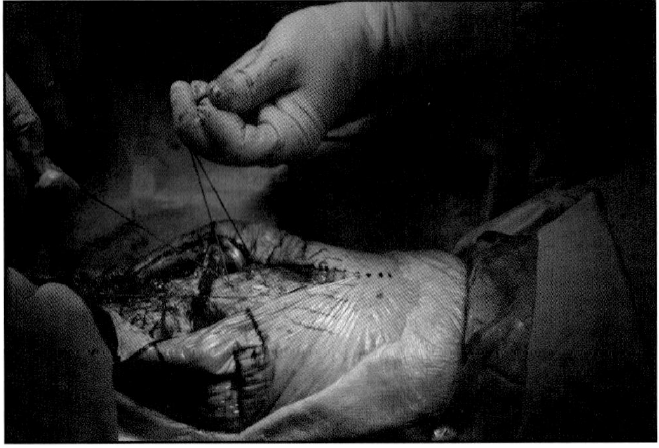

**Figure 17-3.** Primary repair is perfomed with non-absorbable suture. Krackow technique is used on the patella tendon stump.

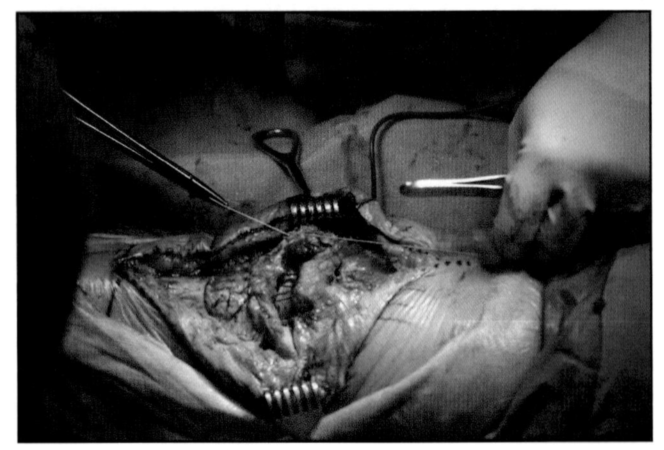

**Figure 17-4.** The repair is tensioned in full-extension as tight as possible and tied over a bone bridge at the superior patella pole.

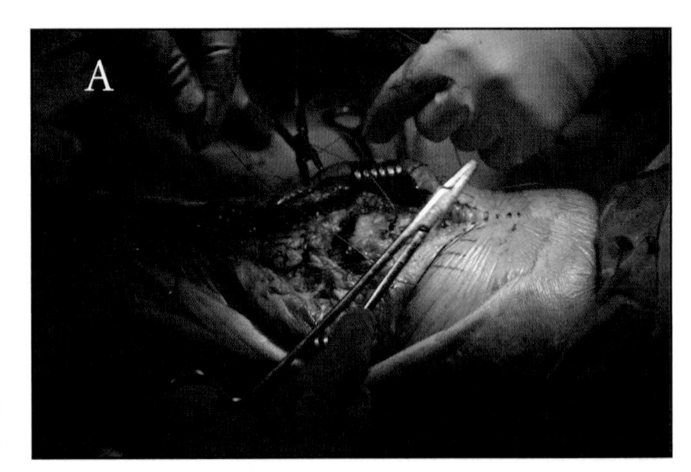



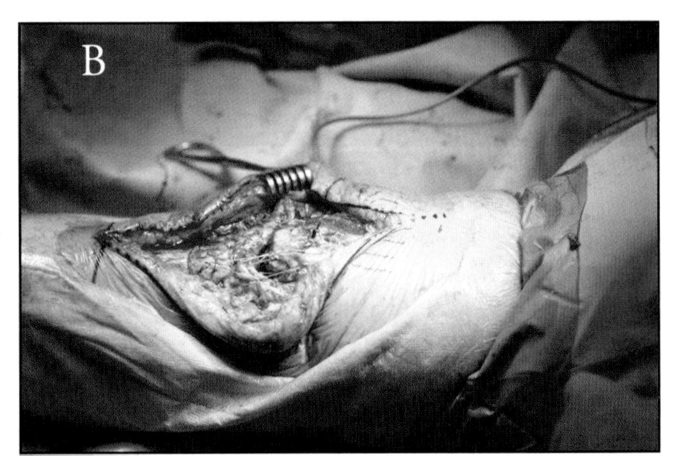



**Figure 17-5.** The repair is augmented with the use of #1 Vicryl in an interrupted figure of eight technique.

1-cm deep in the proximal part of the tibia slightly distal and medial to the original insertion site of the patellar tendon. An osteotome is used to lift out the unwanted bone (Figure 17-6). The prepared tibia is shown in Figure 17-7. The Achilles tendon allograft is then prepared. The calcaneal bone block is cut to match the created rectangular/trapezoidal space in the proximal tibia (Figure 17-8). A "key stone" is created to maximize friction fit and boney contact (Figure 17-9). The bone block is gently impacted into the proximal tibia (Figure 17-10). Two 3.5-mm screws are used. The screws are angled in different planes to avoid the tibial component and lessen the possibility of stress riser formation (Figure 17-11). The most proximal part of the Achilles tendon allograft is cut to obtain a rectangular patch (Figure 17-12). The rectangular patch is used to augment the attempted primary repair and is sutured in place with #1 Vicryl in an interrupted fashion (Figure 17-13). The Achilles tendon is then draped over the anterior tibia and patella. The knee should be positioned in full extension.

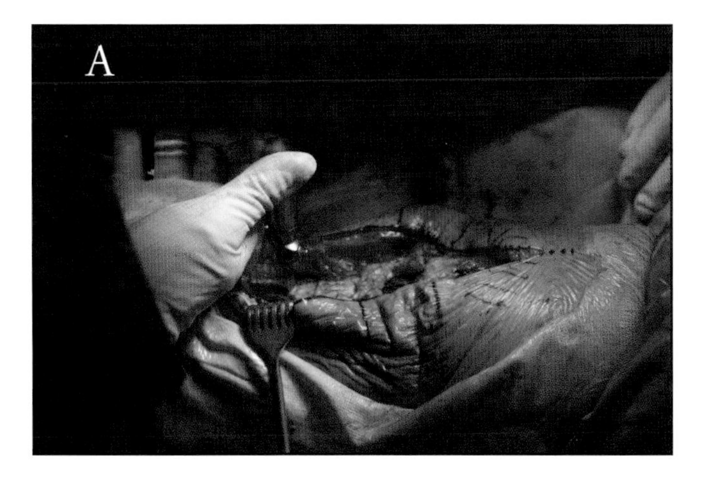


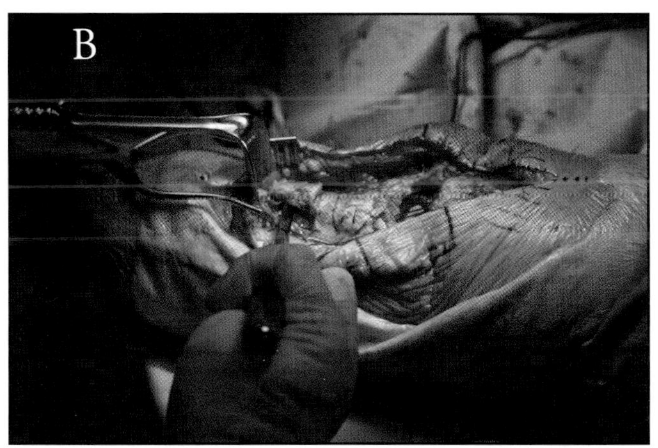


**Figure 17-6.** (A) The proximal part of the tibia is prepared for insertion of the calcaneal bone block. A small saw is used to make a rectangular/trapezoidal cavity. (B) Osteotome is used to lift out the unwanted bone.

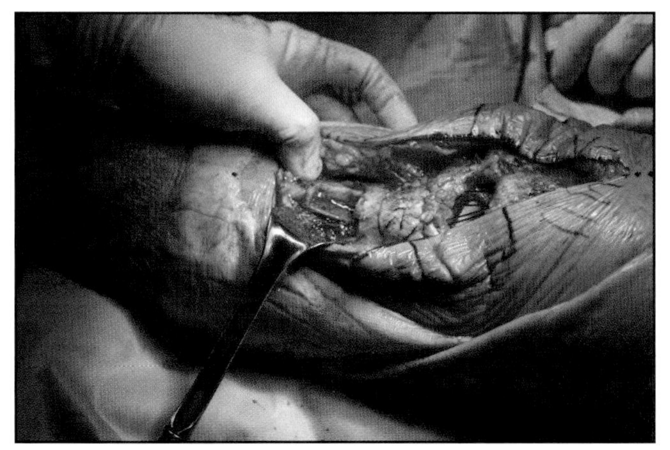

**Figure 17-7.** Prepared proximal tibia cancellous bed.

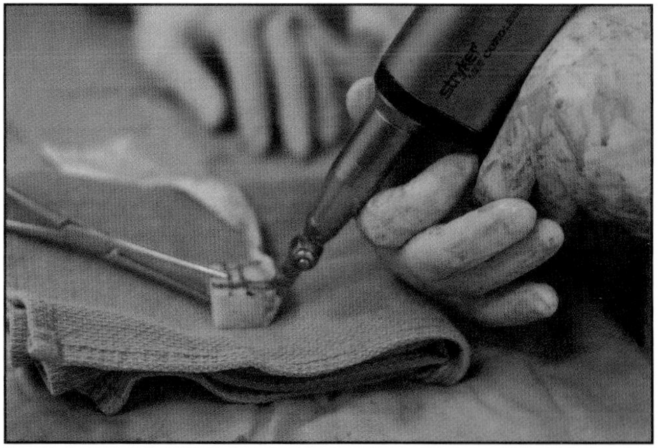

**Figure 17-8.** The calcaneal bone block is cut to match the created rectangular/trapezoidal space in the proximal tibia.

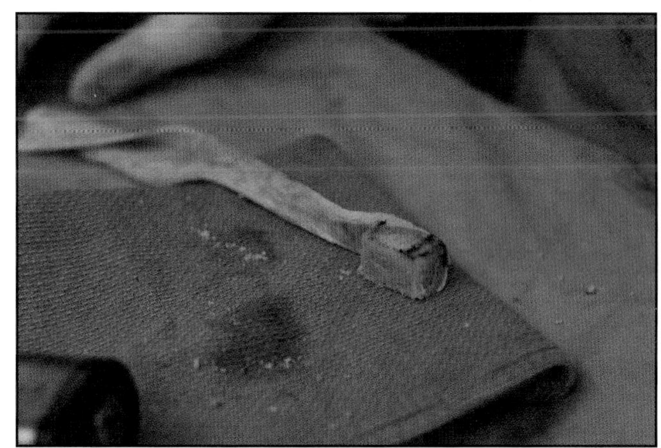

**Figure 17-9.** A "key stone" is created to maximize friction fit and boney contact.

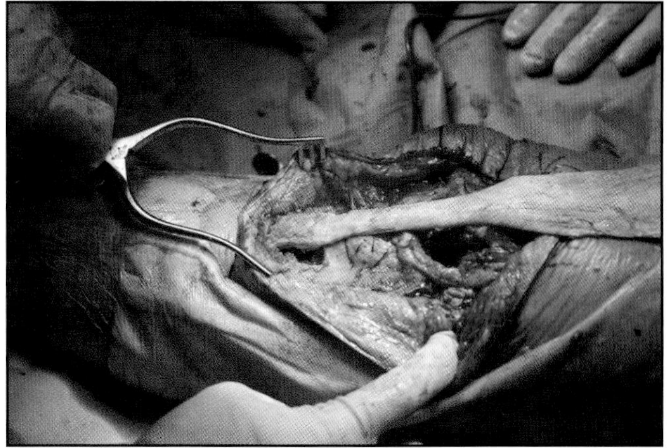

**Figure 17-10.** The bone block is gently impacted into the proximal tibial.

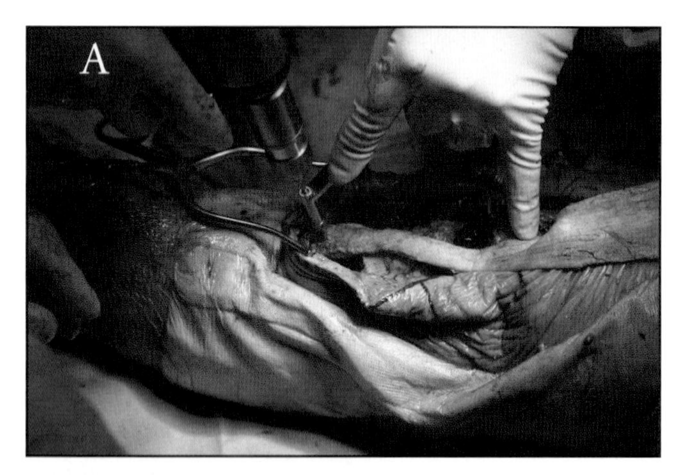


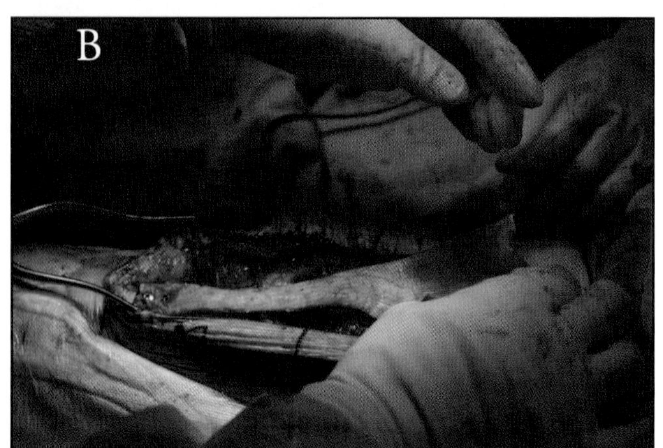


**Figure 17-11.** Two 3.5-mm screws are used. The screws are angled in different planes to avoid the tibial component and lessen the possibility of stress riser formation.

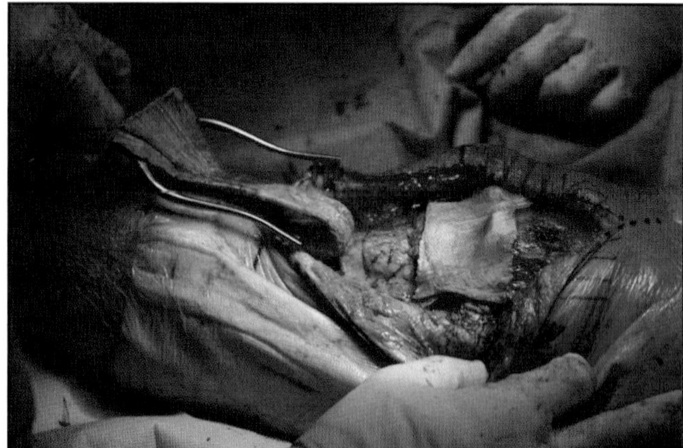

**Figure 17-12.** The most proximal part of the achilles tendon allograft is cut to obtained a rectangular patch.

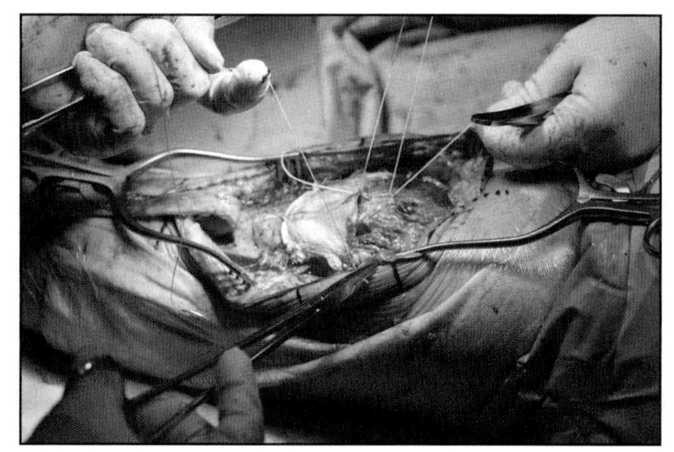

**Figure 17-13.** The rectangular patch is used to augment the primary repair, and is sutured in place with #1 Vicryl, in an interupted fashion.

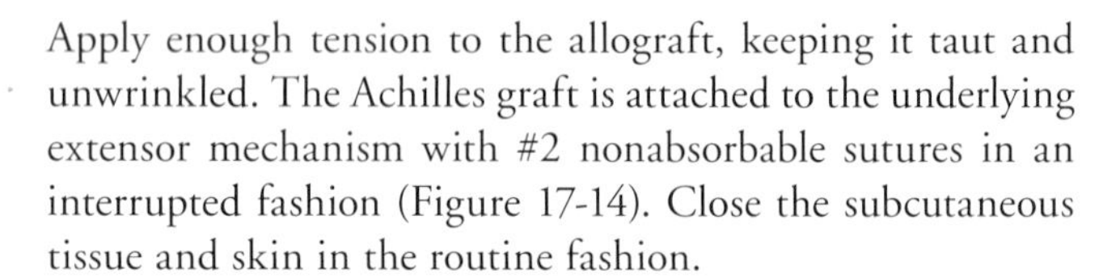

Apply enough tension to the allograft, keeping it taut and unwrinkled. The Achilles graft is attached to the underlying extensor mechanism with #2 nonabsorbable sutures in an interrupted fashion (Figure 17-14). Close the subcutaneous tissue and skin in the routine fashion.

### Postoperative Management

Immobilization in full extension used a hinged-knee brace is recommended for 3 weeks. Touch-down weight bearing is recommended for the first 3 weeks and then partial weight bearing for an additional 3 weeks. Gradual range of motion is begun at 3 weeks postoperatively. The hinged-knee brace is unlocked with the extension stop initially set at 60 degrees. Gradual increase in flexion is allowed over the following 3 weeks until passive flexion is greater than 90 degrees. Most patients will regain preinjury flexion without the need for manipulation under anesthesia.

## *Type IIIb*

Prepare and drape the operative leg with the same technique used for a primary total knee replacement, with the same considerations for anesthesia. The procedure is done under tourniquet to improve visualization. Approach the knee through the pre-existing surgical scar. Skin flaps can be elevated for exposure but should be minimized if possible to decrease the occurrence of wound necrosis. The arthrotomy is performed through a medial parapatellar approach (Figure 17-15). The joint is exposed and evacuated of fluid and/or blood. A scar excision is performed to free-up the extensor mechanism. Scar is excised around the patella to expose the loose patella implant and patella fracture (Figure 17-16). Débridement of the lateral gutter is often necessary to mobilize the patella. A lateral release may be necessary to evert the patella, but lateral release after fracture should be avoided because this can compromise the vascularity to

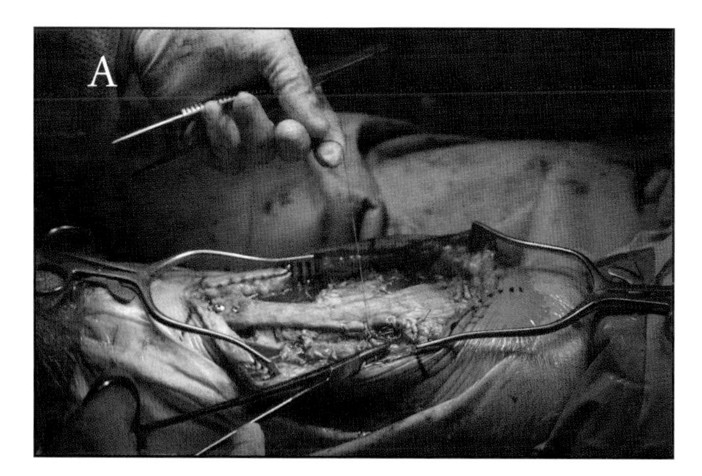


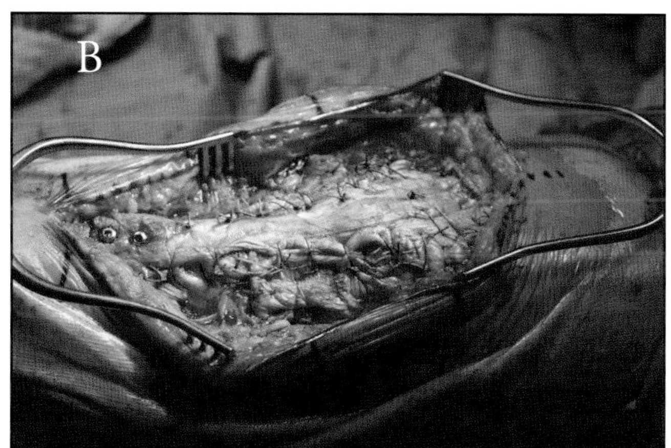


**Figure 17-14.** The Achilles graft is attached to the the underlying extensor mechanism with number-2 nonabsorbable sutures, in an interrupted fashion.

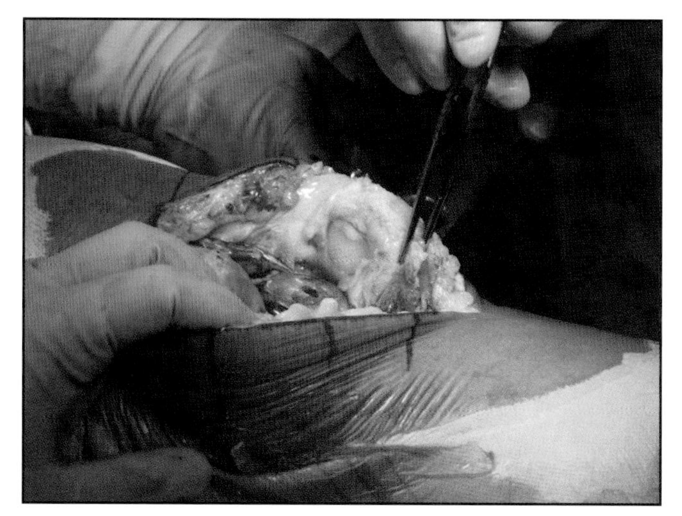

**Figure 17-15.** Joint is exposed through the medial parapatellar arthrotomy.

the remainder of the patella and compromise healing. The knee should be in extension when the patella is everted to minimize stress on the fracture and the patella tendon

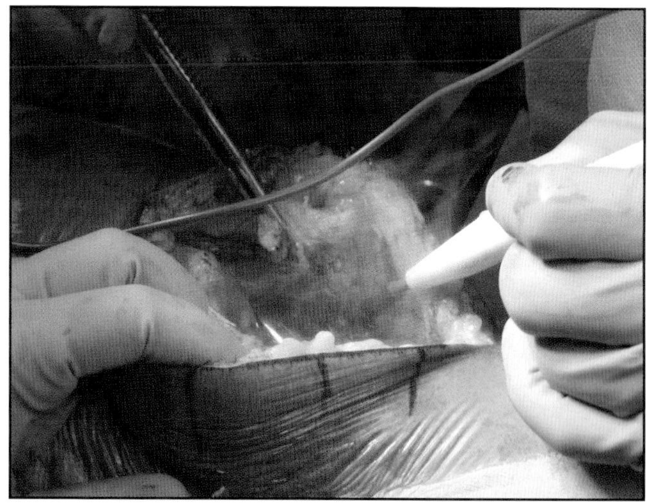

**Figure 17-16.** The scar is excised around the patella for exposure.

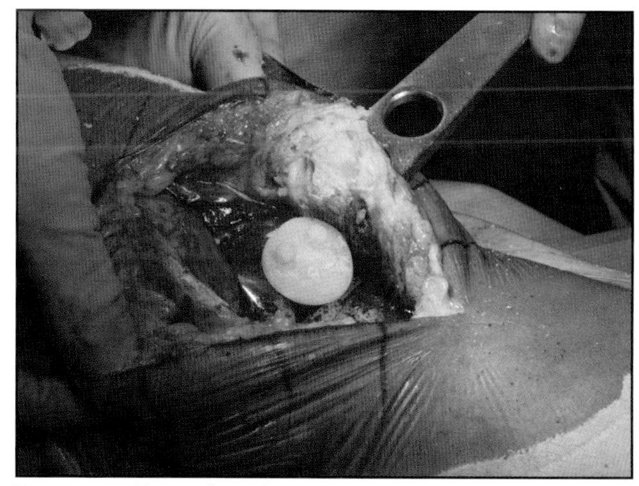

**Figure 17-17.** The patella implant is removed with cement and devitalized bone.

attachment. The patella component is removed (Figure 17-17). Care must be taken to preserve native bone and prevent further displacement of the fracture fragments. Any loose fragments of cement, polyethylene, or necrotic bone are excised. Irrigate the joint copiously with pulsatile lavage. Débride the patella fragments of fibrous scar and devitalized bone (Figure 17-18).

The patella is then prepared to accept the Tantalum metal component. First, determine the most appropriate size using available templates. Once the size is determined, the patella remnant is prepared using special patella hemispherical reamers (Figure 17-19). The reamers are intended to débride the bone to incite bleeding and shape the bed for the Tantalum metal component for maximum bone-to-implant contact. The implant is then placed within the prepared bony bed. Use the existing patella shell of bone

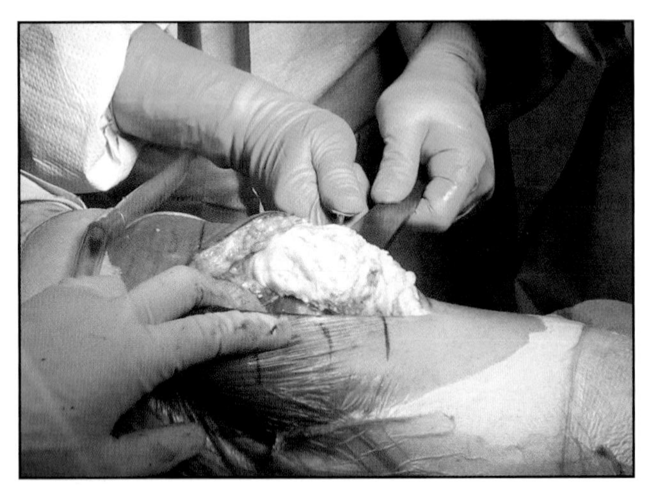

**Figure 17-18.** Débride the patella fragments of fibrous scar and devitalized bone.

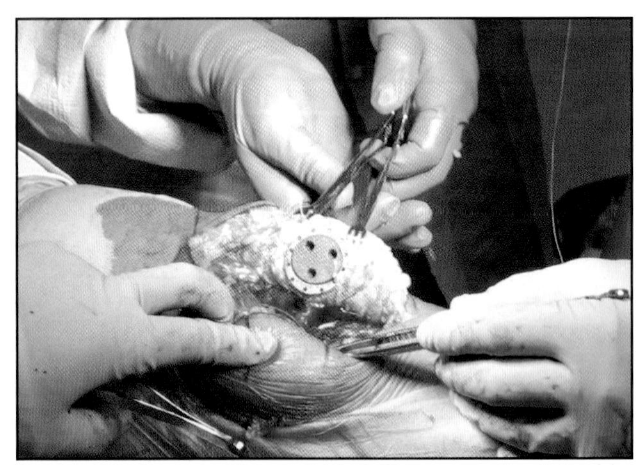

**Figure 17-20.** Use the existing patella shell of bone to assess position of the augment. Place the inferior pole of the patella augment near the joint line.

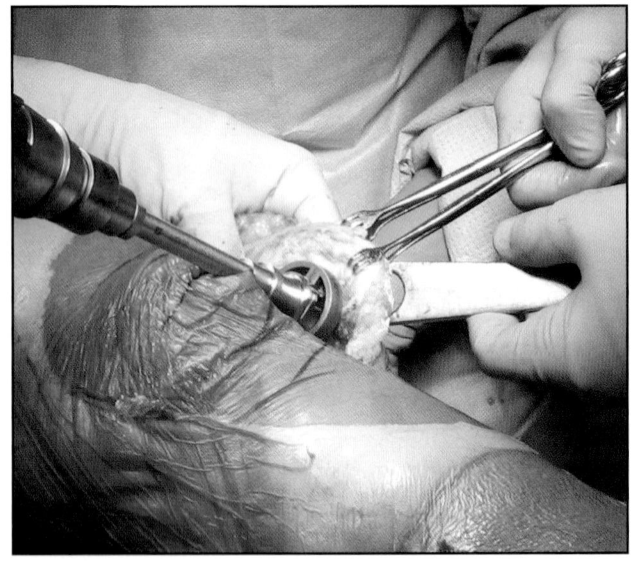

**Figure 17-19.** Once the size is determined, the patella remnant is prepared using special patella hemispherical reamers.

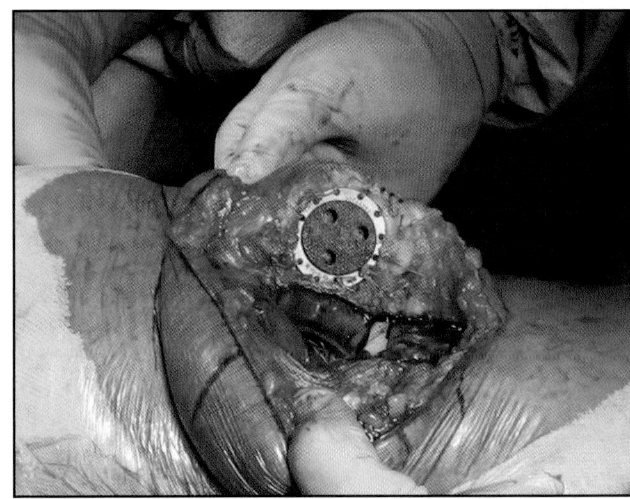

**Figure 17-21.** The trabecular implant is fixed to the remaining bone and soft tissue using nonabsorbable sutures through the peripheral holes on the trabecular implant.

to assess position of the augment. Place the inferior pole of the patella augment near the joint line (Figure 17-20). The Tantalum metal implant is fixed to the remaining bone and soft tissue using nonabsorbable sutures through the peripheral holes on the implant (Figure 17-21). We prefer to use #1 FiberWire (Arthrex, Naples, FL). The sutures can be passed through bone with the aid of 1.6- or 2.0-mm drill and available suture passers. Incorporation of the fragments into the suture construct is preferred. The Tantalum metal implant is used as a scaffolding to fix the fragments together. The final construct should be stable and have intimate contact with the underlying bony fragments. A standard 3-peg polyethylene patella component is then cemented into the Tantalum metal augment (Figure 17-22). Normal patella tracking is key to preventing undue stress on the construct. Patella tracking can be optimized with the use of lateral release.

Repair of the medial retinaculum is performed with interrupted sutures using #1 Vicryl. Close the subcutaneous tissue and skin in the routine fashion. Preoperative and postoperative radiographs are compared in Figure 17-23.

## Postoperative Management

Immobilization in full extension utilizing a hinged-knee brace is recommended for 3 weeks. Touch-down weight bearing is recommended for the first 3 weeks and then partial weight-bearing for an additional 3 weeks. Gradual

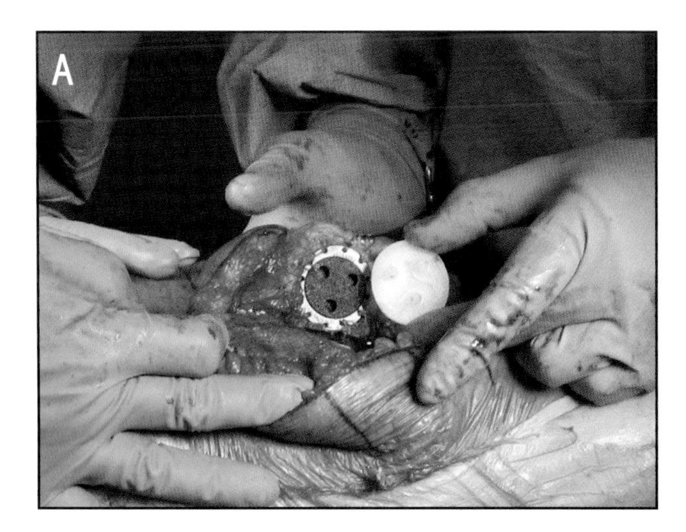


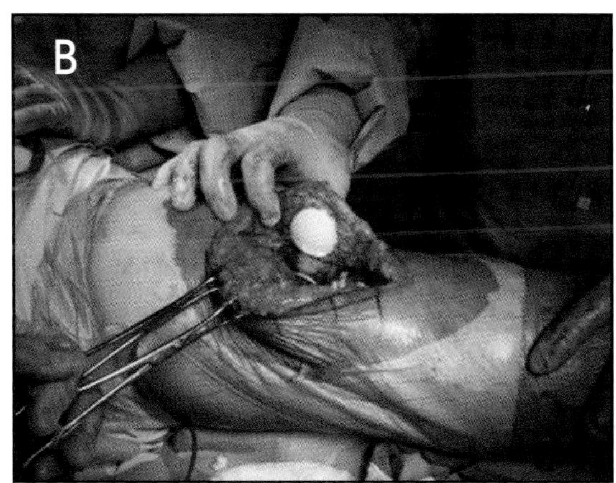


**Figure 17-22.** (A) A standard 3-peg polyethylene patella component is used. (B) The patella is cemented into place.

range of motion is begun at 3 weeks postoperative. The hinged-knee brace is unlocked with the extension stop initially set at 60 degrees. Gradual increase in flexion is allowed over the following 3 weeks until passive flexion is greater than 90 degrees. Most patients will regain pre-injury flexion without the need for manipulation under anesthesia.

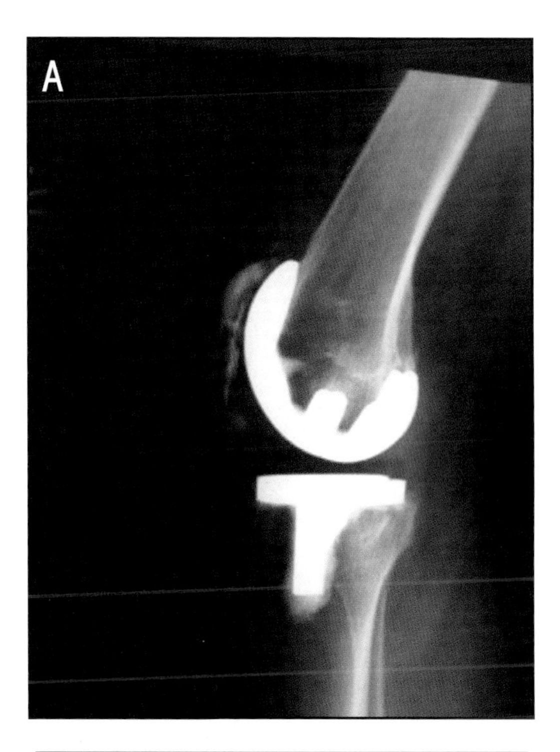


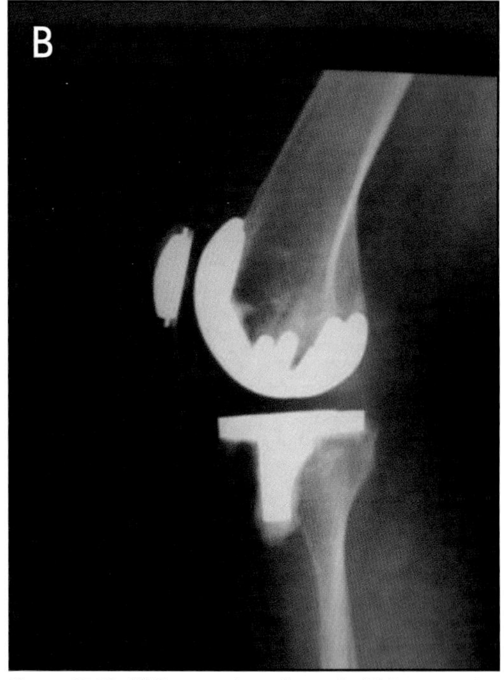


**Figure 17-23.** (A) Preoperative radiograph. (B) Postoperative radiograph.

## References


1. Ortiguera C, Berry D. Patella fracture after TKA. *J Bone Joint Surg Am*. 2002;84:532-540.
2. Zehntner M, Ganz R. Internal fixation of supracondylar fractures total knee arthroplasty. *CORR*. 1999;293:219-224.
3. Rand R. Extensor mechanism complications following TKA. *J Bone Joint Surg Am*. 2004;2062-2069.
4. Crossett L, Sinha R, Sechriest F, Rubash H. Reconstruction of a ruptured patellar tendon with Achilles tendon allograft following total knee arthroplasty. *J Bone Joint Surg Am*. 2002;84:1354-1361.
5. Burnett S, Berger R, Paprosky W, Della Valle C, Jacobs J, Rosenberg A. Extensor mechanism allograft reconstruction after total knee arthroplasty: a comparison of two technique. *J Bone Joint Surg Am*. 2004;86:2694-2699.
6. Nelson C, Lonner J, Lahiji A, Kim J, Lotke P. Use of a trabecular metal patella for marked patella bone loss during revision total knee arthroplasty. *J Arthroplasty*. 2003;18:37-41.

# 18

# Periprosthetic Fractures in Total Knee Arthroplasty

*Garen Daxton Steele, MD and Brian A. Klatt, MD*

Periprosthetic fractures in total knee arthroplasty (TKA) are defined as those fractures that occur within 15 cm of the knee replacement.[1] The incidence of the injuries is estimated to be around 0.3% to 2.5%.[1-8] As the population ages and as more knee replacements are done, the number of periprosthetic fractures continues to rise. Supracondylar femur fractures comprise the majority of these fractures, but the surgeon will also encounter tibia and patella fractures. This chapter will address periprosthetic TKA femur and tibia fractures. Periprosthetic TKA fractures of the patella are discussed in Chapter 16.

Several key factors will determine how these fractures are managed.

- Is the implant well-fixed or loose?
- Is the fracture displaced or nondisplaced?
- Is there adequate bone attached to the implant to allow fixation?

The timing of periprosthetic fractures will also impact the management. Iatrogenic intraoperative fractures are treated differently than postoperative fractures, which can occur decades beyond the implantation.

Management strategies employ a variety of modalities, including nonoperative, internal fixation, and revision. Choosing the correct management strategy requires a thorough patient evaluation and a complete understanding of the treatment armamentarium. The expertise required is that of a surgeon with a good grasp of joint arthroplasty techniques and with an understanding of advanced fracture management techniques. Periprosthetic fractures in the setting of TKA can be a challenge to treat.

## Risk Factors

Any condition that increases the likelihood of osteopenia will put patients more at risk for periprosthetic TKA fractures. Rheumatoid arthritis, chronic steroid use, advancing age, neurological disorders, and female gender are some of the conditions known to be associated with increased risk.[9] Previous revision arthroplasty adds risk due to the relative osteopenia combined with the added stress distribution from the constraint of the components.

Femoral notching is one of the more commonly discussed risk factors for supracondylar fractures (Figure 18-1). Numerous biomechanical studies show the reduction in torsional strength of the bone.[10,11] Clinical evaluation of the effects of notching on supracondylar femur fractures suggests that the risk is not as high as previously thought and osseous remodeling has the potential to reduce the relative risk.[12] Notching should be avoided nonetheless and protected postoperative rehabilitation should be considered should a substantial notching occur. Less than 1 cm has not been shown to increase the risk of fracture.

## Intraoperative Periprosthetic Fractures

Preoperatively, the surgeon can identify which patients are at risk for intraoperative complications. Fractures can occur in patients with severe osteoporosis. The surgeon can evaluate the medical history for risk factors and



Parvizi J, Klatt B.
*Essentials in Total Knee Arthroplasty* (pp 151-160).

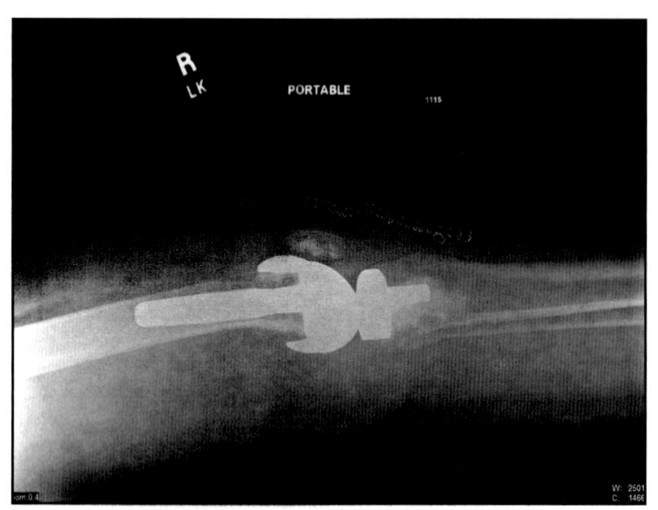


**Figure 18-1.** Femoral notching of the anterior cortex is shown.

identify osteopenia/bone defects on x-ray. On the other hand, patients with extremely brittle bone in the setting of osteonecrosis or osteopetrosis can fracture with overaggressive instrumentation as well. Cysts can create bony defects that can affect the bone's ability to fit guides and prosthetics and surgeons should be aware preoperatively. Previous tibial or femoral osteotomies provide a host of challenges. Especially with concomitant removal of hardware, the surgeon must be aware of areas of weakened bone. After hardware removal, the surgeon may elect to bypass the screw holes with a stemmed component to prevent creation of a stress riser above the knee replacement. Preoperative awareness can be vital to avoidance of intraoperative fractures.

During surgery, the surgeon should have awareness to the quality of the bone and should be alert to recognize any fractures. Bone that is particularly easy to cut or soft should cause the surgeon to exercise caution. The majority of intraoperative fractures will be nondisplaced, therefore careful attention is necessary to avoid discovering them on postoperative radiographs. Understanding the equipment will allow the surgeon to know when a fracture is more likely occur. For example, femoral prostheses with a box are more likely to split the condyles than those without a box. If the bone cut for the box is accidentally undersized for the implant, the bone can split with trial insertion in very poor bone. If resistance is met when impacting the femoral component, the surgeon should reevaluate. Intramedullary (IM) devices can perforate the femoral or tibial cortex and can also fracture through anteriorly if used to elevate the femur. Taking all of the steps into account combined with diligent concentration can hopefully minimize these complications. If one does experience a fracture intraoperatively, the treatment decision must be concise given the relative confines of the situation.

### Femoral Fractures

Some of the more commonly encountered intraoperative fractures are nondisplaced condyle fractures. This fracture can occur as stated before from an improper box cut, which allows the prosthetic or trial to wedge open the condyles. Too deep of a cut can also weaken the condyle. In some prostheses, the box is the same for all knee implant sizes, so a smaller component may weaken the condyles more. In addition, the smaller components are often used in women who, in general, have worse bone quality. If the fracture is incomplete, then cementing the component may suffice as fixation. It is critical that cement not be placed into any fracture site as this will prevent healing of the fracture. If the fracture is complete, then adding screw fixation is an option. Furthermore, if the condyles are displaced, the surgeon may need to add a plate to stabilize the fracture.

Cortical perforations of the femur can occur with the initial drilling of the canal or with the long IM guide. In osteoporotic bone, an IM rod used to lift the femur can pull through the anterior cortex of the femur. Treatment depends on the location and extent of the perforation. The defect can be bone grafted with a strut or may require a stem to bypass the area into intact bone.

Avulsion fractures of the epicondyle via the medial collateral ligament may require screw fixation or possibly suture anchors depending on the size of the bony fragment and associated ligamentous stability. If the sleeve of fracture remains intact, this type of fracture may require no treatment.

### Tibial Fractures

Tibial fractures are much less encountered than the previously defined femoral fractures. More common types of fractures include vertical shear fractures that can occur during impaction of the trial or prosthesis. Depending on the stability of the fracture, screw fixation can be implemented, but most often these can be addressed with protected weight bearing in the postoperative period.

## Postoperative Fracture

Femoral fractures comprise the majority of periprosthetic TKA fractures postoperatively. Supracondylar femur fractures are the most common type of femoral fracture. Numerous criteria have been developed to exactly define the supracondylar region of the femur in relation to arthroplasty. Current convention is 15 cm of the distal femur or 5 cm within the proximal extent of the stem.

## Presentation

Patients should have an adequate trauma evaluation if associated with a significant fall or motor vehicle accident. Mechanism of injury should be assessed to determine if there was significant trauma to cause the associated fracture. In most cases, these occur as a result of a low energy fall in the face of osteoporotic bone. Soft tissue assessment must be made with attention to open fracture, previous incisions, and quality of the tissue envelope. It is difficult to assess the general alignment and extensor mechanism in the face of the fracture. These can be addressed at surgery if they are too painful to evaluate.

Distal neurovascular status must be evaluated as bony fragments can injure the blood vessels where they are tethered over the posterior aspect of the knee.

Radiographic examination should include orthogonal views of both the fracture and the prosthesis with attention to include the entire prosthesis if there is a stem or previous hardware.

History of pain preceding the fracture may indicate that a loose component or osteolysis lead to the fracture. For treatment, the most crucial part of the history is the determination of the type of implant. This can dictate surgical options. To use a retrograde IM nail, the implant must have a large enough open box to allow the nail to enter the femoral canal. Permission should be obtained from the patient to obtain records from the surgeon and hospital where the original surgery was done.

## Classification

Numerous classification schemes have been developed for supracondylar femur fractures. There is no system that is simple to use with a clearly defined treatment based on the classification. The key issues to define treatment are as follows:

- Is the fracture displaced?
- Is the component well-fixed?
- Is there adequate bone attached to the component to fix this to the remainder of the long bone?

The Rorabeck, Chen, and Digioia and Rubash systems are some of the more commonly used systems.[1,2,4] The common feature to these systems is degree of displacement and the Rorabeck system adds the integrity of the prosthesis. These fractures are so complex and there are many variables to take into consideration, therefore a simple classification scheme cannot be used to dictate management, but they have some value for communication and study purposes.

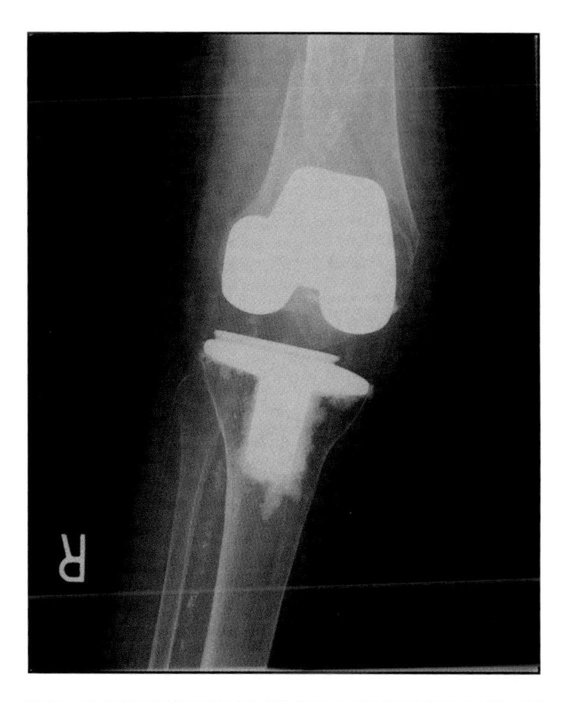


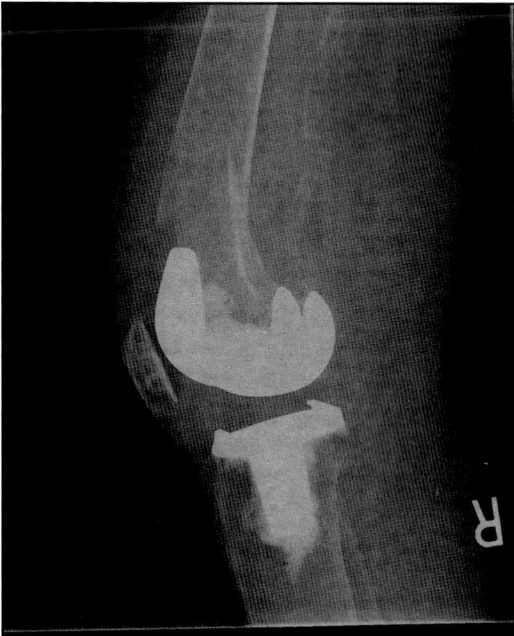


**Figure 18-2.** AP and lateral x-ray of a supracondylar distal femoral periprosthetic fracture. Note that the fracture is displaced and has minimal comminution.

One example classification system can be found in Insall and Scott's Surgery of the Knee. This classification is as follows: Type I, nondisplaced fracture, stable components; Type IIA, displaced fracture, stable components, no comminution (Figure 18-2); Type IIB, displaced fracture, stable components, comminuted; and Type III, displaced or nondisplaced fracture with loose components.

## Treatment

The goal should be early range of motion and return to preoperative status. These goals may not always be possible. An older more debilitated patient may not be able to tolerate extensive surgery but will also have a difficult time with nonoperative management.

### Nonoperative Management

Historically, nonoperative management was a popular treatment option.[4,13] Studies have shown some success when used for nondisplaced fractures or stable fractures after adequate reduction. Casting, bracing, and skeletal traction are the main modalities used. Infections and surgical complications are minimized, but prolonged immobilization can lead to stiffness and the myriad of problems associated with recumbency in elderly patients. Modern studies suggest increased evidence for eventual surgical management, and nonoperative management should be reserved for stable, nondisplaced fractures or patients who are poor surgical candidates.

These patients can be managed in a cast or brace non-weight bearing for 8 to 12 weeks. Range of motion in the knee can be allowed if the fracture is stable.

### Operative Management

Fixation and revision are the 2 main choices of management and there are many options within these categories. The integrity of the prosthesis will determine which option is best. If the implant is loose, then revision is the only option. If the implant is well fixed, fixation may be possible depending on the amount of distal bone. There needs to be adequate distal bone for the implant to hold the prostheses stable until healing occurs. If there is a hip stem proximally, then do not end fixation just short of the stem. This creates a stress riser, which can lead to an interprosthetic fracture. An interprosthetic fracture is extraordinarily difficult to treat.

## Fixation

Fixation can be done with external fixation, fixed angle devices, plating, or IM rodding. Each option has relative merits and drawbacks.

### External Fixation

External fixation devices have a limited utility in these fractures. As more surgeons begin to use thin wire frames for fracture management, they may find a role in periprosthetic fractures, but there is a paucity of information at this time. Concern here is for a high rate of infection with the pin tracts. A pin tract infection in the vicinity of a TKA could result in a septic TKA.

### Buttress Plating

Buttress plating refers to standard plates without the locking option. This allows screws to be placed in multiple planes and directed in multiple directions, but these screws provide no axial stability. Therefore, the fixation is less rigid with these plates. With these plates, the technique calls for extensive exposure. The operative dissection allows for excellent visualization and anatomic reduction, but the soft tissue stripping disrupts the periosteal biology. Fixation may be difficult in highly osteopenic bone because the screws must obtain purchase in the bone.

### Fixed Angle Devices

Both the dynamic condylar screw and the blade plate are fixed angle devices. With these 2 implants, there is a rigid connection between the lateral plate and the distal device that attaches to the distal fragment. The rigid angle provides an axial stability that is not found with the use of traditional plating.

The alignment of these devices limits where they can be placed on and in the distal bone. Either the blade or the condylar screw must be able to gain adequate fixation while still allowing proper proximal femoral alignment. The screw or blade has to be planned well so that the proper angle will be recreated with the fixation of the plate to the proximal bone. An understanding of the fixation device and the intact femoral component determine the utility of these devices. Both require a large amount of distal bone to gain fixation. This can be more challenging with posterior stabilized knees, because the box will interfere with distal placement of the blade plate or condylar screw.

### Locked Plating

Introduction of locked plating has greatly changed the approach to the fixation options (Figure 18-3). Unlike the traditional buttress plating and like fixed angle devices, locked plates provide axial stability. Compared to the classic fixed angle devices, locking plates are more versatile in placement and can achieve fixation with less distal bone. The screws can be placed in various locations and angles in the distal fragment. Combination plates allow for compression screws, which help in reduction of the plate to the bone.

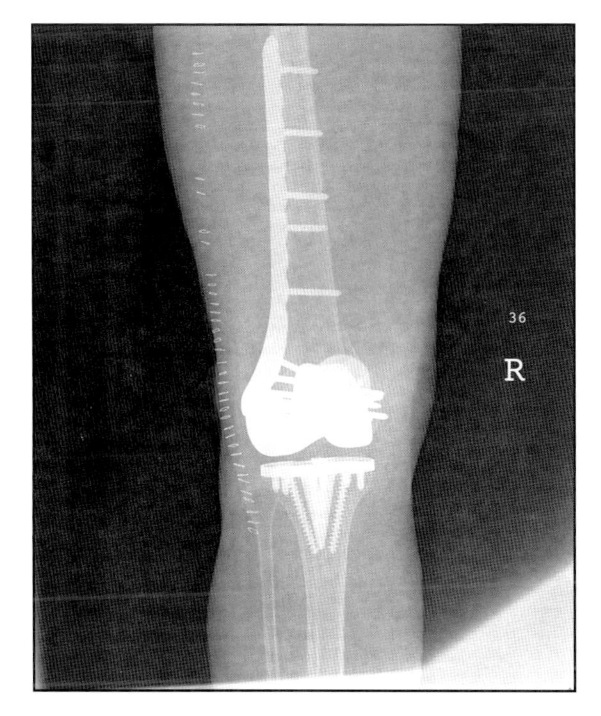


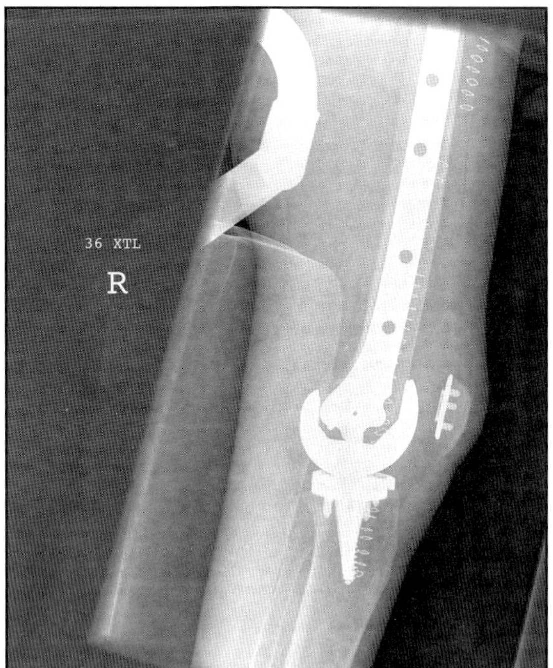


**Figure 18-3.** Fixation of a supracondylar fracture with a locked plate is demonstrated. Note the multiple screws in the distal fragment.

The locking plates can be inserted with very limited biological disruption. Techniques can be used to leave periosteum intact and to place screws percutaneously. Indirect reduction techniques can be used in many cases, but open reduction must be used if adequate fixation is not possible via an indirect means. The plates remain an outstanding fixation option even if indirect reduction cannot be used.[14-16]

## IM Rods

IM devices are a viable option in patients with an open box that will allow collinear access to the IM canal (Table 18-1).

It is important to "know" the knee implant. Make and size of the implant will allow the surgeon to determine the size of the open box, if there is one (Figure 18-4). This will determine what size nail can be used.

Supracondylar or standard retrograde femoral nails can be used for these fractures (Figure 18-5). The fracture site can be indirectly reduced with a rigid construct, preventing any biological disruption. There must be adequate screw options for distal fixation with the chosen device. Some manufacturers have multidirectional screws, which may be necessary depending on the prosthetic parameters. The surgeon must also be aware of ipsilateral hip prosthesis, which can limit proximal fixation. Disadvantages of nails include accelerated metallosis especially if the box is created or altered. Antegrade nails can be used for proximal fractures in the setting of a closed box.[8,18-20]

## Flexible IM Nails

Flexible IM nails are another option, but their use is limited. These can be used with a closed box when an IM nail cannot be used. Morbidity is low due to minimal dissection. Flexible nails are much less rigid and will occasionally result in malunion due to shortening and rotation. A small review by Ritter et al[21] revealed 100% union rates.

## Additional Modalities

Cement and structural bone graft can be used to assist in fixation with all of these devices. If screws have poor purchase in bone that is severely osteopenic, a cortical window can be use to add cement, which will provide better screw fixation. Strut grafts such as fibular or tricortical iliac crest can be interpositioned or onlayed to add fixation. These fractures usually occur in patients with compromised healing capability. Bone grafting with autograft, allograft, or demineralized bone graft can be used to promote healing. bone morphogenic protein can be considered in cases where biological healing is severely impaired.

Table 18-1

**INTERCONDYLAR OPENING OF FEMORAL TOTAL KNEE COMPONENT BY MANUFACTURER AND MODEL[17]**

| *Company* | *Model* | *Smallest Intercondylar Diameter (M/L or A/P) (mm)* |
|---|---|---|
| Biomet (Warsaw, IN) | AGC sizes 55 to 80 | 17.0 to 22.0 |
| | Maxim PCR sizes 55 to 80 | 13.0 to 15.0 |
| | Maxim PCS open box sizes 55 to 80 | 14.0 |
| | Ascent PCR sizes XS - XXL | 17.0 to 23.0 |
| | Ascent PCS open box sizes XS - XXL | 20.0 |
| Kirschner | Performance | 14.0 |
| DePuy/Johnson & Johnson (Warsaw, IN) | AMK Cruciate Retaining 1488, 1688 sizes 1 to 5 | 14.2 to 21.5 |
| | AMK 1489 Series sizes 1 to 5 | 14.5 to 20.6 |
| | AMK Congruency Posterior Stabilized 1956 sizes 1 to 5 | 13.2 to 17.2 |
| | AMK Posterior Stabilized (diverging box) 1866 | 13.25 |
| | AMK Universal 1489 | 14.5 |
| | AMK Coordinate Ultra | Closed box |
| | LCS sizes Small - Large+ | 13.6 to 22.0 |
| | LCS Complete sizes Small - Large+ | 14.4 to 21.9 |
| | PFC Sigma Cruciate Retaining | 17.4 |
| | PFC Sigma Posterior Stabilized | 11.9 |
| | PFC Sigma TC3 Cruciate Substituting | 11.9 |
| | PFC Modular Cruciate Retaining | 19.9 |
| | PFC Modular Cruciate Substituting | 9.3 |
| | PFC TC3 | Closed box |
| Wright Medical (Arlington, TN) | Advantim PCR | 19.0 |
| | Advantim Open Housing Posterior Stabilized | 16.0 |
| | Advantim Closed Housing Posterior Stabilized | Closed box |
| | Advance Medial Pivot (PCR) | 18.0 |
| | Advance Posterior Stabilized | Closed box |
| | Axiom (PCR) sizes 55 to 85 | 14.0 to 22.0 |
| | Axiom (Posterior Stabilized) sizes 55 to 85 | 16.0 to 24.0 |
| Howmedica/Osteonics (Now Stryker Orthopaedics, Mahway, NJ) | PCA sizes Small - X-large | 12.0 to 16.0 |
| | Duracon | 18.5 |
| | Omnifit | Closed box |
| | Scorpio CR sizes 3 to 13 | 17.0 to 21.0 |
| | Scorpio PS sizes 3 to 13 | 17.0 to 21.0 |
| | Scorpio TS | Closed box |
| Centerpulse (Intermedics/Sulzer) (Now owned by Zimmer [Warsaw,IN[) | Natural, NKII | 14.0 |
| | Apollo PCR | 18.5 |
| | Apollo Posterior Stabilized | Closed box |

(continued)

Table 18-1 (continued)

**INTERCONDYLAR OPENING OF FEMORAL TOTAL KNEE COMPONENT BY MANUFACTURER AND MODEL**[17]

| COMPANY | MODEL | SMALLEST INTERCONDYLAR DIAMETER (M/L OR A/P) (MM) |
|---|---|---|
| Zimmer (Warsaw, IN) | Insall/Burstein I sizes 55 to 72 | 15.5 to 18.8 |
| | Insall/Burstein II sizes 54 to 74 | 15.3 to 21.0 |
| | Miller/Galante I sizes Small - Large++ | 10.6 to 17.4 |
| | Miller/Galante II sizes 1 to 8 | 11.9 |
| | Nex Gen LPS sizes A - H Open Box | 14.1 to 21.6 |
| Smith & Nephew (London, United Kingdom) | Genesis | 20.0 |
| | Genesis II | 16.5 |

Su ET, DeWal H, Di Cesare PE. Periprosthetic femoral fractures above total knee replacements. *J Am Acad Orthop Surg.* 2004;12(1):12-20.

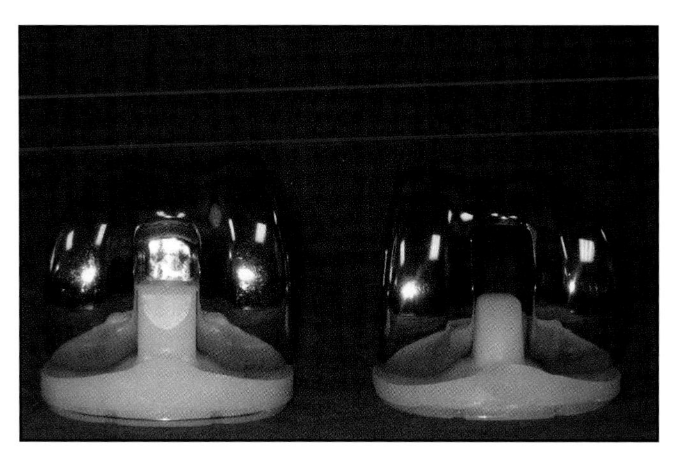

**Figure 18-4.** Closed box of the Scorpio TS implant is shown on the left. Open box of the Scorpio NRG is demonstrated on the right.

## Fixation Around Stemmed Components

In patients with pre-existing well-fixed stemmed components, a challenge exists for fixation near the stem. IM devices are usually not an option. If a plate is used, the stem will preclude the use of bicortical screws and either cerclage wires or a combination of unicortical screws and wires will need to be used.

## REVISION ARTHROPLASTY

If the prosthesis is determined to be loose or if the fracture characteristics preclude operative fixation, the arthroplasty must be revised. Revision arthroplasty also may be necessary for previous failed nonoperative or operative fixation. One advantage of revision arthroplasty is earlier range of motion and weight bearing. It allows quicker resumption of normal activities because weight bearing is usually allowed immediately.

An initial period of nonoperative management can be used in rare cases. If adequate reduction can be maintained and the patient can tolerate the stabilization, the revision surgery may be easier in the face of a healed fracture.

Removal of the failed prosthesis is the first step during the revision. After this, an assessment is made of the remaining bone and ligaments for reconstruction. If there remains adequate distal bone for the ligamentous attachments, a nonconstrained component can be used. If the remaining ligamentous attachments are decreased, the revision may do well with a more constrained polyethylene. If there are no remaining ligamentous attachments, the revision will need a hinge mechanism to provide stability. Although premature failure rates may be high, use of constrained components is often necessary.

All revisions should have a stemmed component because the original metaphyseal bone that was used for fixation of the primary knee is now compromised. The canals are reamed to either press fit or cement stems.

Defects can be managed with augments, allograft/autograft, or cement depending on the size and location of the defect. No defect more than 5 mm should be filled with cement. If the defect is greater than 5 mm, an augment should be used. A new innovation in revision surgery allows for the use of ingrowth metaphyseal sleeves (Figure 18-6). These implants are ideal to fill the metaphyseal defects, and they give a great degree of fixation to the knee components.

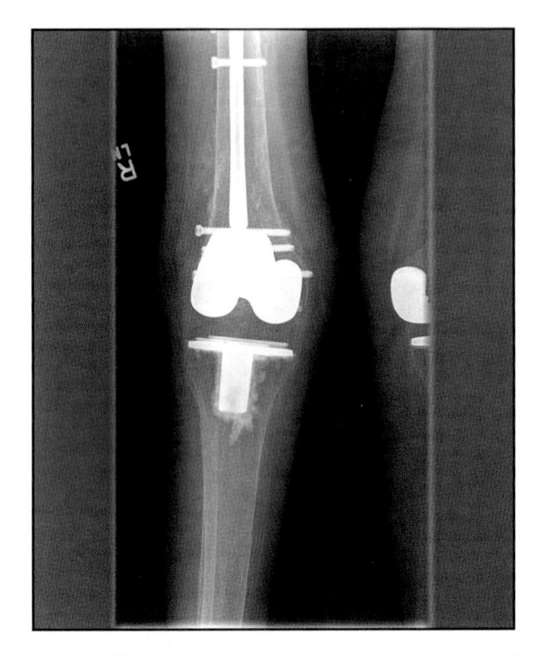


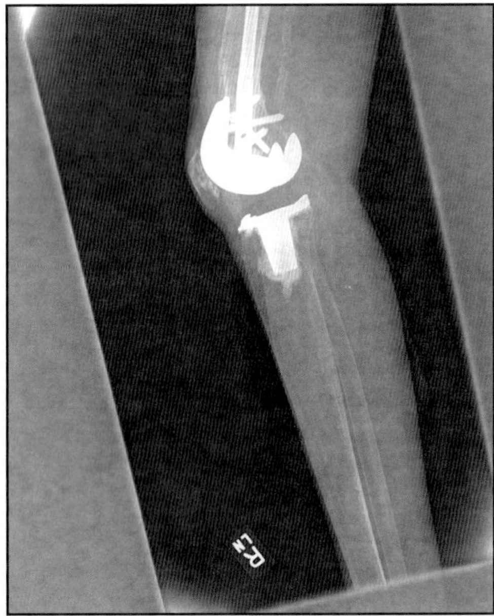

Figure 18-5. Fixation of the fracture shown in Figure 18-2 with a retrograde IM nail.

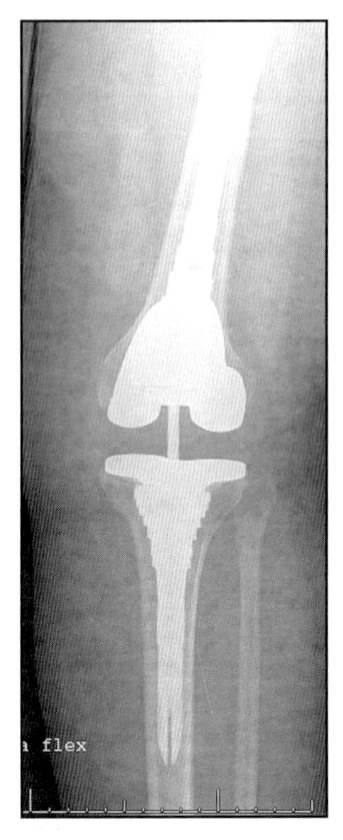


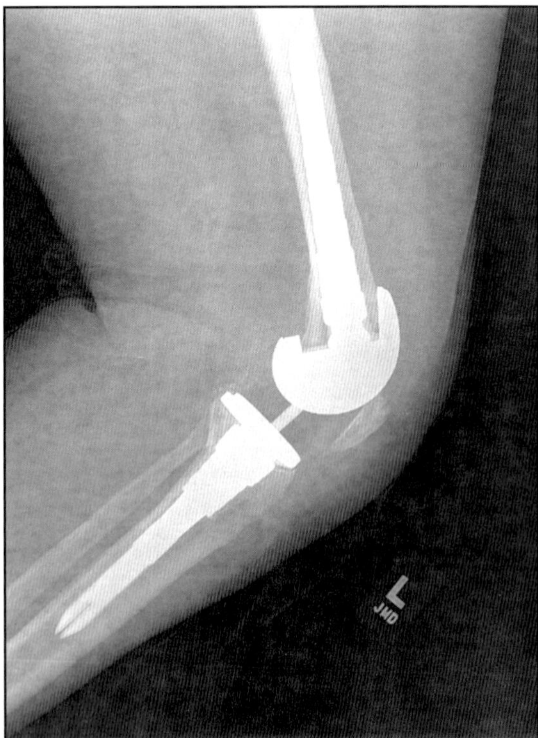


**Figure 18-6.** Depuy PFC Sigma revision is shown with the use of ingrowth sleeves to replace metaphyseal bony loss.

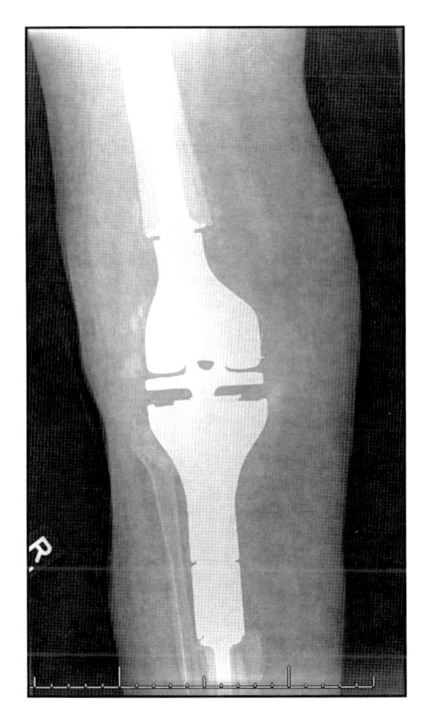

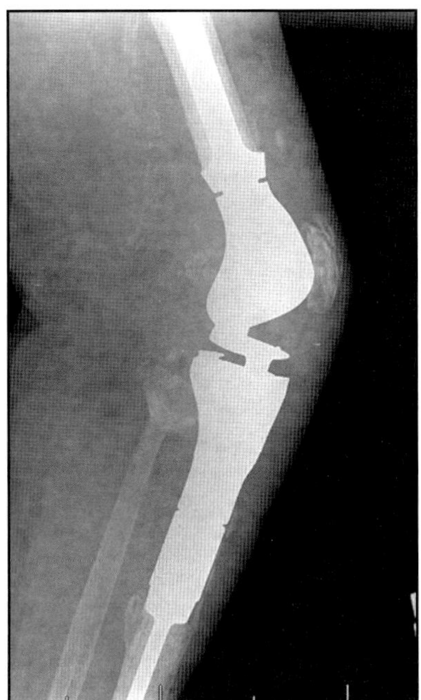

**Figure 18-7.** Megaprosthesis with hinge is shown.

If a significant amount of bone loss is encountered, an allograft prosthesis composite, distal femoral allograft, or tumor prosthesis (aka megaprosthesis) may be required (Figure 18-7). Megaprostheses are useful in the event where extensive distal bone is lost. These systems are designed to replace the distal femur and proximal tibia when extensive bone is lost. They require the use of a hinge at the knee, as there is complete loss of the distal bone at the level of the knee. With no bone, there are no remaining ligaments to stabilize the knee.

## Tibia Fractures

Periprosthetic tibia fractures are much less common than femur or patellar fractures. The basic treatment guidelines are the same as femur fractures. Felix et al[7] classified these fractures as Type I, tibial plateau; Type II, adjacent to stem; Type III, distal to stem; and Type IV, tibial tubercle. The modifier is A, well fixed; B, loose prosthesis; and C, intraoperative. The degree of displacement is not taken into account this system, so treatment recommendations are not directly based on class. Many type A fractures can be treated nonoperatively with protected weight bearing with immobilization based on the fracture. If the fracture is displaced, unstable operative fixation may be necessary. Screw fixation with modern plates will provide adequate fixation. Keel and stem design will determine what type of screws can be used for the plateau. Most Type B fractures will require revision with a stemmed prosthesis.

## Postoperative Management and Complications

Treatment modality and patient factors will dictate the postoperative management. Early range of motion should be considered for all patients. If good stability of the fracture can be achieved, this will allow for early motion. Weight bearing should be advanced based on fracture healing, but full weight bearing should be achieved by 6 months. Weight bearing can start at 8 weeks if there is evidence of fracture healing. Many of these patients have poor biology and they often require a longer period of protected weight bearing. If healing is not evident, further surgery for bone grafting to encourage healing may be needed. Nutrition labs in these patients should also be assessed, and supplements should be provided for deficiencies. Little data exist to quantify the complication rate following treatment of periprosthetic fractures, but revision data report higher complication rates. Patients must be followed diligently in the early postoperative setting until union is achieved. Total joint surgeons will continue to see more periprosthetic fractures and must be fully aware of the preoperative risk factors and evaluation, intraoperative treatment options, and postoperative management.

## REFERENCES


1. DiGioia AM 3rd, Rubash HE. Periprosthetic fractures of the femur after total knee arthroplasty: a literature review and treatment algorithm. *Clin Orthop Relat Res.* 1991;(271):135-142.
2. Rorabeck CH, Taylor JW. Classification of periprosthetic fractures complicating total knee arthroplasty. *Orthop Clin North Am.* 1999;30(2):209-214.
3. Rorabeck CH, Angliss RD, Lewis PL. Fractures of the femur, tibia, and patella after total knee arthroplasty: decision making and principles of management. *Instr Course Lect.* 1998;47:449-458.
4. Chen F, Mont MA, Bachner RS. Management of ipsilateral supracondylar femur fractures following total knee arthroplasty. *J Arthroplasty.* 1994;9(5):521-526.
5. Rorabeck CH, Taylor JW. Periprosthetic fractures of the femur complicating total knee arthroplasty. *Orthop Clin North Am.* 1999;30(2):265-277.
6. Backstein D, Safir O, Gross A. Periprosthetic fractures of the knee. *J Arthroplasty.* 2007;22(4 Suppl 1):45-49.
7. Felix NA, Stuart MJ, Hanssen AD. Periprosthetic fractures of the tibia associated with total knee arthroplasty. *Clin Orthop Relat Res.* 1997;(345):113-124.
8. Ayers DC. Supracondylar fracture of the distal femur proximal to a total knee replacement. *Instr Course Lect.* 1997;46:197-203.
9. Dennis DA. Periprosthetic fractures following total knee arthroplasty. *Instr Course Lect.* 2001;50:379-389.
10. Lesh ML, Schneider DJ, Deol G, et al. The consequences of anterior femoral notching in total knee arthroplasty: a biomechanical study. *J Bone Joint Surg Am.* 2000;82-A(8):1096-1101.
11. Zalzal P, Backstein D, Gross AE, et al. Notching of the anterior femoral cortex during total knee arthroplasty characteristics that increase local stresses. *J Arthroplasty.* 2006;21(5):737-743.
12. Ritter MA, Faris PM, Keating EM. Anterior femoral notching and ipsilateral supracondylar femur fracture in total knee arthroplasty. *J Arthroplasty.* 1988;3(2):185-187.
13. Sochart DH, Hardinge K. Nonsurgical management of supracondylar fracture above total knee arthroplasty: still the nineties option. *J Arthroplasty.* 1997;12(7):830-834.
14. Healy WL, Siliski JM, Incavo SJ. Operative treatment of distal femoral fractures proximal to total knee replacements. *J Bone Joint Surg Am.* 1993;75(1):27-34.
15. Zehntner MK, Ganz R. Internal fixation of supracondylar fractures after condylar total knee arthroplasty. *Clin Orthop Relat Res.* 1993;(293):219-224.
16. Marti A, Fankhauser C, Frenk A, et al. Biomechanical evaluation of the less invasive stabilization system for the internal fixation of distal femur fractures. *J Orthop Trauma.* 2001;15(7):482-487.
17. Su ET, DeWal H, Di Cesare PE. Periprosthetic femoral fractures above total knee replacements. *J Am Acad Orthop Surg.* 2004;12(1):12-20.
18. Smith WJ, Martin SL, Mabrey JD. Use of a supracondylar nail for treatment of a supracondylar fracture of the femur following total knee arthroplasty. *J Arthroplasty.* 1996;11(2):210-213.
19. Weber D, Pomeroy DL, Schaper LA, et al. Supracondylar nailing of distal periprosthetic femoral fractures. *Int Orthop.* 2000;24(1):33-35.
20. Maniar RN, Umlas ME, Rodriguez JA, et al. Supracondylar femoral fracture above a PFC posterior cruciate-substituting total knee arthroplasty treated with supracondylar nailing: a unique technical problem. *J Arthroplasty.* 1996;11(5):637-639.
21. Ritter MA, Keating EM, Faris PM, et al. Rush rod fixation of supracondylar fractures above total knee arthroplasties. *J Arthroplasty.* 1995;10(2):213-216.

19

# Total Knee Infection

*Michael Williamson, MD and Javad Parvizi, MD*

Periprosthetic infection is a potentially devastating complication of total knee arthroplasty (TKA). Although the incidence has improved significantly to the current rates of approximately 1% for primary procedures and 7% for revision surgeries, infection remains one of the major complications of TKA.[1-3] Technical improvements such as vertical laminar flow operating theaters, body exhaust systems, and perioperative antibiotics along with expeditious surgical technique have helped to reduce the incidence of infection.[4] However, periprosthetic infection remains a costly burden for patients, physicians, and the health care system.[5]

## Classification

The nature and subsequent treatment of periprosthetic infections differs according to the timing of and circumstance of their presentation.[6] Patients with acute postoperative infections present within 6 weeks of surgery, frequently with complaints of pain, local inflammation, and constitutional symptoms (eg, fever, chills).[7] Late chronic infections present after the 6-week postoperative period, often with more insidious onset of symptoms.[1] Acute hematogenous infections present late as the result of hematogenous delivery of the offending organism to the joint from an infection at a remote site.[8] Finally, some periprosthetic infections are diagnosed only by intraoperative cultures obtained during revision surgery performed for other reasons.[9]

## Risk Factors

Multiple medical comorbidities may increase the risk of periprosthetic infection following TKA. Diabetic patients have demonstrated higher rates of infection following TKA, with some series reporting an incidence as high as 7%.[10,11] Morbid obesity (ie, body mass index above 35) has also been shown to significantly increase the risk for postoperative infection.[12] Other risk factors include rheumatoid arthritis, psoriasis, immunosuppressive therapy, prior open surgery, and poor nutritional status.[1,13]

## History and Physical Examination

The most important first step in identification of periprosthetic infection is a thorough clinical history and physical examination. Signs such as fever, local inflammation, draining periarticular sinus tract, and severe joint pain with range of motion are highly suggestive of infection. However, clinical history and examination alone may not accurately diagnose infection.[14] Indeed, periprosthetic infection may have a subtle presentation that is similar to that of other conditions such as aseptic loosening or hematoma, requiring the employment of additional diagnostic modalities to confirm or exclude its presence.[7]



Parvizi J, Klatt B.
*Essentials in Total Knee Arthroplasty* (pp 161-166).

## Serologic Tests

The serologic tests of white blood cell count (WBC) with differential, erythrocyte sedimentation rate (ESR), and C-reactive protein (CRP) are routinely obtained in the patient with suspected periprosthetic infection. WBC count has not been shown to be a reliable marker for periprosthetic infection in the absence of systemic infection.[15] CRP and ESR are nonspecific inflammatory markers that normally rise rapidly after TKA and then return to baseline postoperatively in approximately 3 weeks and 3 months, respectively.[16-19] Conditions other than periprosthetic infection may cause elevations in ESR and CRP, including other infections, metastatic disease, and chronic inflammatory diseases such as rheumatoid arthritis or gout.[16] In the absence of these confounding factors, new or persistent elevation of CRP beyond 3 weeks or ESR beyond 3 months postoperative should raise concern of possible periprosthetic infection. In a study of revision total hip arthroplasty, Spangehl et al reported that an ESR of more than 30 mm/hr had a sensitivity of 82%, a specificity of 85%, and negative predictive value of 95% in detection of periprosthetic infection.[20] In that study, they also reported that CRP of more than 1 mg/dL had a sensitivity of 96%, specificity of 92%, and negative predictive value of 99%.[20] More recently, Greidanus et al reported in a prospective study of revision TKA that the optimal positivity of ESR is 22.5 mm/hr, with sensitivity of 93% and specificity of 83%, and that of CRP is 13.5 mg/L, with sensitivity of 91% and specificity of 86%.[21] While ESR and CRP are not in themselves diagnostic of infection, they are useful screening tools in the diagnosis of periprosthetic infection. Serum measurement of interleukin-6 (IL-6) may become another useful test for periprosthetic infection. IL-6 levels peak within 12 hours of surgery and return to baseline within 2 to 3 days postoperatively.[22] One study showed that an elevated IL-6 (> 12pg/mL) had 100% sensitivity, 95% specificity, 89% positive predictive value, and 100% negative predictive value for diagnosis of periprosthetic infection.[23]

## Joint Fluid Aspiration

Evaluation of synovial fluid is one of the most important elements in diagnosis of periprosthetic infection. Measurement of the concentration of leukocytes and the relative proportion of polymorphonuclear cells (PMNs) can provide useful information to that end. Synovial fluid WBC counts of more than 50,000 cells/uL and PMN percentage more than 80% are believed to be suggestive of infection in native joints,[24] and similar figures have been supported in some studies of total joint arthroplasty.[20] However, more recent studies suggest that these criteria are inaccurate for prosthetic joints. Trampuz et al reported in a prospective study of TKA that a joint fluid cell count of 1700 cells/uL had a PPV of 73% and a NPV of 98%; percentage of PMNs more than 65% yielded a PPV of 94% and NPV of 99%.[25] Parvizi et al reported a similar fluid cell count cutoff of 1760 cells/uL with PPV of 99% and NPV of 88%.[26] Their PMN percentage cutoff was slightly higher at 73%, and had a PPV of 96% and NPV of 91%.[26] These results suggest that joint fluid aspirates with cell counts of 1700 cells/uL and PMNs of more than 70% should be regarded as suggestive of periprosthetic infection.

Culture of aspirated joint fluid may be used to confirm the diagnosis of infection, as well as to identify the offending organism and direct antibiotic therapy. Aspirate should be sent for aerobic, anaerobic, mycobacterial, and fungal cultures. Although some studies have shown high accuracy for diagnosis of infection with aspirate culture,[27] the predictive value of the test may depend on the prevalence of infection in the group tested.[28] In a study by Barrack et al, the positive predictive value of a positive culture was enhanced when performed on patients suspected to have periprosthetic infection by clinical presentation or laboratory abnormality.[28] Aspiration should be performed 2 weeks after any antibiotic administration if possible and should be repeated for negative cultures in the presence of high clinical suspicion.[28] Aspirate culture should be used as a confirmatory rather than a screening test in patients with clinical features or laboratory abnormalities that suggest periprosthetic infection.[20,26,28]

Joint aspiration is best performed from the superior lateral portal of the knee with the knee in extension. The superior pole of the patella is palpated and the patella is manually subluxed laterally. After sterile preparation of the skin, a large bore needle (18 gauge) is introduced under the quadriceps tendon at the superior aspect of the patella. For larger patients, a spinal needle may be required. A minimum of several milliliters of fluid is required for complete analysis. The fluid should be inspected with gross inspection at the time of aspiration and the findings noted. Cloudy fluid is more likely infectious. Clear fluid or bloody fluid can suggest other causes. If a dry tap is encountered, this is noted in the chart. A dry tap can indicate the absence of an infection if there is truly no synovial fluid in the joint.

## Radiographic Studies

Plain x-rays should be obtained on any patient presenting with a painful TKA. Certain nonspecific findings such as periosteal reaction, osteolysis, and bone resorption may appear in patients with periprosthetic infection; however, these patients will more likely have no radiographic changes. Therefore, plain x-rays are more useful to rule out other etiologies, such as fracture or aseptic loosening.[27]

Technicium-99m (Tc-99) bone scan, which identifies areas of high metabolic activity, is frequently used as a screening test for periprosthetic infection, given its high negative predictive value.[29] Indium-111 (I-111) radiolabeled leukocyte scan may have higher sensitivity and NPV by comparison.[30] The accuracy of these scans may be enhanced when used in combination. In the combined test, uptake of Tc-99 and I-111 in the same location indicates aseptic changes, whereas I-111 uptake without Tc-99 uptake suggests an infectious process.[31] The sensitivity and specificity of the combined scans have been reported to be as high as 100% and 95%, respectively.[31] A sulfa colloid scan can be added to the indium scan to improve the accuracy of the evaluation.

Fluorodeoxyglucose positron emission tomography (FDG-PET) has more recently been utilized in the detection of periprosthetic infection. FDG-PET detects increased glucose uptake by activated macrophages and neutrophils in areas of infection. Although one study reported relatively poor accuracy of FDG-PET when compared to combined Tc-99 and tagged WBC scans,[31] other investigators have shown promising results for FDG-PET, at least in THA.[26,32] This modality may be less amenable to TKA, however. One study reported only 91% sensitivity and 72% specificity for infection around TKA due to a large number of false positives.[33]

## Intraoperative Diagnosis

Intraoperative examination of tissue for the presence or absence of purulence may serve as an adjunct modality in the detection of periprosthetic infection. However, it is not necessarily accurate, with reported PPV and NPV of 78% and 89%, respectively.[26] Intraoperative Gram stain has high specificity (97% to 100%), but it has been shown to be ineffective for detection of periprosthetic infection, with poor reported sensitivities of 12% to 20%.[20,35]

In cases in which infection is not confirmed or organism isolated preoperatively, intraoperative analysis of frozen sections of joint capsule or periprosthetic membrane may be used for detection of infection. However, different authors have used different criteria to define infection in these sections. Mirra et al reported criteria of more than 5 PMNs in more than 5 high-power fields (using 500x).[36,37] A later study using 400x as high power showed that these criteria had sensitivity of 84% and specificity of 96%.[38] Another author reported more than 5 inflammatory cells in more than 10 fields as 90% sensitive and 96% specific when compared to intraoperative culture.[39] Still another concluded that one PMN in 10 or more high power fields was consistent with septic failure in 97.8% of cases.[40]

Intraoperative fluid and tissue culture are considered the gold standard for identification of periprosthetic infection. However, the accuracy of this test may be limited by false-positive (contamination) and false-negative results.[7] Although some authors have shown high culture positivity in joints not clinically infected, others have reported negative cultures in the presence of clinical infection.[7,41] Atkins et al reported 65% sensitivity for intraoperative cultures and advocated taking 5 to 6 samples per patient with 3 or more positive cultures required for confirmation of infection.[35] Other authors documented 89% agreement when an organism was isolated from 3 samples.[40] Intraoperative culture does have high specificity (97% to 100%) and positive predictive value (98% to 100%), making it effective for confirmation of infection.[26] As a practical matter, the surgeon treating a periprosthetic infection should obtain multiple tissue or fluid samples and make effort to minimize the risk of contamination of those samples. In addition, antibiotics should be withheld for 2 weeks prior to surgery and perioperative antibiotics should not be administered until after cultures are obtained.[7]

## Treatment

### Irrigation and Débridement

TKA infections may be treated with débridement and retention of components in select patients.[42] Such an approach may be preferred in patients whose comorbidities make a 2-stage resection and reimplantation prohibitive.[43-45] It may also be used in acute postoperative or hematogenous infections.[46,47] In general, an acute infection is one of less than 30 days duration, but this time period is still somewhat controversial. If an infection is acute, it is possible to resolve this infection with irrigation, retention of components, and antibiotics. If the infection is chronic in nature, the best chance to eradicate infection is to do a 2-stage reimplantation. Some studies have shown failure rates for irrigation and débridement with retention of components as high as 40% to 70%.[48,49] Risk factors identified for failure include advanced age, prolonged duration of symptoms prior to treatment, and type of infecting organism.[46,49,50] Susceptible gram-positive organisms have a higher chance of success with débridement and retention. *S. aureus* has a particularly low success rate with irrigation and retention of components. Resistant and gram-negative infections are less likely to resolve with retention and will be better served with a 2-stage revision. However, better results may be expected in immunocompetent patients with acute postoperative or acute hematogenous infections with minimal delay to treatment and less virulent infecting organisms.[46,47] A host that is unable to mount a good immune response should be treated with a 2-stage revision. Multiple débridements may ultimately improve rates of component retention.[46]

## Single-Stage Revision Arthroplasty

Single-stage revision arthroplasty is a less frequently employed technique to eradicate infection. It involves removal of all components, irrigation and débridement, and reimplantation of all components in a single surgical procedure. Single stage revision arthroplasty followed by a 6-week course of intravenous (IV) antibiotics has been reported to have low rates of recurrence, similar to 2-stage resection arthroplasty.[51,52] However, some studies have shown improved failure rates and implant survival in 2-stage revision.[53,54]

## Two-Stage Revision Arthroplasty

In most cases of infected TKA, the treatment of choice is a 2-stage revision arthroplasty, in which the infected prosthesis is débrided, an antibiotic-laden cement spacer is placed while the patient undergoes a 6-week regimen of IV antibiotics, and a reimplantation is performed thereafter when deemed clinically appropriate. Although 6 weeks of IV antibiotics has been used as the standard for duration of antibiotic therapy, the appropriate timing of reimplantation may vary.[55,56] Resolution of infection prior to reimplantation should be assessed using clinical exam and diagnostic laboratories (eg, CRP, ESR) as previously described, and some authors recommend clearance of joint aspirate culture as well.[56]

Outcomes following 2-stage revision have been generally positive for eradication of infection and survival of prostheses. Hart and Jones reported an 88% rate of eradication of infection in TKAs treated with staged revision at 4 years follow-up.[57] Other authors have reported similar results of 82% to 93% infection clearance with 2-stage revision.[47,58] As with irrigation and débridement, the virulence of the infecting organism may be a factor in the success of staged revision. Although some authors have found similar reinfection rates with antibiotic-resistant and nonresistant organisms,[59] other investigators have shown poorer survivability of TKAs infected with resistant organisms.[60]

Some authors have favored using articulating spacer blocks to ameliorate soft tissue stiffness and thus facilitate exposure at the time of reimplantation and patient function postoperatively.[58,61] One comparison of revision arthroplasty with static versus articulating spacers demonstrated similar reinfection rates between the groups but significantly improved postoperative motion in the articulating spacer group.[62] Another study reported improvement in infection rates, postoperative knee motion, and retention of bone stock using articulating spacers.[58]

## Antibiotic Suppression

Antibiotic treatment alone should only be considered for cases in which staged revision arthroplasty is not feasible. Some authors have reported reasonable success rates for antibiotic suppression. Rao et al reported an 86% success rate for operative débridement with retention of components followed by chronic antibiotic suppression.[63] Other studies have demonstrated much poorer results, with success rates on the order of 18% to 24%.[3,48,64] Chronic suppression should be reserved for the patient with a single, well-fixed prosthesis who cannot practically undergo staged revision and who is infected with an organism of low virulence that is susceptible to a tolerable oral antibiotic.[6,65]

## References


1. Peersman G, Laskin R, Davis J, Peterson M. Infection in total knee replacement: a retrospective review of 6489 total knee replacements. *Clin Orthop Rel Res.* 2001;392:15-23.
2. Phillips JE, Crane TP, Noy M Elliott TS, Grimer RJ. The incidence of deep prosthetic infections in a specialist orthopaedic hospital: a 15-year prospective survey. *J Bone Joint Surg Br.* 2006;88(7):943-948.
3. Hanssen AD, Rand JA. Evaluation and treatment of infection at the site of a total hip or knee arthroplasty. *Instr Course Lect.* 1999;48:111-122.
4. Hanssen AD, Osmon DR. The use of prophylactic antimicrobial agents during and after hip arthroplasty. *Clin Orthop Rel Res.* 1999;369:124-138.
5. Jain NB, Higgins LD, Ozumba D, et al. Trends in epidemiology of knee arthroplasty in the United States, 1990-2000. *Arthritis Rheum.* 2005;52(12):3928-3933.
6. Tsukayama DT, Goldberg VM, Kyle R. Diagnosis and management of infection after total knee arthroplasty. *J Bone Joint Surg Am.* 2003;85(suppl 1):S75-S80.
7. Bauer TW, Parvizi J, Kobayashi N, Krebs V. Diagnosis of periprosthetic infection. *J Bone Joint Surg Am.* 2006;88(4):869-882.

8. Cook JL, Scott RD, Long WJ. Late hematogenous infections after total knee arthroplasty: experience with 3013 consecutive total knees. *J Knee Surg.* 2007;20(1):27-33.
9. Marculescu CE, Berbari EF, Hanssen AD, Steckelberg JM, Osmon DR. Prosthetic joint infection diagnosed postoperatively by intraoperative culture. *Clin Orthop Rel Res.* 2005;439:38-42.
10. Meding JB, Reddleman K, Keating ME, et al. Total knee replacement in patients with diabetes mellitus. *Clin Orthop Rel Res.* 2003;416:208-216.
11. England SP, Stern SH, Insall JN, Windsor RE. Total knee arthroplasty in diabetes mellitus. *Clin Orthop Rel Res.* 1990;260:130-134.
12. Namba RS, Paxton L, Fithian DC, Stone ML. Obesity and perioperative morbidity in total hip and total knee arthroplasty patients. *J Arthroplasty.* 2005;20(7 suppl 3):46-50.
13. Wilson MG, Kelley K, Thornhill TS. Infection as a complication of total knee replacement arthroplasty: risk factors and treatment in sixty-seven cases. *J Bone Joint Surg Am.* 1990;72(6):878-883.
14. Fitzgerald RH Jr. Diagnosis and management of the infected hip prosthesis. *Orthopedics.* 1995;18(9):833-835.
15. Rand JA, Morrey BF, Bryan RS. Management of the infected total joint arthroplasty. *Orthop Clin North Am.* 1984;15:491-504.
16. Shih LY, Wu JJ, Yang DJ. Erythrocyte sedimentation rate and C-reactive protein values in patients with total hip arthroplasty. *Clin Orthop Rel Res.* 1987;225:238-246.
17. White J, Kelly M, Dunsmuir R. C-reactive protein level after total hip and total knee replacement. *J Bone Joint Surg Br.* 1998;80(5):909-911.
18. Moreschini O, Greggi G, Giordano MC, Nocente M, Marghertini F. Postoperative physiopathological analysis of inflammatory parameters in patients undergoing hip or knee arthroplasty. *Int J Tissue React.* 2001;23:151-154.
19. Bilgen O, Atici T, Durak K, Karaeminogullari O, Bilgen MS. C-reactive protein values and erythrocyte sedimentation rates after total hip and knee arthroplasty. *J Int Med Res.* 2001;29:7-12.
20. Spangehl MJ, Masri BA, O'Connell JX, Duncan CP. Prospective analysis of preoperative and intraoperative investigations for the diagnosis of infection at the sites of two hundred and two revision total hip arthroplasties. *J Bone Joint Surg Am.* 19999:81(5):672-683.
21. Greidanus NV, Masri BA, Garbuz DS, et al. Use of erythrocyte sedimentation rate and c-reactive protein level to diagnose infection before revision total knee arthroplasty. *J Bone Joint Surg Am.* 2007;89:1409-1416.
22. Kragsbjerg P, Holmberg H, Vikerfors T. Serum concentrations of interleukin-6, tumor necrosis factor-alpha, and C-reactive protein in patients undergoing major operations. *Eur J Surg.* 1995;161(1):17-22.
23. DiCesare PE, Chang E, Preston CF, Liu CJ. Serum interleukin-6 as a marker of periprosthetic infection following total hip and knee arthroplasty. *J Bone Joint Surg Am.* 2005:87(9):1921-1927.
24. Krey PR, Bailen DA. Synovial fluid leukocytosis: a study of extremes. *Am J Med.* 1979;67(3):436-442.
25. Trampuz A, Hanssen AD, Osmon DR, Mandrekar J, Steckelberg JM, Patel R. Synovial fluid leukocyte count and differential for the diagnosis of prosthetic knee infection. *Am J Med.* 2004;117(8):556-562.
26. Parvizi J, Ghanem E, Menashe S, Barrack RL, Bauer TW. Periprosthetic infection: what are the diagnostic challenges? *J Bone Joint Surg Am.* 2006;88:138-147.
27. Duff GP, Lachiewicz PF, Kelley SS. Aspiration of the knee joint before revision arthroplasty. *Clin Orthop Rel Res.* 1996:132-139.
28. Barrack RL, Jennings RW, Wolfe MW, Bertot AJ. The value of preoperative aspiration before total knee revision. *Clin Orthop Rel Res.* 1997;345:8-16.
29. Levitsky KA, Hozack WJ, Balderston RA, et al. Evaluation of the painful prosthetic joint: relative value of bone scan, sedimentation rate, and joint aspiration. *J Arthroplasty.* 1991;6(3):237-244.
30. Scher DM, Pak K, Lonner JH, Finkel JE, Zuckerman JD, DiCesare PE. The predictive vale of indium-111 leukocyte scans in the diagnosis of infected total hip, knee, or resection arthroplasties. *J Arthroplasty.* 2000;15(3):295-300.
31. Love C, Marwin SE, Tomas MB, et al. Diagnosing infection in the failed joint replacement: a comparison of coincidence detection 18F-FDG and 111In-labeled leukocyte/99mTc-sulfur colloid marrow imaging. *J Nucl Med.* 2004;45(11):1864-1871.
32. Pill SG, Parvizi J, Tang PH, et al. Comparison of fluorodeoxyglucose positron emission tomography and (111) indium-white blood cell imaging in the diagnosis of periprosthetic infection of the hip. *J Arthroplasty.* 2006;21(6 suppl 2):91-97.
33. Zhuang H, Duarte PS, Pourdehnad M, et al. The promising role of 18F-FDG PET in detecting infected lower limb prosthesis implants. *J Nucl Med.* 2001;42(1):44-48.
34. Feldman DS, Lonner JH, Desai P, Zuckerman JD. The role of intraoperative frozen sections in revision total joint arthroplasty. *J Bone Joint Surg Am.* 1995;77:1807-1813.
35. Atkins BL, Anthanasou N, Deeks JJ, et al. Prospective evaluation of criteria for microbiological diagnosis of prosthetic-joint infection at revision arthroplasty. The OSIRIS Collaborative Study Group. *J Clin Microbiol.* 1998;36:2932-2939.
36. Mirra JM, Amstutz HC, Matos M, Gold R. The pathology of the joint tissues and its clinical relevance in prosthesis failure. *Clin Orthop Rel Res.* 1976;117:221-240.
37. Mirra JM, Marder RA, Amstutz HC. The pathology of failed total joint arthroplasty. *Clin Orthop Rel Res.* 1982;170:175-183.
38. Lonner JH, Desai P, DiCesare PE, Steiner G, Zuckerman JD. The reliability of analysis of intraoperative frozen sections for identifying active infection during revision hip or knee arthroplasty. *J Bone Joint Surg Am.* 1996;78(10):1553-1558.
39. Athanasou NA, Pandey R, de Steiger R, Crook D, Smith PM. Diagnosis of infection by frozen section during revision arthroplasty. *J Bone Joint Surg Br.* 1995;77(1):28-33.
40. Pandey R, Berendt AR, Athanasou NA. Histological and microbiological findings in non-infected and infected revision arthroplasty tissues. The OSIRIS Collaborative Study Group.

Oxford Skeletal Infection Research and Intervention Service. *Arch Orthop Trauma Surg.* 2000;120(10):570-574.

41. Padgett DE, Silverman A, Sachjowicz F, Simpson RB, Rosenberg AG, Galante JO. Efficacy of intraoperative cultures obtained during revision total hip arthroplasty. *J Arthroplasty.* 1995;10:420-426.
42. Bernard L, Hoffmeyer P, Assal M, Vaudaux P, Schrenzel J, Lew D. Trends in the treatment of orthopaedic prosthetic infections. *J Antimicrob Chemother.* 2004;53(2):127-129.
43. Fisman DN, Reilly DT, Karchmer AW, Goldie SJ. Clinical effectiveness and cost-effectiveness of 2 management strategies for infected total hip arthroplasty in the elderly. *Clin Infect Dis.* 2001;32(3):419-430.
44. Morrey BF, Westholm, Schoifet S, Rand JA, Bryan RS. Long-term results of various treatment options for infected total knee arthroplasty. *Clin Orthop Rel Res.* 1989;248:120-128.
45. Rand JA. Alternatives to reimplantation for the salvage of the total knee arthroplasty complicated by infection. *J Bone Joint Surg Am.* 1993;75(2):282-289.
46. Mont MA, Waldman B, Banerjee C, Pacheco IH, Hungerford DS. Multiple irrigation, débridement, and retention of components in infected total knee arthroplasty. *J Arthroplasty.* 1997;12(4):426-433.
47. Segawa H, Tsukayama DT, Kyle RF, Becker DA, Gustilo RB. Infection after total knee arthroplasty: a retrospective study of the treatment of eighty-one infections. *J Bone Joint Surg Am.* 1999;81(10):1434-1445.
48. Schoifet S, Morrey BF. Treatment of infection after total knee arthroplasty by débridement with retention of the components. *J Bone Joint Surg Am.* 1990;72(9):1383-1390.
49. Marculescu CE, Berbari EF, Hanssen AD, et al. Outcome of prosthetic joint infections treated with débridement and retention of components. *Clin Infect Dis.* 2006;42(4):471-478.
50. Burger RR, Basch T, Hopson CN. Implant salvage in infected total knee arthroplasty. *Clin Orthop Rel Res.* 1991;273:105-112.
51. Buechel FF, Femino FP, D'Alessio J. Primary exchange revision arthroplasty for infected total knee replacement: a long-term study. *Am J Orthop.* 2004;33(4):190-198.
52. Callaghan JJ, Katz RP, Johnston RC. One-stage revision surgery of the infected hip: a minimum 10-year follow-up study. *Clin Orthop Rel Res.* 1999;369:139-143.
53. Elson RA. Exchange arthroplasty for infection: perspectives from the United Kingdom. *Orthop Clin North Am.* 1993;24(4):761-767.
54. Garvin KL, Fitzgerald RH Jr, Salvati EA, et al. Reconstruction of the infected total hip and knee arthroplasty with gentamicin-impregnated Palacos bone cement. *Instr Course Lect.* 1993;42:293-302.
55. Hoad-Reddick DA, Evans CR, Norman P, Stockley I. Is there a role for extended antibiotic therapy in a two-stage revision of the infected knee arthroplasty? *J Bone Joint Surg Br.* 2005;87(2):171-174.
56. Mont MA, Waldman BJ, Hungerford DS. Evaluation of preoperative cultures before second-stage reimplantation of a total knee prosthesis complicated by infection: a comparison-group study. *J Bone Joint Surg Am.* 2000;82-A(11):1552-1557.
57. Hart WJ, Jones RS. Two-stage revision of infected total knee replacements using articulating cement spacers and short-term antibiotic therapy. *J Bone Joint Surg Br.* 2006;88(8):1011-1015.
58. Fehring TK, Odum S, Calton TF, Mason JB. Articulating versus static spacers in revision total knee arthroplasty for sepsis. *Clin Orthop Rel Res.* 2000;380:9-16.
59. Volin SJ, Hinrichs SH, Garvin KL. Two-stage reimplantation of total joint infections: a comparison of resistant and non-resistant organisms. *Clin Orthop Rel Res.* 2004;427:94-100.
60. Kilgus DJ, Howe DJ, Strang A. Results of periprosthetic hip and knee infections caused by resistant bacteria. *Clin Orthop Rel Res.* 2002;404:116-124.
61. Hofmann AA, Kane KR, Tkach TK, Plaster RL, Camargo MP. Treatment of infected total knee arthroplasty using an articulating spacer. *Clin Orthop Rel Res.* 1995;321:45-54.
62. Emerson RH Jr, Muncie M, Tarbox TR, Higgins LL. Comparison of a static with a mobile spacer in total knee infection. *Clin Orthop Rel Res.* 2002;404:132-138.
63. Rao N, Crossett LS, Sinha RK, LeFrock JL. Long-term suppression of infection in total joint arthroplasty. *Clin Orthop Rel Res.* 2003;414:55-60.
64. Bengston S, Knutson K. The infected knee arthroplasty: a 6-year follow-up of 357 cases. *Acta Orthop Scand.* 1991;62(4):301-311.
65. Hanssen AD. Managing the infected knee: as good as it gets. *J Arthroplasty.* 2002;17(4 suppl 1):98-101.

# 20

# Aseptic Loosening

*Zachary Post, MD*

Total knee arthroplasty (TKA) by almost any measure is extremely successful at relieving pain and restoring function for patients debilitated with knee arthritis. Patient satisfaction rates are generally reported above 90%.[1] Failure of knee arthroplasty is, for the most part, an infrequent event. General studies show the incidence of revision for any reason to be 3% or less at 5 and 10 years.[2] However, given the large number of knee replacements done in the United States every year, even a small percentage results in a large number of revision surgeries. The cost to society of revision knee replacement is difficult to accurately estimate but is generally regarded to be in the hundreds of millions of dollars.[3,4] More importantly, the effect on the revision knee surgery patient can be devastating. For this reason, it is imperative that orthopedic surgeons performing knee arthroplasty understand the mechanisms of failure and know how to minimize that risk.

The most common causes of knee arthroplasty failure include infection, aseptic loosening and wear, arthrofibrosis, and instability.[3] In the study by Sharkey et al,[3] the participants were broken down into groups needing revision sooner than 2 years and those needing revision after 2 years. Most revisions (55.6%) were done before 2 years, and 25% of those were done for infection. In fact, the most common reason for revision prior to 2 years was infection. However, in that same study, looking at the group needing revision at greater than 2 years, wear and aseptic loosening were the most common causes. Of those late revisions, nearly 60% showed evidence of either wear or aseptic loosening. Although not stratified, most had evidence of both. Looking at the entire group needing revision at any time, wear and aseptic loosening were the most common finding at revision overall (Figure 20-1). Instability was also noted as a common reason for revision.[3] Decreasing the amount of aseptic loosening could help reduce the need for revision knee surgery. However, the causes of aseptic loosening are multifactorial and difficult to pin down. Understanding the known ways to avoid aseptic loosening and the revision of knee replacements that goes with it could pay large dividends to any aspiring joint surgeon.

## Particle Disease

The concept of aseptic loosening has been described and explained in many ways over the past 30 years. During the early years of arthroplasty, Harris et al ascribed the localized bone resorption, and subsequent component loosening, seen in artificial joints to "cement disease."[5] He felt that particles of cement were somehow related to the loss of bone seen around artificial joints. It was in no small part that this idea lead to cementless implants, which are commonly used in hip arthroplasty today. However, when cementless implants showed similar patterns of bone loss and loosening, it became clear that the explanation was far more complicated. This idea of cement particle-mediated bone loss was expanded to include polyethylene particles by the late 1980s. In his landmark study, Howie injected a solution containing polyethylene particles into the knee joint of rats. He noted bone resorption around a stable bone cement plug in the knees with particles and none in the knees without.[6]



Parvizi J, Klatt B.
*Essentials in Total Knee Arthroplasty* (pp 167-174).

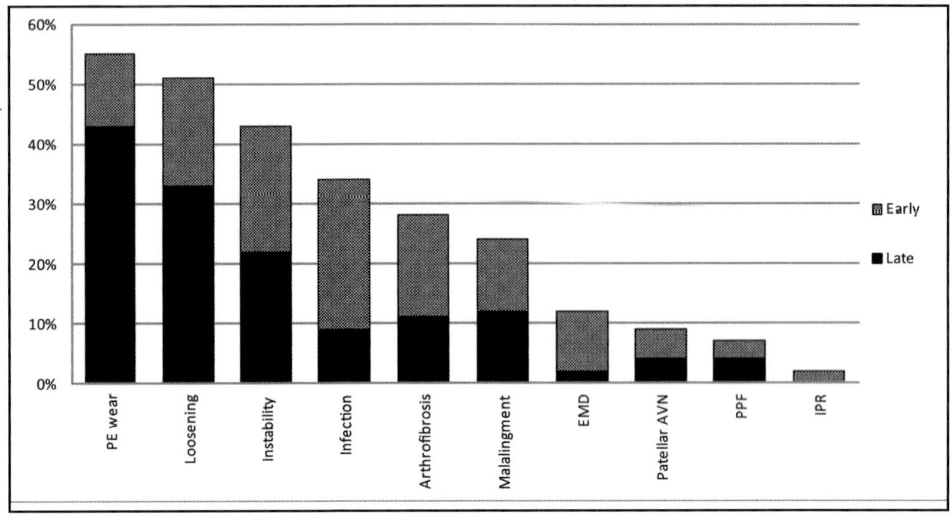


**Figure 20-1.** Causes of TKA failure. (Adapted from Sharkey PF, Hozack WM, Rothman RH, Shanstri S, Jacoby BA. Why are total knee arthroplasties failing today? *Clin Orthop Relat Res.* 2002;404:7-13.)

Schmalzried et al helped further clarify what was going on with their paper on the effective joint space in 1992.[7] They showed that small polyethylene particles were present in macrophages in the periprosthetic region, particularly at the prosthesis/cement and bone interface. The implication was that all areas of the prosthesis that could be exposed to joint fluid were susceptible to osteoclast-mediated bone resorption. As the cement bone interface deteriorated more, small particles of cement and bone would be released into the joint fluid. These particles would then cause third body wear, leading to more polyethylene particle generation. As the interface is broken down by osteolysis, the joint fluid gains even more access to the bone/prosthesis interface (Figure 20-2). This cycle could ultimately play a role in loosening of the prosthesis.[7] While the original study was done using total hip arthroplasty, the concept of polyethylene-mediated loosening certainly applies to TKA.

Our understanding of the process of bone resorption has become more complete recently. It is now recognized that small particles, be they polyethylene, bone cement, or metal, around an artificial joint can stimulate an inflammatory response from the body. Particles smaller than 1 µm are phagocytized by macrophages, which then stimulate osteoclasts or themselves differentiate into osteoclasts.[8] These activated osteoclasts then resorb bone around the prosthesis. This process, in combination with other factors, can lead to loosening of the implant. Although there are several small particles in the fluid surrounding joint implants, the primary source of these small particles is now recognized as polyethylene wear.

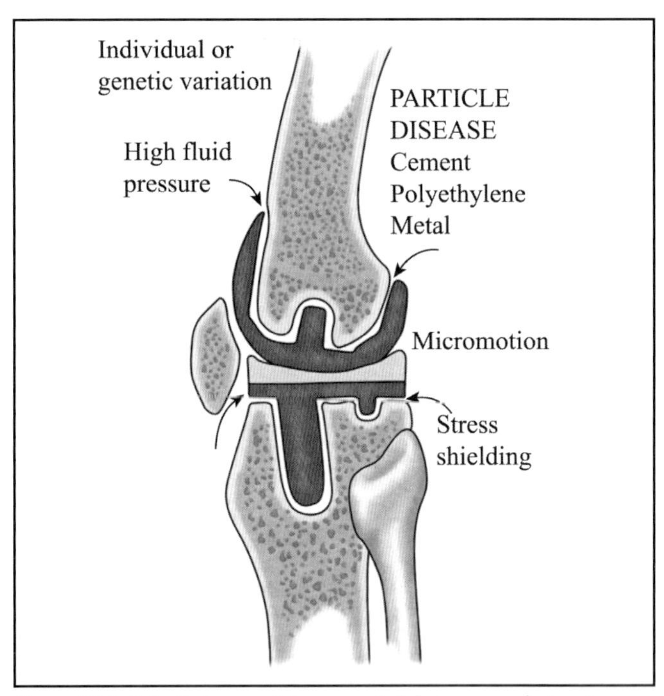


**Figure 20-2.** Polyethylene particles generated during wear elicit an immune response and expose the entire bony-cement interface to potential osteolysis and loosening.

## A Question of Wear

One question that routinely comes up when meeting with preoperative knee arthroplasty patients is, “How long will my new knee last?” Trying to answer this question can be daunting for the surgeon and confusing for the patient.

Most orthopedic surgeons know that there are several factors that will influence the answer, most having to do with wear of the polyethylene. First is the age of the patient. Age, which indirectly implies activity level, can have a huge impact on the expected lifespan of a hip or knee replacement.[9] In our clinic, we frequently make the comparison of a 45-year-old male laborer and an 85-year-old nursing home resident. The first will be using his new knee extensively and under a multitude of loads. The second may not do anything more than get up to use the bathroom several times per day. The difference in the amount of wear each will experience can be dramatic. Collier et al found that age was one of only 3 factors that was significantly related to loss of thickness of the polyethylene in total knee replacements.[10] More wear equates to more particle generation and the potential for osteolysis and eventual loosening of the prosthesis.[11]

In a modern knee replacement, wear particles can come from 2 sources. Most modern knee designs have a modular polyethylene component. In addition to the rolling, sliding, and rotational motions on the articular side of the polyethylene, there can be some "back side" wear on the nonarticular surface. Wear from the bearing surface has been shown to generate large, flake-shaped particles.[12] These larger particles are not taken up by macrophages. However, the particles generated by back-sided wear are smaller (submicron) and it has been suggested that this mode of wear could be more important in terms of osteolysis than articular wear.[13,14] The longer the components are in place and the more motion they see, the more wear and polyethylene particles generated.

Another important factor closely associated with wear is the method of manufacturing and thickness of the polyethylene component. All polyethylene components are composed of long polymer chains of individual ethylene monomers. Polyethylene components are then made by either machining previously formed polyethylene or by compression molding polyethylene powder. Studies have shown that components made by compression molding have better wear characteristics.[13,15] The cause of the difference in wear is likely small cracks or imperfections introduced during machining. The wide variety of motions that a knee replacement is exposed to can lead to shearing and crack propagation at these imperfections. Compression-molded components are not exposed to the machining process and therefore less likely to have imperfections that could become cracks.

The stress the polyethylene component experiences is proportional to the thickness of the component. Most knee arthroplasty systems use a metal tibial component that supports a modular polyethylene. The forces associated with weight bearing are transferred down the femur, through the femoral component, across the polyethylene, and then distributed across the rigid tibial plate. A thinner polyethylene provides a more linear force transmission as opposed to distributing the forces throughout the poly. With a more linear force transmission, there are higher point stresses across the component. When the thickness of the polyethylene decreases to less than 6 mm, the contact stresses that the component experience go up dramatically.[16] With less material to distribute the force, the component will experience more stress, and ultimately more wear. In their article, Bartel et al recommend that polyethylene thickness be kept above 8 to 10 mm when possible to minimize this effect.[16]

When polyethylene has been formed, either by machining or compression molding, it must be sterilized before it can be implanted. Historically, polyethylene was sterilized with gamma radiation in air. Once sterilized, the component would then be packaged in air as well. In addition to sterilizing a component, the exposure of polyethylene to radiation generates free radicals on the polymer chains. These free radicals can then do one of two things. The first is to cross-link with another polymer chain. This reaction strengthens the bonds between the monomers of the polyethylene and can have a beneficial effect on the polyethylene. Specifically, it is theorized to increase the wear resistance of the component. However, in an oxygen-rich environment, the free radicals on the polyethylene chain can react to form free oxygen radicals (Figure 20-3). These highly reactive compounds then cause oxidative damage to the poly.

Oxidative damage can continue to occur even after a component is sterilized. Storage in an oxygen-rich environment allows the process of free radical formation and degradation to continue until the polyethylene is implanted. The longer the component sits on the shelf before implantation, the more damage is done. Because the surface of the polyethylene is most exposed to the oxygen, the oxidative damage is most significant in the superficial 2 mm. The effect is the formation of a thin layer of unstable polyethylene at the articular surface. This damaged layer can shear and flake off during normal wear, leading to a massive inflammatory response and rapid failure (Figure 20-4). During the late 1980s and early 1990s, hundreds of cases of catastrophic polyethylene failure were discovered. In 1996, Collier et al showed that this catastrophic failure could be due to gamma irradiation in air.[17]

Even without catastrophic failure, the time that a polyethylene component was exposed to this oxidative environment had a detrimental effect on the performance and ultimate longevity of a total knee. Collier et al showed that shelf age was one of just 3 factors significantly associated with

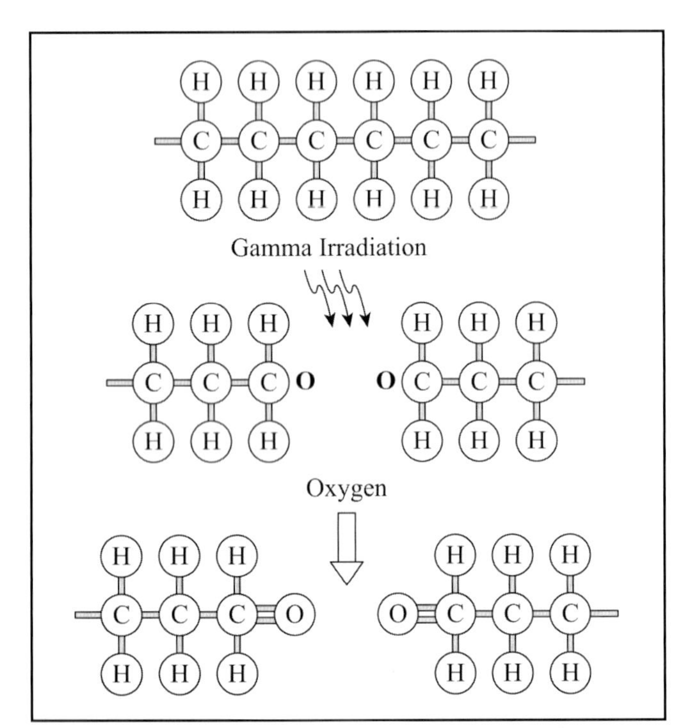


**Figure 20-3.** The effect of gamma irradiation in the presence of oxygen is to form free radicals that can then cause degradative oxidation of the polyethylene chains.

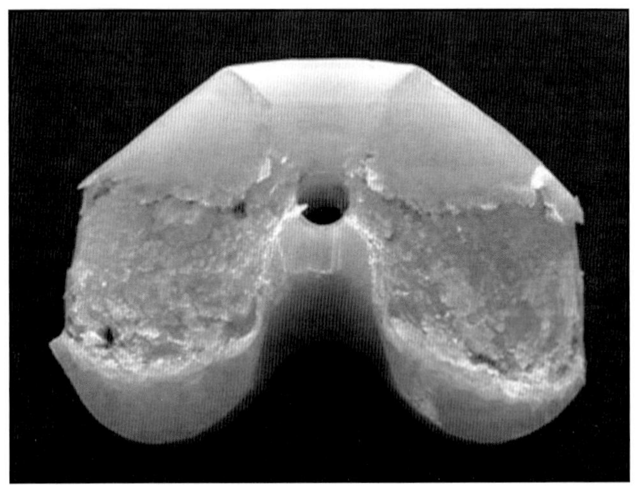

**Figure 20-4.** Oxidation damage at the surface of polyethylene tibial implants can lead to massive osteolysis and early failure. (From © American Academy of Orthopaedic Surgeons. Reprinted from the *Journal of the American Academy of Orthopaedic Surgeons*, Volume 15(1), p. 55 with permission.)

polyethylene wear. In fact, just 1 year of additional shelf age was equivalent to 10 years of patient age or 5 degrees more varus in initial mechanical alignment.[10]

As mentioned previously, exposure of polyethylene to gamma irradiation can generate cross-linking of the polymer chains. In hip arthroplasty, it has been shown that increased cross-linking of the polymer chains leads to decreased wear in vitro.[13,18] However, to date, no study has shown that increasing the level of cross-linking has a beneficial effect on wear rates of TKA in vivo.

The process of highly cross-linking polyethylene involves a procedure to quench the free radicals that are generated. There are several ways of accomplishing this. Each manufacturer uses a slightly different approach and most are proprietary. The most common method involves exposure of the polyethylene to radiation followed by remelting in an oxygen-free environment. The heat from remelting destroys the remaining free radicals, thereby avoiding future oxidative damage. The down side, and there is always a down side, is that the process of eliminating the free radicals decreases the mechanical properties of the component.[19] It is yet to be shown if this decrease in mechanical properties will have a negative impact on the clinical outcomes of total knees with highly cross-linked polyethylene. Because no studies have shown a beneficial effect of highly cross-linked polyethylene in knee arthroplasty, caution should be used when using this new technology.

Not only does the method of manufacturing and sterilization have an effect on the wear characteristics of polyethylene, the actual component design can play a roll as well. Knee replacements are generally of 3 basic designs: cruciate retaining, posterior stabilized, and rotating platform. The esoteric details of the differences between them are beyond the scope of this chapter; however, the amount of conformity of each can affect the wear and, theoretically, the rate of aseptic loosening.

In simplified terms, a component that retains the posterior cruciate ligament (PCL) retains more of the natural stability of the native knee. As a result, the arthroplasty does not rely on inherent stability from the components. The consequence is that, historically, PCL-retaining designs have used a more flat polyethylene insert. Theoretically, PCL retaining knees give more natural knee kinematics. With less component constraint, again theoretically, the femoral component is free to "rollback" on the polyethylene, much the same way a native knee does. Whether that actually happens is subject to much debate. What does result, however, is less contact area during standing and in the stance phase of gait. The definition of pressure is force divided by area. With less area for distribution of force, the pressure at the small area of contact in PCL retaining knees can be high (Figure 20-5). This increased pressure can lead to increase linear wear of the polyethylene.

Posterior stabilized (PS) knee designs use a post-cam mechanism to affect rollback. During implantation of a

PS knee, the PCL is sacrificed. This sacrifice of a native knee stabilizer must be compensated for by the component. One of the ways to increase the stability of the component is to increase conformity or the contact area of the femoral component and the poly. A more "dished" polyethylene will more evenly distribute force transmission, leading to lower pressure and theoretically, less wear (see Figure 20-5). However, the effect of increased constraint is to translate more of the coronal and rotational stress to the bone-cement interface, which can also lead to loosening. Also, the addition of the post-cam interface introduces another wear surface. While not a major source of wear, this interface does generate some wear particles.

The rotating platform TKA design is purported to combine the advantages of PCL retaining and PS knees. The post-cam mechanism replaces the PCL as in a PS knee, but the interface of the polyethylene and tibial component is not fixed. The polyethylene is allowed to rotate around a post in the tibial portion of the poly. The idea is that by allowing rotational freedom of the poly, the rotational forces are not translated to the tibial interface. However, there have been no convincing studies that show any clinical difference between the rotating platform knee and the traditional PS knee. There are the additional interfaces between the undersurface of the polyethylene and tibial tray as well as the tibial post and the tibial tray that could increase the volume of wear particles. Again, there are no studies in the literature that show a significant increase in the aseptic loosening associated with the rotating platform design.

Ultimately, all of the design factors and processing methods used to make knee components can have an impact on wear and subsequent aseptic loosening. The only study that has looked at several of these issues in any meaningful way and over a meaningful period of time is the paper by Collier et al.[10] As mentioned before, they looked at loss of polyethylene thickness and its association with several factors, including gender, age, postoperative hip-knee-ankle angle, polyethylene shelf age, weight, tibial component varus, initial polyethylene thickness, and manufacturing method. Of those, only polyethylene shelf age, postoperative hip-knee-ankle angle, and patient age were significant.[10]

## More Than Just Wear

Of the 3 significant factors associated with polyethylene wear, according to Collier et al,[10] only hip-knee-ankle angle is dependent on surgeon technique. It has long been taught and generally accepted that the mechanical axis following TKA should be within 3 degrees of varus and 5 degrees of valgus. It is said that one of the commandments of hip arthroplasty is, "Thou shalt not varus." This is also true of knee arthroplasty, perhaps more so.

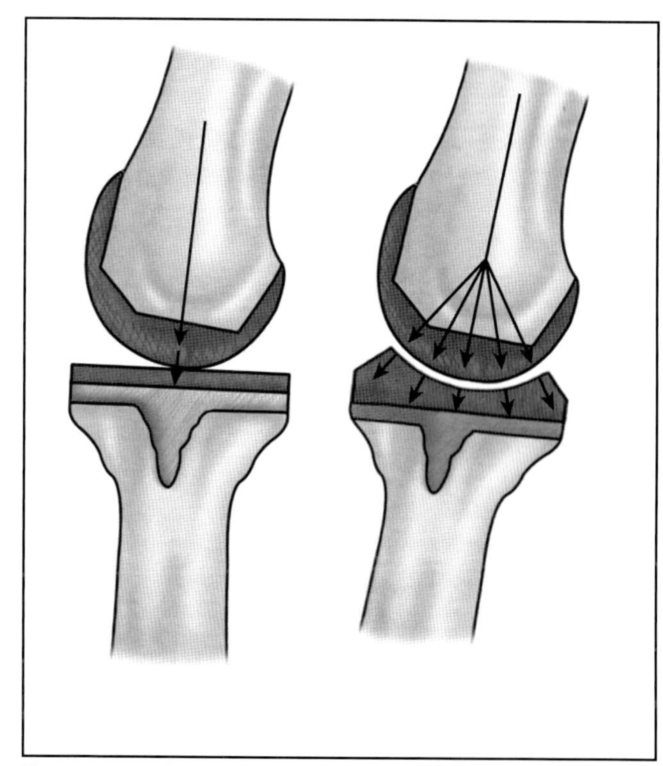

**Figure 20-5.** With a more conforming polyethylene tray, there is a more even distribution of the force associated with weight bearing.

Failure to obtain proper alignment in the coronal plane can be detrimental in several ways. The first is unequal load transmission during weight bearing. The mechanical axis of a native knee passes through the middle of the knee. Most arthritic knees have fallen into a varus alignment, causing the mechanical axis to lie more in the medial compartment. The result is increased medial side arthritis. Failure to correct this alignment at TKA will continue the pathologic wear state. The paper by Collier et al found that simply placing a TKA in 5 degrees more varus could lead to 0.11 to 0.14 mm/year more polyethylene wear.[10] They also found that less varus alignment decreased the amount of medial tibial polyethylene wear 2 to 3 times as much as it increased the lateral polyethylene wear.[10]

Malalignment, in addition to increasing the amount of wear and subsequent loosening of a total knee, can contribute to aseptic loosening in a mechanical sense as well. The ideal alignment after TKA would have a mechanical axis of zero. In this situation, the force associated with weight bearing is nearly all compression. Bone cement, used for fixation in most TKA systems, is strongest in compression. Deviations from a zero degree mechanical axis begin to introduce more shear and tension forces at the bone cement interface. Bone cement is much more likely to fail in situations involving shear and tension. In addition to loosening of the prosthesis independently, as bone cement fails, small particles of bone and cement are released into the periarticular environment. As discussed earlier, these small particles contribute to third body wear as well as macrophage activation. Each factor will lead to increased loosening of the prosthesis.[7]

Theories about the cause of aseptic loosening of knee replacements have evolved over the years. Although wear is well established as an important contributor to the process of loosening, more less-studied factors have recently been shown to be important as well. One of the emerging theories is high pressure fluid disruption of the interface. While not a new idea, Schmalzried mentions it as early as 1992, and while not the sole cause, fluid pressure likely plays some role.[7] Another theory is that of bacterial endotoxin activation of the periarticular macrophages. While sterilization of components kills all bacteria on an implant, there may still be remnants of the cell wall and other factors capable of stimulating the immune system.[20] Another intriguing theory is that of low grade infection. Overt infection of total knee replacements is less than 1% in most studies. However, one study out of Sweden showed that the risk of aseptic loosening of cemented total hips was less when the cement used contained gentamicin compared to when the cement contained no gentamicin.[20,21] This is likely true of total knees also.

The more our understanding of aseptic loosening deepens, the less we seem to know about it. What we do know is that it is well established as the most common indication for revision of total knee replacements. It is associated with wear of polyethylene. It involves activation of the immune system. Mechanical malalignment increases the risk of loosening. There are potentially dozens of other contributing factors to this complex mechanism of knee arthroplasty failure.

## Diagnosis of Aseptic Loosening

Most patients who have aseptic loosening of their knee replacement will present complaining of pain. Unfortunately, this is a common complaint after knee replacement and not at all specific for aseptic loosening. The longer the components have been implanted, the more likely they are to be loose, but this is not a guarantee. Some patients presenting relatively soon after knee replacement will have loose components and some presenting several years later will not. Most describe an ill-defined ache that seems to be worse with activity. Others will say that their pain is worse when getting up after sitting or resting for a period of time. Almost all describe the pain as diffuse and not well localized to one side or the other of the knee. Usually the pain is insidious in onset and has been present for several weeks to months.

The examination of a patient with aseptic loosening can vary from normal to grossly abnormal. The majority of patients will have some effusion. The irritation of a loose component will generally cause a proliferation of the synovium surrounding the joint. This proliferation leads to increased fluid production and subsequent swelling. The inflamed synovium is also a likely cause of the pain with which patients present. There may or may not be instability on exam. However, most patients will note a decreased range of motion from before they had symptoms. An important part of the examination of any patient presenting with knee replacement pain is the alignment of the knee. Patients will report their knee seems to "go in" more or they seem to be more "knock kneed." Some will say their knee seems to "give out" more that it used to. The presence of a clinical malalignment different from a previous alignment is nearly pathognomonic for loosening of some sort.

The most important part of the work-up for aseptic loosening of a knee replacement is to rule out infection. All patients presenting with pain after total knee replacement should be worked up for infection before exploration of any other cause is undertaken. The first step in this process should include evaluation of inflammatory markers including CRP and ESR. Any elevation in these markers should prompt an aspiration of the knee. The complete evaluation and diagnosis of an infected total knee is beyond the scope of this chapter. However, it should be emphasized again that making sure there is not an infection present is critical before a thorough evaluation for aseptic loosening.

A standard part of the work-up for knee pain after knee replacement is obtaining x-rays. Evaluating the fixation status of a total knee by x-ray alone can be difficult. Depending on the type of knee replacement used, as well as the manufacturer, the interface between the component and the bone-cement is often obscured. Components from a posterior stabilized system with a closed box make it difficult to see the femoral interface. In addition, a less-than-perfect lateral of the components will make seeing the interface impossible. As opposed to the femur, the tibial interface is generally well visualized. The presence of a continuous radiolucent line at either the femoral or tibial interface is strongly suggestive of a loose component. Unfortunately, this line is rarely seen.

The best radiographic indication of loosening is settling or change in alignment of one of the components (Figure 20-6). Occasionally, this change can be very subtle. Because of this reason, it is important to compare previous x-rays to current ones. Often a change in alignment will be seen without an obvious radiolucent line. This finding in combination with a convincing clinical picture is strongly suggestive of loosening. A bone scan (technetium) can be used to rule out loosening of an implant. If the scan is negative, then it is very unlikely that the implant is loose. However, positive bone scans in TKA are an extremely nonspecific test. An elevated scan can be seen with a normal knee, an infection, a loose implant, a knee with complex regional pain syndrome, and other pathology.

## Management

Once the diagnosis of aseptic loosening is relatively certain, revision knee arthroplasty is the only way to alleviate symptoms and return function to the patient. Several chapters could be written on the technical aspects of revision knee surgery, and a complete discussion is beyond the scope of this chapter. Although the details of revision arthroplasty are esoteric, the principles are straightforward. In fact, they are the same principles that apply to primary knee reconstruction and include restoration of the mechanical axis and joint line, equal flexion and extension gaps, and balanced collateral ligaments. However, unlike primary knee arthroplasty, revisions often present multiple challenges, including bone loss, ligament incompetence, and stiffness, among others.

In dealing with aseptic loosening, the old adage that an ounce of prevention is worth a pound of cure could well apply. Understanding the ways to prevent the early development of loosening is critical to avoiding this difficult-to-manage complication.

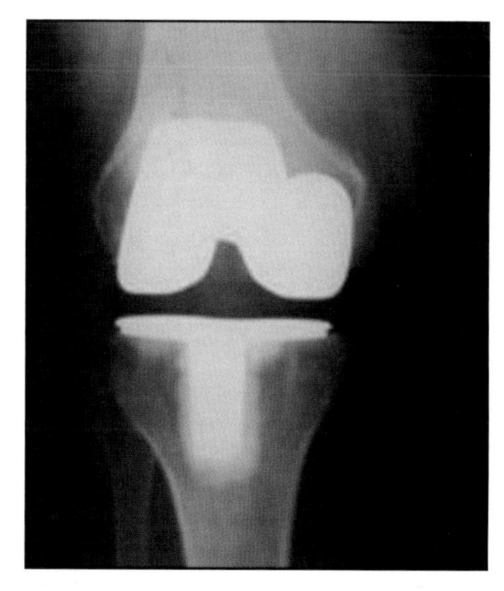

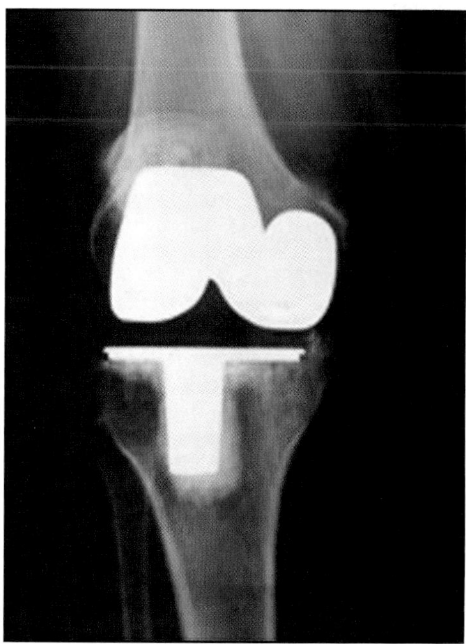

**Figure 20-6.** (A) X-ray of 54-year-old patient 1 year after right TKA. (B) 7 years postoperative x-ray of same knee. Note the surrounding osteolysis and increased varus of the tibial component.

## Summary

Our understanding of aseptic loosening of knee replacements continues to evolve. It is clear that there is not one cause of all loosening but rather a myriad of contributors. Of these, wear seems to be the most important factor. However, other lesser-known factors play a large role. In fact, there may still be more causes of loosening that we do not understand. As our knowledge of the causes of aseptic loosening increases, the numerous ways by which total knees can fail will become clearer. As the list of potential causes gets longer, the ways to prevent it will also increase. It may well be that we still do not completely understand the most important way to prevent aseptic loosening. Attention to minor details of the physical exam as well as radiographic findings can help make the diagnosis of aseptic loosening. Management of the loose knee is fraught with difficulty, but ultimately, revision knee arthroplasty is the only way to restore patient function. Failure rates after total knee replacement are already very low. The pursuit to decrease aseptic loosening promises less morbidity for patients. Ultimately, that is the goal of all medicine.

## References


1. Emmerson KP, Moran CG, Pinder IM. Survivorship analysis of the kinematic stabilizer total knee replacement: a 10-14 year follow-up. *J Bone Joint Surg Br.* 1996;78:441-445.
2. Rand JA, Ilstrup DM. Survivorship analysis of total knee arthroplasty: cumulative rates of survival of 9200 total knee arthroplasties. *J Bone Joint Surg Am.* 1991;73:397-409.
3. Sharkey PF, Hozack WM, Rothman RH, Shanstri S, Jacoby BA. Why are total knee arthroplasties failing today? *Clin Orthop Relat Res.* 2002;404:7-13.
4. Igenix: Data Analyst Group. Columbus, OH, Ingenix 1999.
5. Harris WH, Schiller AL, Scholler JM, Freiberg RA, Scott R. Extensive localized bone resorption in the femur following total hip replacement. *J Bone Joint Surg Am.* 1976;58:612-618.
6. Howie DW, Vernon-Roberts B, Oakeshott R, Manthey B. A rat model of resorption of bone at the cement-bone interface in the presence of polyethylene wear particles. *J Bone Joint Surg Am.* 1988;70:257-263.
7. Schmalzried TP, Jasty M, Harris WH. Periprosthetic bone loss in total hip arthroplasty: polyethylene wear debris and the concept of the effective joint space. *J Bone Joint Surg Am.* 1992;74:849-863.
8. Green TR, Fisher J, Stone M, Wroblewski BM, Ingham E. Polyethylene particles of a "critical size" are necessary for the induction of cytokines by macrophages in vitro. *Biomaterials.* 1998;19:2297-2302.
9. Schmalzried TP, Shepherd EF, Dorey FJ, et al. Wear is a function of use, not time. *Clin Orthop Relat Res.* 2000;381:36-46.
10. Collier MB, Engh CA Jr, McAuley JP, Engh GA. Factors associated with the loss of thickness of polyethylene tibial bearings after knee arthroplasty. *J Bone Joint Surg Am.* 2007;89:1306-1314.
11. Sochart DH. Relationship of acetabular wear to osteolysis and loosening in total hip arthroplasty. *Clin Orthop Relat Res.* 1999;363:135-150.
12. Schmalzried TM, Callaghan JJ. Wear in total hip and knee replacements. *J Bone Joint Surg Am.* 1999;81:115-136.
13. Naudie DDR, Ammeen DJ, Engh GA, Rorabeck CH. Wear and osteolysis around total knee arthroplasty. *J Am Acad Orthop Surg.* 2007;15:53-64.
14. Wasielewski RC, Parks N, Williams I, Surprenant H, Collier JP, Engh GA. Tibial insert undersurface as a contributing source of polyethylene wear debris. *Clin Orthop Relat Res.* 1997;345:53-59.
15. Won CH, Rohatgi S, Kraay MJ, Goldberg VM, Rimnac CM. Effect of resin type and manufacturing method on wear of polyethylene tibial components. *Clin Orthop Relat Res.* 2000;376:161-171.
16. Bartel DL, Bicknell VL, Wright TM. The effect of conformity, thickness, and material on stresses in ultra-high molecular weight components for total joint replacement. *J Bone Joint Surg Am.* 1986;68:1041-1051.
17. Collier JP, Sperling DK, Currier JH, Sutula LC, Saum KA, Mayor MB. Impact of gamma sterilization on clinical performance of polyethylene in the knee. *J Arthroplasty.* 1996;11:377-389.
18. McKellop H, Shen FW, Lu B, Campbell P, Salovey R. Development of an extremely wear-resistant ultra high molecular weight polyethylene for total hip replacements. *J Orthop Res.* 1999;17:157-167.
19. Puértolas JA, Medel FJ, Cegoñino J, Gomez-Barrena E, Ríos R. Influence of the remelting process on the fatigue behavior of electron beam irradiated UHMWPE. *J Biomed Mater Res B Appl Biomater.* 2006;76:346-353.
20. Sundfeldt M, Carlsson LV, Johansson CB, Thomsen P, Gretzer C. Aseptic loosening, not only a question of wear: a review of different theories. *Acta Orthopaedica.* 2006;77:177-197.
21. Malchua H, Herberts P, Soderman P, Oden A. Prognosis of total hip replacement. Presented at annual meeting of the American Academy of Orthopaedic Surgeons; March 17, 2000; Orlando, FL.

# 21

# Complex Primary Total Knee Arthroplasty

*Benjamin Bender, MD; Luis Pulido, MD; and Javad Parvizi, MD*

Patients with complex primary total knee arthroplasty (TKA) are patients with extra-articular deformity, post-traumatic arthrosis, neuropathic arthritis, severe varus or valgus knees, postosteotomy patients, or patient with medical comorbidities. In these complex primary cases, it can be a challenge to restore the mechanical axis, to balance the periarticular soft tissues, and to accurately position the individual prosthetic components. The patients with medical comorbidities can present another challenge. Treatment of the complex primary TKA often requires modification of the surgical approach, technique, or prosthesis to appropriately perform TKA and optimize outcome.

## Extra-Articular Varus or Valgus Deformity

Osteoarthritis with an extra-articular deformity of the knee is defined by an arthritic process of the knee with an extra-articular varus or valgus deformity. Usually, these patients have intact joint space kinematics and stable collateral ligaments. This type of knee deformity usually occurs after an overcorrected tibial osteotomy, a tibial fracture malunion, or a congenital deformity of the tibia. Although more rare, the deformity may be located in the femur. Causes of femoral deformity may be fracture nonunion or malunion, previous osteotomy, or a metabolic disease (eg, rickets, osteomalacia, Paget's disease).

Restoration of limb alignment during TKA normalizes the distribution of forces across the knee and the implant, therefore enhancing implant survival and performance. An extra-articular, extra-ligamentous deformity may not be amenable to routine techniques of intra-articular bone resection and ligamentous balancing. In such situations, the treatment alternatives include adjustment of resurfacing cuts with ligamentous release or advancement or corrective extra-articular osteotomy in conjunction with, or staged with, TKA. Fixed angular deformities and contractures need to be released at the time of surgery either through soft tissue or bony maneuvers. The stiff knee can present a challenge for exposure alone. Any knee with gross ligamentous instability, particularly in the medial-lateral plane, may need to have specially stabilized components or ligamentous augmentation for a successful procedure.

Previous incisions performed for prior medial or lateral meniscectomy, which are either oblique or behind the midline, as well as cross transverse incisions for patellectomy or high tibial osteotomy at 90 degrees can be ignored. Parapatellar incisions in the line of the main incision should be included if useful. The most lateral longitudinal incision should be used if it will allow adequate access to the knee for arthroplasty. If a longitudinal incision is placed too close to a longitudinal scar from a previous surgery, the skin between these 2 incisions may necrose from disruption of the vascular supply. Special consideration should be given to patients with local skin problems such as psoriasis to reduce the risk of infection.

Patients may present late for surgery with severe deformity because of a combination of several factors. These include ignorance, fear of surgery, access to alternative



Parvizi J, Klatt B.
*Essentials in Total Knee Arthroplasty* (pp 175-186).

medicine, and the high cost of treatment. Patients with a severe knee axis deformity tend to have increased posterior knee instability. Insufficient correction of the axis is more common in a severe axis deviation and is usually associated with a poor clinical outcome. The management of a tibial bone defect with bone, cement, or metal wedges gives rise to further problems. Ligamentous stability can be achieved in the majority of difficult knee arthroplasties with attention to proper extremity alignment, proper prosthesis positioning, careful balancing of the extension and flexion spaces, and use of a posterior stabilized knee design.

Correction of large axis deformities by a wide soft tissue release and large bony reconstruction leads to collateral ligament destabilization and subsequent knee instability. An unconstrained TKA can be used without a soft tissue release but with an addition of tibial osteotomy to preserve the collateral ligaments and to correct the axis deviation. This modality of treatment was recommended by several authors as an alternative method of correction of extra-articular deformity of > 15 degrees varus or valgus.

In the presence of extra-articular deformity of 10 degrees or more in the coronal plane or 20 degrees or more in the sagittal plane, complex imbalance of the collateral ligaments may result when the deformity is addressed solely with modified intra-articular bone resection and soft-tissue releases. To limit such ligament imbalance and to reduce the need for constrained implants, these patients can be treated with simultaneous or staged femoral osteotomy and resurfacing knee arthroplasty. The femoral osteotomy site should be secured with a plate or a locked intramedullary nail, depending on the location of the deformity and the subsequent osteotomy. A different technique for correction of the deformity with intramedullary nail combined with TKA was also described. Retrograde nailing of the femoral osteotomy or femoral nonunion was completed first. Once proper alignment and fixation were achieved, a custom-made rod extension was screwed into the threaded portion of the distal nail. The rod extension served as the intramedullary alignment guide for the distal femoral jig of the knee prosthesis system. TKA was performed using standard instruments and technique.

The preferred technique of Insall was the subject of a report to treat a series of deformities that were associated with arthrosis of the knee. Deformities were adequately addressed with modified intra-articular bone resection and ligament balancing, obviating the need for additional osteotomy. Coronal plane deformities averaged 14 degrees (range, 5 to 22 degrees), and sagittal plane deformities averaged 12 degrees (range, 0 to 38 degrees). The authors reported marked improvement in scores, according to the system of The Hospital for Special Surgery after a minimum of 2 years of follow-up; however, there were radiolucent lines in 3 knees. None of the lines were considered progressive and only one knee required a revision because of failure of a metal-backed patellar component. This technique may be reasonable if the function and balance of the collateral ligaments are not compromised. The risk with this technique is that it may alter joint-line position and the femoral component may not always rest flush on the cut bone surfaces. Oblique gaps left between the prosthesis and the bone on the concavity side of the deformity may need to be filled with polymethylmethacrylate (PMMA), structural bone graft, or wedges. The theoretical concerns in such cases are that structural support may be insufficient and oblique shear forces may make the bone-cement interfaces vulnerable to early demarcation and perhaps lead to long-term failure.

## Varus Deformity

Severe preoperative deformities have long been a challenge for surgeons performing TKA. Returning the knee alignment to an angular anatomic norm of 5 degrees valgus may be difficult and may require intraoperative ligament releases and/or ligament tensioning to achieve proper ligament balance.

Mild to moderate varus deformity of the knee is frequently encountered in primary TKA. Varus deformity in osteoarthritis of the knee is associated with significant rotational deformity. The tibia tends to locate in an externally rotated position in the knees with severe varus deformity. Some of the axes used as a reference during the assessment of the femoral rotation are not reliable during advance arthritic changes; for example, the posterior condyles can be affected by the arthritic changes and thus can lead to an incorrect measurement. Femorotibial rotation is difficult to quantify even on computed tomography (CT) scans because of the intrinsic uncertainty of the reference line for each bone. The pathomechanism of this rotational deformity has not been elucidated although impingement of the anterior cruciate ligament (ACL) and subsequent insufficiency may be important. CT assessment of the knee prior to surgery may be used to determine appropriate rotational alignment in TKA, such as the relationship between varus deformity and rotational deformity in knees with OA.

Sacrificing the posterior cruciate ligament (PCL) and using a PCL-substituting prosthesis for the correction of a severe varus deformity is widely accepted, it is associated with better postoperative alignment, flexion, and residual flexion contracture using when compared to a

PCL-retaining prosthesis. Insall et al's technique for correction of varus deformity by progressively releasing the medial soft tissues until they equal the length of the lateral ligamentous structures is widely used.[1] However, in severe varus deformity with a tibiofemoral angle of more than 15 degrees, this may require releasing of the superficial medial collateral ligament, the semimembranosus, the posteromedial capsule, and the pes tendons, leaving the medial side barren. This extensive direct medial soft tissue release increases the likelihood of overcorrection and may necessitate use of a thicker polyethylene insert or even a more-constrained prosthesis. To overcome this problem, a technique using downsizing and lateralizing the tibial component and removing the exposed medial proximal tibial bone has been proposed. This technique increases the length of the medial ligamentous structures by shortening the distance between their origin and insertion without the need for an extensive medial soft tissue release. The same concept can be applied if the tibia is between sizes. The smaller size is used and shifted laterally to allow the uncapped medial bone to be resected. With this technique, the PCL can be retained whenever present with excellent clinical and radiographic midterm results. Preoperative alignment has no impact on the outcome of TKA at intermediate follow-up times.

The results of treating severe intra- and extra-articular varus deformity to restore alignment and stability without the need for constrained implants using posterior stabilized fixed-bearing implants with selective posteromedial release and reduction osteotomy of posteromedial tibial flare was also reported. Proximal tibial osteotomy was used to correct severe extra-articular deformity. A total of 86% knees were in 4 to 10 degrees valgus postoperatively. Mean Knee Society score improved from 22.8 to 91.1, and function score from 22.8 to 72.1 at 2 to 9 years. Twenty-eight of 30 bone grafts for tibial defects were successfully incorporated. No significant instability was noted postoperatively. Three knees out of 171 showed tibial component loosening. Theoretical disadvantage of reduction osteotomy is potential weakening of the posteromedial cortex. When substantial bone is removed, it is prudent to use a metal-back component and a tibial stem extender to prevent overloading of the posteromedial tibial bone.

Significant bone defect on the posterior part of the medial tibial condyle usually accompanies severe varus deformity. Many methods have been reported to address this problem. Among these are cement filling for defects that are smaller than 1 cm, bone grafts, and often used metallic augmentation for defects that are larger than 1 cm. Another method consists of producing a step-cut defect, the horizontal floor of which is gently sloping downward on the lateral side (to lock the graft in place). After removal of sclerotic and avascular bone (using a burr or gouge) from the floor and sidewalls of the defect, autologous resected bone usually from the intercondylar notch is fashioned to fit snugly into the defect, it is impacted into place. When the tibial component is placed on it, the sloping floor ensures that the graft is locked in place. This obviates the need for any fixation and also places the graft under a compressive force, which is more suitable for graft incorporation.

## Valgus Deformity

About 17% of patients undergoing TKA have valgus knee deformity characterized by specific bone and soft tissue changes. Valgus knee is encountered in patients with hypoplasia of the lateral condyle, which is often seen in post-traumatic injury to the knee, rheumatoid patients, and in patients with developmental dysplasia of the hip (DDH). Bone changes include lateral femoral condyle hypoplasia and erosion in its distal and posterior aspect. Furthermore, femoral as well as tibial diaphyseal bowing can be present, making the proper component alignment more demanding to achieve. Soft tissue abnormalities often include laxity of the medial structures and retraction of the lateral and posterior structures (usually more evident in extension) as well as the lateral retinaculum. Precise ligament balancing is mandatory to obtain equal and symmetric flexion and extension gaps. Posterior cruciate ligament substitution has been advocated for severe deformities; particularly in valgus arthritic knees in which the posterior cruciate is part of the deformity and its secondary varus rotation restraining effect would increase valgus recurrence. Lateral retinaculum tightness results in lateral patellar subluxation, erosion, and maltracking. The combination of these features makes valgus deformity challenging to correct, and different strategies in terms of approach, bone cuts, soft tissue management, and implant type have been proposed. Extensive releases of the lateral structures were introduced in the 1980s and presented the risk of complications, including lateral condyle avascularity and residual lateral instability.

Lateral structures have relative contribution to varus stability. The iliotibial band and the posterolateral capsule restrain varus rotation mainly in extension and are less effective in flexion. The lateral collateral ligament has a major stabilizing effect in extension but acts as a varus stabilizer in flexion as well. Popliteus tendon cutting affects mainly flexion stability with minimal effects in extension. When the cumulative effect of sequential releases is investigated, a major increase in varus opening occurs in flexion when the popliteus tendon is excised.

Several authors have recently introduced more conservative selective releases. One of the methods described in the literature is a "pie-crusting" multiple-puncture technique, which has the distinguishing feature of being a gradual release of the tight structures under maximal extension space distraction using laminar spreaders until gap symmetry is achieved. Selective release of the tight lateral structures (pie-crusting technique), and of the lateral retinaculum in cases of patellar maltracking, obtains and maintains correction of the frontal plane deformity, restores patellar tracking and function, and avoids the complications of the extensive releases, including lateral condyle avascularity and residual lateral instability. Transient postoperative peroneal nerve was observed in one patient out of 48. In 96% of patients, alignment was achieved within 5 degrees from neutral. No component was revised. The pie-crusting technique reliably corrects moderate to severe fixed valgus deformities with a low complication rate and reasonable midterm results. The multiple punctures allow gradual stretching of the lateral soft tissues and preservation of the popliteus tendon, reducing the risk of posterolateral instability. A lesion of the peroneal nerve after severe valgus deformities and tibial osteotomies is thought to occur in 0% to 11%, and extra-articular correction of the deformity is thought to reduce the stress put on the peroneal nerve and thus cause less peroneal injury.

## Severe Ligamentous Laxity and Massive Bone Loss

TKA associated with severe ligamentous laxity or massive loss remains a significant challenge. Condylar constrained total knee prostheses provide an acceptable solution for revision and complex primary total knee replacements (TKRs) when there is partial compromise of the collateral ligament(s) or an inability to achieve satisfactory stability of the flexion space. Current indications for use of hinged knee prosthesis, excluding the resection of malignant neoplasms about the knee, include AP instability with a very large flexion gap, complete absence of the collateral ligaments, and complete absence of a functioning extensor mechanism. Severe bone loss and ligamentous insufficiency may be encountered during complex primary or revision TKA because of various etiologic factors. The treatment of severe bone deficiency without ligamentous insufficiency can be addressed successfully with the use of allograft-prosthetic constructs using standard knee prostheses. Hinged knee designs occasionally are necessary as salvage procedures for patients with low physical demands who have severe ligamentous insufficiency but should not be used purely for the treatment of bone loss. Modular and segmental replacement allows for maintenance of motion and functional restoration. Alternative options include reconstruction with a large segmental allograft, arthrodesis, or amputation. Massive allografts have 75% to 77% success rate. In one study with middle- to long-term results using structural allograft for uncontained defects in 52 knees, 13 were failures, defined as an increase in the Hospital for Special Surgery knee scores by less than 20 points or reoperation. Twenty-three percent of knees required revision. Allograft survival was 93% at 5 years and 72% at 10 years.

Patients with massive bone loss or ligamentous instability or both with non-neoplastic disorders may require a linked articulated implant to maintain skeletal continuity. Prosthetic knee designs with articular constraint typically are used to restore knee stability. The high failure rates of fixed hinged knee designs, attributed to high transmission forces at the bone-cement interface, lead to the development of rotating hinge implant designs. The rotational freedom of these rotating hinge designs theoretically reduces the joint forces and moments by allowing soft tissue and muscular structures to absorb energy. Although the primary indication for this prosthetic design (modular and segmental replacement) has been for reconstruction of the distal femur or proximal tibia after skeletal resection of malignancy, it has also been used for complex primary or salvage revision knee arthroplasty. Rotating hinge implant designs have been associated with 16% rate of deep infection, 22% rate of patellar instability, and a 6% rate of implant breakage. Massive exposure, long operative time, multiple comorbidities, and compromised soft tissue all lead to an increased risk of postoperative infection. Patients treated with a hinged knee prosthesis after a previous infection seem to be at higher risk than patients who have revision surgery for other indications. It is recommended that implants of this kind be used only in knees with functional absence of a collateral ligament that cannot be treated by soft tissue reconstruction. Previous studies using a rotating hinge design have shown variable results. One study on a series of 38 knees found a 90% satisfaction result for primary and 83% satisfaction result for revision arthroplasty with a minimum of 25 months follow-up. However, another study on 50 standard Kinematic Rotating Hinge prostheses concluded that the results were not significantly improved over those for the older hinge-type implants. Only 80% of primary surgeries and 74% of revision surgeries had satisfactory results.

## Total Knee Arthroplasty in Young Active Patients

Arthritic disease in active, younger patients (≤ 55 years) is not uncommon and its prevalence is expected to increase. The application of knee arthroplasty to a younger, more active population was initially discouraged out of concern for accelerated failure rates due to component loosening, polyethylene wear, and the presumed difficulty in performing subsequent revision surgery due to bone loss as well as the increased complications seen in revision TKA. However, delaying knee arthroplasty indefinitely in the younger patient with marked pain and restricted function appears to lead to worse outcomes. Operative options for the younger patient with an arthritic knee remain controversial. A number of surgical options for the arthritic knee exist for these patients. Arthroscopic débridement, realignment osteotomy, and arthrodesis are all surgical options that have been proposed for this difficult problem. These techniques are addressed in Chapter 5. Many of these treatments, however, provide only short-term relief of symptoms or compromise function. More recently, there has been a trend of offering knee arthroplasty as an option to provide pain relief and improve function in the active, younger patient with knee osteoarthritis. Several studies suggest that knee arthroplasty in younger patients is a reasonable option. Many authors have reported their series of TKA in younger patients and the results have been quite acceptable at intermediate follow-up, with survival ranging from 87% to 96.5% at 8 to 20 years. The longevity of total knees in young patients with rheumatoid arthritis has been reported to be excellent; one study reported long-term results in 32 patients (47 knees) younger than 55 years with rheumatoid arthritis, and these patients had a survival rate of 93.7% at 20 years. Another study reported on the long-term survivorship of cemented TKA in 52 young patients, where average follow-up was 12 years (range 10 to 15 years). Fifteen percent (8 patients) were revised, 2 revisions (one for sepsis and one for instability) were before 10 years, and all were associated with polyethylene wear and osteolysis. Implant survival rate was estimated to be 96% at 10 years and 85% at 15 years of follow-up.

Some studies suggest cementless fixation with current techniques results in a lower migration rate after 5 years and fewer radiolucent lines than are found in cemented TKA. Augmentation of fixation with peripheral tibial screws is considered important for immediate fixation, biomechanical studies demonstrate less micromotion when screws are used, and fewer radiolucent lines under those components that were fixed with 4 screws than in identical implants fixed without screws was also documented. A study with cementless TKA using a total knee system designed for porous-ingrowth fixation showed that young, heavy patients fare as well as older, lightweight patients when this implant is used with the osteointegration technique. Patients younger than 55 years and whose weight was greater than 90 kg were compared with gender-matched patients who were 65 years of age or older and who weighed less than 80 kg. The mean Knee Society scores and pain scores were similar for both groups. Function scores were better for the young, heavy patients. None of the knees in either group loosened.

A prospective review of 1047 patients 55 years old or younger who underwent knee arthroplasty in a community joint registry over a 14-year period showed that 85% of cemented TKA implants survived at 14 years in the population under 55 years of age (mean 49.8 years) in this specific community registry. Cementless designs and unicondylar knee arthroplasty (UKA) increased revision risk independently. Patients were implanted with 1047 joints of 3 predominant designs by 48 surgeons in 4 hospitals associated with a community joint registry. There were a total of 73 revisions performed: 5.6% (37/653) in women and 9.2% (36/394) in men. Cemented TKAs performed best, with a cumulative revision rate of 15.5%, compared to 32.3% in UKA patients and 34.1% in cementless designs. Men had a higher cumulative revision rate than women: 31.9% compared to 20.6%. Adjusting for implant type and gender, there was no difference in cumulative revision rate based on diagnosis (OA versus other) or age group or between cruciate-retaining and cruciate-substituting designs.

The choice to continue with TKA in the younger patient is a difficult one. Nonoperative management should be tried first (physical therapy and modification of activities to limit those that involve impact and anti-inflammatory medications), and more conservative operative management such as proximal tibial osteotomy may be considered in patients with unicompartmental disease and malalignment, mainly in those patients with high demand activities. Appropriate patient selection for high tibial osteotomy (HTO) is mandatory since patient satisfaction after HTO tends to decline over time (Table 21-1). Patients who have undergone this procedure before TKA may be at higher risk of complications with subsequent arthroplasty.

## Total Knee Arthroplasty Following Osteotomy

In general, varus deformity is corrected with a closing wedge osteotomy, which can correct to about 9 to 10 degrees of valgus. Severe varus deformity >15 degrees can be

Table 21-1

**CONTRAINDICATION TO HIGH TIBIAL OSTEOTOMY**

| *ABSOLUTE CONTRAINDICATION TO HIGH TIBIAL OSTEOTOMY* |
|---|
| • Inflammatory arthritis (rheumatoid, crystalline deposition, inflammatory) |
| • Tricompartmental arthritis |
| • Flexion arc < 90 degrees |
| • Previous meniscectomy in the contralateral compartment |
| • Flexion contracture > 10 degrees |
| *RELATIVE CONTRAINDICATION TO HIGH TIBIAL OSTEOTOMY* |
| • Age > 60 |
| • Patellofemoral arthritis |
| • Collateral ligament insufficiency (MCL, LCL) |
| • ACL insufficiency |
| • Medial bone loss > 1 cm |
| • Correction needed > 20 degrees |

Table 21-2

**INDICATIONS FOR POSTERIOR STABILIZED TOTAL KNEE PROSTHESIS**

- Patellectomy
- High tibial osteotomy
- Severe angular deformity (varus, valgus > 15 degrees)
- Rheumatoid arthritis
- Fixed flexion > 20 degrees

corrected with proximal dome osteotomy, maintaining the joint line and minimizing the amount of bone resected. Valgus deformity can be corrected with medial proximal tibial closing wedge osteotomy; this procedure in more severe deformities can lead to joint line obliquity and tibiofemoral subluxation. That is the reason why severe valgus deformity with lateral unicompartmental involvement is addressed with distal femoral medial closing wedge osteotomy, which allows for correction to about 2 degrees of valgus. TKA following femoral or tibial osteotomy can be challenging.

## Prior High Tibial Osteotomy

HTO is often used for the treatment of unicompartmental osteoarthritis of the knee, typically as a time-buying procedure to delay eventual TKA. Patient selection is crucial for the success of a HTO, and the surgeon should be familiar with the indications and the contraindications for this procedure (see Table 21-1). The patient satisfaction rate following HTO decreases over the years, 73% to 95% of patients at 5 years after surgery report good outcome, whereas only 30% to 46% report the same outcome 10 years following surgery. Causes of failure of HTO are primarily undercorrection with subsequent return of deformity and progressive arthritis in the unaffected compartment. Although HTO one time was thought to bear no effect on the outcome of eventual TKA, multiple studies have demonstrated less favorable outcomes after HTO, in addition to expected surgical challenges. There are reports of lower total knee scores for patients with HTO prior to TKA when compared with similar patients without prior osteotomy, and decreased postoperative ranges of motion. Patella infera, a known complication of HTO, is correlated with a poor clinical outcome. Patella infera is believed to be a consequence of the osteotomy surgery and subsequent immobilization in a long leg cast. Technical difficulties of TKA in patients with prior HTO result from patella infera, periarticular scarring, preoperative malalignment because of undercorrection or overcorrection, proximal tibial bone deficiency, and retained hardware. Other have studied TKA after HTO and found no difference in postoperative knee function or complications when compared with primary TKA without previous osteotomy. More favorable results in these studies may be attributed to lesser degrees of pre-TKA deformity. Surgical challenges following HTO include skin incisions. Although transverse skin incisions may be ignored, lateral longitudinal skin incisions must be respected and an adequate intervening skin bridge of at least 7 cm must be left between the 2 incision sights. Also, scarring over the lateral compartment and infrapatellar region may be encountered, making patellar eversion and lateral compartment exposure more difficult. Lateral retinacular release, quad snip, V-Y quadricepsplasty, or a tibial tubercle osteotomy may be necessary for exposure. Medial subperiosteal exposure must also be carefully performed to maintain the continuous soft tissue sleeve necessary for closure and medial soft-tissue stability. It is likely that technical difficulties with exposure led to suboptimal component positioning, soft-tissue balancing, and limb alignment. Because ligamentous balancing may be difficult, a PCL-substituting prosthesis is routinely used (Table 21-2). Another common problem after previous HTO is the medial offset of the intramedullary canal of the tibia relative to the center of the tibial tray. Extramedullary alignment usually is advocated in this situation, and medialization of the tibial tray or an offset tibial stem may also be needed to accommodate the deformity. Rotational deformity also may be encountered with previous HTO, because the proximal fragment may be rotated relative to the tibial shaft. The tibial tray must be inserted carefully to avoid internal rotation and subsequent patellar tracking problems. A study reported on the long-term clinical and radiographic outcome of TKA in patients who had undergone a previous proximal tibial osteotomy to identify the risk factors that may result in an inferior outcome. One hundred sixty-six cemented condylar total knee prostheses were implanted in 118 patients who had a previous proximal tibial osteotomy for the treatment of osteoarthritis. The average interval between the osteotomy and the TKA was 8.6 years. The mean Knee Society pain score improved from 34.5 to 82.9 points, and the mean function score improved from 44.6 to 88.1 points. There was also a substantial improvement in the mean arc of motion. Thirteen knees (8%) were revised at a mean of 5.9 years. At the time of the final follow-up, progressive complete radiolucent lines indicating a loose prosthesis were present around 17 tibial components and 7 femoral components. The authors concluded their study by stating that there was a very high rate of radiographic evidence of loosening in this patient population as compared with knees without previous tibial osteotomy. Male gender, increased weight, young age at the time of TKA, coronal laxity, patella baja (extensor mechanism maltracking), and preoperative limb malalignment were identified as risk factors for early failure. Despite these findings, TKA can provide reliable and durable pain relief and improvement in function for patients who have had a previous proximal tibial osteotomy.

## Prior Varus Femoral Osteotomy

The reports of TKA following femoral osteotomy are sparse in the literature. Varus distal femoral osteotomy is an entirely different procedure from proximal tibial osteotomy. Rigid internal fixation is nearly always employed during varus distal femoral osteotomy, and patella infera has not been reported as a consequence of this procedure. TKA following distal femoral varus osteotomy addresses pain and knee function, but the procedure is technically challenging and is associated with inferior results when compared with those of primary arthroplasty performed in a patient without a prior femoral osteotomy. Understanding the effects of a previous distal femoral varus osteotomy on the knee is critical to the surgical decision making. The extra-articular varus deformity of the femur following varus distal femoral osteotomy often results in a situation in which the femoral anatomical axis intersects the lateral femoral condyle rather than the intercondylar notch. Therefore, when intramedullary alignment is used, the starting hole should be placed where the femoral anatomic axis intersects the distal part of the femur at the knee. The use of an intramedullary femoral alignment guide increases the tendency to place the femoral component in relative varus angulation (in < 5 degrees of valgus). Therefore, in knees with previous distal femoral varus osteotomy, it is better to access the alignment of the femoral component with an extramedullary guide. Following distal femoral osteotomy, intra-articular correction during TKA may lead to ligamentous instability, which may in some cases not be correctable with ligament releases. Careful preoperative templating and determination of the appropriate location of the starting hole when using an intramedullary guide is significant for obtaining best femoral alignment in these cases. The other option is to use extramedullary femoral alignment. Whether intramedullary or extramedullary alignment guides are used for positioning of the cutting blocks, an extramedullary assessment of alignment with localization of the femoral head should be performed prior to distal femoral resection in an effort to obtain optimal coronal alignment. The extra-articular deformity that results from distal femoral osteotomy presents additional problems. To create a neutral mechanical axis (an axis through the center of the hip, knee, and ankle joints in the coronal plane) in a patient who has a varus extra-articular deformity, resection of relatively more bone from the distal aspect of the lateral femoral condyle than from the distal aspect of the medial femoral condyle is often necessary. This is opposite to the typical surgical preparation. As a consequence, lateral ligamentous instability that is not correctable with the use of standard medial releases may result, thus there is a frequent need to use constrained condylar knee prostheses. Despite the technical difficulties encountered during TKA following varus distal femoral osteotomy, the results were reported to be good to excellent for 7 of the 11 knees in one study. In the same study, 4 patients (4 knees) who had a fair result had only mild pain but had additional problems due either to malalignment or instability. In another study, 8 cases of TKR following supracondylar varus femoral osteotomy were reviewed. The distal femur was offset medially on the femoral diaphysis, the outcome was excellent and it was measured both by the clinical result as well as by the alignment.

In summary, malposition rate is relatively high in patients undergoing TKR after distal femoral osteotomy, the procedure is technically challenging, and the results are not as good as reported for primary knee arthroplasty and for knee arthroplasty after proximal tibial osteotomy

# Previous Patellectomy

Most patients following TKA after patellectomy report persistent pain and functional disability because of quadriceps weakness. The type of prosthesis that is most advantageous in this setting was earlier debated. The results of TKA after patellectomy in patients treated with PCL-retaining and PCL-substituting prostheses were compared in one study, with a control group of TKA patients without previous patellectomy. Knee Society scores at 5 years averaged 89 for the PCL-substituting knees and 67 for the PCL-retaining knees. Twelve of 13 PCL-retaining knees demonstrated more than 1 cm of anteroposterior instability in 90 degrees of flexion compared with only 1 of 9 PCL-substituting knees. The 4-bar linkage of the quadriceps tendon, the patellar tendon, and the cruciate ligaments is disrupted by patellectomy, and the PCL and posterior capsule are incapable of maintaining long-term sagittal plane stability. PCL-substituting prostheses are currently recommended for these patients (see Table 21-2). Patients with multiple previous knee surgeries may experience less reliable pain relief with TKA.

## Neuropathic Arthropathy

Although neuropathic arthropathy generally is considered a relative contraindication to TKA, reasonable outcomes have been reported following arthroplasty for Charcot arthropathy. Neuropathic arthropathy, or Charcot joint as it is better known, is a progressive degenerative disease of the joint that may lead to severe deformity and dysfunction. The exact pathomechanism for this disease is not known. The attenuation or lack of nociception resulting in poor joint protection and unnoticed microtrauma is believed to be responsible for development of bone destruction and attenuation of ligaments. Charcot arthropathy can be caused by any condition causing sensory or autonomic neuropathy. The number one cause in the United States is diabetic neuropathy. Some other causes are alcohol, intra-articular steroid injections, tabes dorsalis, spinal cord injury, syringomyelia, and leprosy. The reported results regarding arthroplasty in neuropathic patients have been diverse, with some studies showing encouraging outcomes whereas another study argued against TKA in patients with a Charcot joint because of a high complication and failure rate. A recent study of 40 modern design condylar total knee arthroplasties in 29 patients, with a follow-up averaged 7.9 years (range, 2 to 15 years) for clinical and 6.4 years (range, 2 to 15) for radiographic surveillance, showed significant improvement in Knee Society pain and function scores and range of motion after knee arthroplasty. Extensive bone fragmentation and bone defect were present in 38 knees (95%). Metal wedge augments (10 knees, 8 patients), autologous bone grafting (17 knees, 13 patients), and bone allografts (2 knees, 2 patients) were used to reinforce the bony defects. Ligamentous instability necessitated the use of long-stem components in 27 knees and rotating hinge prostheses in 5 knees. There were 6 reoperations for periprosthetic fracture (2 knees, 2 patients), aseptic loosening (2 knees, 2 patients), instability (1 knee, 1 patient), and deep infection (1 knee, 1 patient). The markedly improved outcome of patients with neuropathy is contributed to the modification in surgical techniques, medical treatment, and anesthesia care of the patients and the introduction of condylar design prostheses with the fact that the incidence of neurosyphilis has been declining.

In general, TKA may be offered to a select group of patients with end-stage neuropathic arthropathy. In this specific group of patients, the basic principles of knee arthroplasty in restoring limb alignment, reinforcing bony defects by bone grafting or augmented prostheses, careful ligamentous balancing, and appropriate selection of constrained prostheses particularly are of great importance. The technical challenges encountered during TKA in patients with neuropathic arthropathy usually are reserved for complex revision arthroplasty. The outcome of TKA in patients with end-stage Charcot joint, although somewhat inferior, is not significantly different to the results of arthroplasty in other patients particularly because of the degree of destruction and deformity encountered in Charcot joints.

## Total Knee Arthroplasty in Hemophilic Patients

Knee arthroplasty can relieve pain and restore alignment in patients with hemophilic arthropathy, but restoration of motion is suboptimal and the risk of perioperative complications is significant. Perioperative complications include hemorrhage, superficial skin necrosis, nerve palsies, deep infection, and progressive radiolucencies in the tibia. Perioperative factor VIII level of $< 80\%$ has a greater probability of complications and in the patient undergoing TKA, the perioperative factor VIII level should be maintained at 100%. A hematologist should be consulted for perioperative care to make certain that the factor is properly dosed. Several patients with hemophilic arthropathy have been infected with human immunodeficiency virus (HIV) contracted from contaminated transfusions of coagulation factors. HIV-infected hemophiliac patients with an average CD4 lymphocyte count of 463 cells/μL had no infections and 88% good or excellent results. However, for HIV-infected hemophiliac patients with CD4 lymphocyte counts of less than 200 mm,[3] 30% were complicated by postoperative infection.

Despite the anatomical challenges, the mechanical survival of TKRs in patients with hemophilia is quite good. However, the prevalence of infection after the TKRs is high. The prevention of late infection would substantially improve the long-term outcome of TKRs in this patient population.

## Total Knee Arthroplasty in Diabetic Patients

TKA in diabetic patients results in an increased wound complication rate (up to 12%), increased infection rate (up to 7%), and frequent revisions (up to 7%). The rate of deep joint infections in diabetic patients is statistically higher than the reported incidence of sepsis in nondiabetic patients. Strict control of serum glucose levels seems to reduce perioperative complications for diabetic patients. Nineteen percent of the diabetic patients in one study were found to have unsatisfactory outcomes compared with 4% of the control group. Diabetes mellitus and advanced age are risk factors for admission to a rehabilitation facility after total joint arthroplasty; muscle weakness or peripheral neuropathy associated with diabetes could account for this association. As mentioned previously, diabetes is the number one reason for Charcot arthropathy in the Unites States. Utmost safety measures should be in use for diabetic patients having TKA to minimize both wound complications and joint sepsis.

## References

1. Insall JN, Binazzi R, Soundry M, Mestriner LA. Total knee arthroplasty. *Clin Orthop.* 1985;192:13.

## Bibliography

### Extra-Articular Deformity

Incavo SJ, Kapadia C, Torney R. Use of an intramedullary nail for correction of femoral deformities combined with total knee arthroplasty: a technical tip. *J Arthroplasty.* 2007;22(1):133-135.

Karachalios T, Sarangi PP, Newman JH. Severe varus and valgus deformities treated by total knee arthroplasty. *J Bone Joint Surg Br.* 1994;76:938.

Krackow KA, Holtgrewe JL. Experience with a new technique for managing severely overcorrected valgus high tibial osteotomy at total knee arthroplasty. *Clin Orthop.* 1990;258:213.

Lonner JH, Siliski JM, et al. Simultaneous femoral osteotomy and total knee arthroplasty for treatment of osteoarthritis associated with severe extra-articular deformity. *J Bone Joint Surg.* 2000;82A:342.

Mann JW III, Insall JN, Scuderi GR. Total knee arthroplasty in patients with associated extra-articular angular deformity. *Orthop Trans.* 1997;21:59.

Uchinou S, Yano H, Shimizu K, Masumi S. A severely overcorrected high tibial osteotomy: revision by osteotomy and a long stem component. *Acta Orthop Scand.* 1996;67:193.

Whiteside LA. Correction of ligament and bone defects in total arthroplasty of the severely valgus knee. *Clin Orthop Relat Res.* 1993;(288):234-245.

### Varus Deformity

Aglietti P, Buzzi R, Baldini A, Lup D, De Luca L. Comparison of mobile-bearing and fixed-bearing total knee arthroplasty: a prospective randomized study. *J Arthroplasty.* 2005;20:145-153.

Aglietti P, Lup D, Cuomo P, Baldini A, De Luca L. Total knee arthroplasty using a pie-crusting technique for valgus deformity. *Clin Orthop Relat Res.* 2007;464:73-77.

Dixon MC, Parsch D, Brown RR, Scott RD. The correction of severe varus deformity in total knee arthroplasty by tibial component downsizing and resection of uncapped proximal medial bone. *J Arthroplasty.* 2004;19(1):19-22.

Faris PM, Herbst SA, Ritter MA, Keating EM. The effect of preoperative knee deformity on the initial results of cruciate-retaining total knee arthroplasty. *J Arthroplasty.* 1992;7:527.

Karachalios T, Sarangi PP, Newman JH. Severe varus and valgus deformities treated by total knee arthroplasty. *J Bone Joint Surg Br.* 1994;76:938.

Laskin RS. Total knee replacement with posterior cruciate ligament retention in patients with a fixed varus deformity. *Clin Orthop.* 1996;331:29.

Laskin RS, Rieger M, Schob C, Turen C. The posterior stabilized total knee prosthesis in the knee with a severe fixed deformity. *Am J Knee Surg.* 1988;1:199.

Matsuda Y, Ishii Y, Noguchi H, Ishii R. Varus-valgus balance and range of movement after total knee arthroplasty. *J Bone Joint Surg Br.* 2005;87:804-808.

Matsui Y, Kadoya Y, Uehara K, Kobayashi A, Takaoka K. Rotational deformity in varus osteoarthritis of the knee: analysis with computed tomography. *Clin Orthop Relat Res.* 2005;(433):147-151.

Mihalko WM, Krackow KA. Anatomic and biomechanical aspects of pie crusting posterolateral structures for valgus deformity correction in total knee arthroplasty: a cadaveric study. *J Arthroplasty.* 2000;15:347-353.

Mullaji A, Marawar S, Sharma A. Correcting varus deformity. *J Arthroplasty.* 2007;22(4 Suppl 1):15-19.

Ritter MA, Faris GW, Faris PM, Davis KE. Total knee arthroplasty in patients with angular varus or valgus deformities of > or = 20 degrees. *J Arthroplasty.* 2004;19(7):862-866.

Teeny SM, Krackow KA, Hungerford DS, Jones M. Primary total knee arthroplasty in patients with severe varus deformity: a comparative study. *Clin Orthop.* 1991;273:19.

Yasgur DJ, Scuderi GR, Insall JN. Medial release for fixed varus deformity. In: Scuderi GR, Tria AJ, eds. *Surgical Technique in Total Knee Arthroplasty.* New York, NY: Springer; 2002:189.

## Valgus Deformity

Aglietti P, Buzzi R, Baldini A, Lup D, De Luca L. Comparison of mobile-bearing and fixed-bearing total knee arthroplasty: a prospective randomized study. *J Arthroplasty.* 2005;20:145-153.

Aglietti P, Lup D, Cuomo P, Baldini A, De Luca L. Total knee arthroplasty using a pie-crusting technique for valgus deformity. *Clin Orthop Relat Res.* 2007;464:73-77.

Matsuda Y, Ishii Y, Noguchi H, Ishii R. Varus-valgus balance and range of movement after total knee arthroplasty. *J Bone Joint Surg Br.* 2005;87:804-808.

Mihalko WM, Krackow KA. Anatomic and biomechanical aspects of pie crusting posterolateral structures for valgus deformity correction in total knee arthroplasty: a cadaveric study. *J Arthroplasty.* 2000;15:347-353.

## Severe Ligamentous Laxity and Massive Bone Loss

Clatworthy MG, Ballance J, Brick GW, Chandler HP, Gross AE. The use of structural allograft for uncontained defects in revision total knee arthroplasty: a minimum five-year review. *J Bone Joint Surg.* 2001;83A:404-411.

Cuckler JM. Revision total knee arthroplasty: how much constraint is necessary? *Orthopedics.* 1995;18:932-936.

Ghazavi MT, Stockley I, Yee G, Davis A, Gross AE. Reconstruction of massive bone defects with allograft in revision total knee arthroplasty. *J Bone Joint Surg.* 1997;79A:17-25.

Harris AI, Poddar S, Gitelis S, et al. Arthroplasty with a composite of an allograft and a prosthesis for knees with severe deficiency of bone. *J Bone Joint Surg.* 1995;77A:373-386.

Hartford JM, Godman SB, Schurman DJ, et al. Complex primary and revision total knee arthroplasty using the condylar constrained prosthesis: an average 5-year follow-up. *J Arthroplasty.* 1998;13:380-387.

Kabo JM, Yang RS, Dorey FJ, et al. In vivo rotational stability of the kinematic rotating hinge knee prosthesis. *Clin Orthop.* 1997;336:166-176.

Rand JA, Chao EY, Stauffer RN. Kinematic rotating-hinge total knee arthroplasty. *J Bone Joint Surg.* 1987;69A:489-497.

Shaw JA, Balcom W, Greer III RB. Total knee arthroplasty using the kinematic rotating hinge prosthesis. *Orthopedics.* 1989;12:647-654.

Spriner BD, Sim FH, Hanssen AD, Lewallen DG. The modular segmental kinematic rotating hinge for non-neoplastic limb salvage. *Clin Orthop Relat Res.* 2004;(421):181-187.

Walker PS, Emerson R, Potter T, et al. The kinematic rotating hinge: biomechanics and clinical application. *Orthop Clin North Am.* 1982;13:187-199.

## Total Knee Arthroplasty in Young Active Patients

Crowder AR, Duffy GP, Trousdale RT. Long-term results of total knee arthroplasty in young patients with rheumatoid arthritis. *J Arthroplasty.* 2005;7 (Suppl 13):12.

Duffy GP, Crowder AR, Trousdale RR, Berry DJ. Cemented total knee arthroplasty using a modern prosthesis in young patients with osteoarthritis. *J Arthroplasty.* 2007;22(6 Suppl 2):67-70.

Gioe TJ, Novak C, Sinner P, Ma W, Mehle S. Knee arthroplasty in the young patient: survival in a community registry. *Clin Orthop Relat Res.* 2007;464:83-87.

McCaskie AW, Deehan DJ, Green TP, et al. Randomised, prospective study comparing cemented and cementless total knee replacement: results of press-fit condylar total knee replacement at five years. *J Bone Joint Surg Br.* 1998;80:971-975.

Morgan M, Brooks S, Nelson RA. Total knee arthroplasty in young active patients using a highly congruent fully mobile prosthesis. *J Arthroplasty.* 2007;22(4):525-530.

Nilsson KG, Karrholm J. Increased varus-valgus tilting of screwfixated knee prostheses: stereoradiographic study of uncemented versus cemented tibial components. *J Arthroplasty.* 1993;8:529-540.

Whiteside LA, Viganò R. Young and heavy patients with a cementless TKA do as well as older and lightweight patients. *Clin Orthop Relat Res.* 2007;464:93-98.

## Total Knee Arthroplasty Following Osteotomy

Beyer CA, Lewallen DG, Hanssen AD. Total knee arthroplasty following prior osteotomy of the distal femur. *Am J Knee Surg.* 1994;7:25-30.

Cameron HU, Park YS. Total knee replacement after supracondylar femoral osteotomy. *Am J Knee Surg.* 1997;10(2):70-71.

Gill T, Schemitsch EH, Brick GW, Thornhill TS. Revision total knee arthroplasty after failed unicompartmental knee arthroplasty or high tibial osteotomy. *Clin Orthop.* 1995;327:10.

Jackson M, Sarangi PP, Newman JH. Revision total knee arthroplasty: comparison of outcome following primary proximal tibial osteotomy or unicompartmental arthroplasty. *J Arthroplasty.* 1994;9:539.

Katz MM, Hungerford DS, Krackow KA, Lennox DE. Results of knee arthroplasty after failed proximal tibial osteotomy for osteoarthritis, *J Bone Joint Surg.* 1987;69A:225.

Laskin R, Palleta G. Total knee replacement in the post patellectomy patient. *J Arthroplasty.* 1994;9:109.

Nelson CL, Saleh KJ, Kassim RA, et al. Total knee arthroplasty after varus osteotomy of the distal part of the femur. *J Bone Joint Surg Am.* 2003;85-A(6):1062-1065.

Parvizi J, Hanssen AD, Spangehl MJ. Total knee arthroplasty following proximal tibial osteotomy: risk factors for failure. *J Bone Joint Surg Am.* 2004;86-A(3):474-479.

Staeheli JW, Cass JR, Morrey B. Condylar total knee arthroplasty after failed proximal tibial osteotomy, *J Bone Joint Surg.* 1987;69A:28.

## Neuropathic Arthropathy

Kim YH, Kim JS, Oh SW. Total knee arthroplasty in neuropathic arthropathy. *J Bone Joint Surg.* 2002;84A:216-219.

Parvizi J, Marrs J, Morrey BF. Total knee arthroplasty for neuropathic (Charcot) joints. *Clin Orthop Relat Res.* 2003;(416):145-150.

Soudry M, Binazzi R, Johanson NA, Bullough PG, Insall JN. Total knee arthroplasty in Charcot and Charcot-like joints. *Clin Orthop Relat Res.* 1986;(208):199-204.

## Total Knee Arthroplasty in Hemophilic Patients

Figgie MP, Goldberg VM, Figgie HE 3rd, Heiple KG, Sobel M. Total knee arthroplasty for the treatment of chronic hemophilic arthropathy. *Clin Orthop Relat Res.* 1989;(248):98-107.

Silva M, Luck JV Jr. Long-term results of primary total knee replacement in patients with hemophilia. *J Bone Joint Surg Am.* 2005;87(1):85-91.

## Total Knee Arthroplasty in Diabetic Patients

England SP, Stern SH, Insall JN, Windsor RE. Total knee arthroplasty in diabetes mellitus. *Clin Orthop Relat Res.* 1990;(260):130-134.

Yang K, Yeo SJ, Lee BP, Lo NN. Total knee arthroplasty in diabetic patients: a study of 109 consecutive cases. *J Arthroplasty.* 2001;16(1):102-106.

# 22

# Total Knee Arthroplasty Revision

*Matthew S. Austin, MD and Eric L. Grossman, MD*

There are approximately 450,000 total knee arthroplasty (TKA) procedures performed in the United States annually.[1] This number is projected to increase over 6-fold to 3.48 million by the year 2030. These figures, coupled with an increasing life expectancy, lead to the expectation that the number of total knee revisions (TKR) will grow exponentially. In 2005, there were approximately 38,200 TKA revisions performed, and this number is projected to increase to 268,200 by 2030.[1]

## Preoperative Evaluation and Indications for Revision Surgery

A clear objective cause for failure of the prior arthroplasty must be identified before revision surgery. Sharkey et al delineated the most common reasons for failure of modern TKA.[2] The etiologies of failure (in descending order of prevalence) were polyethylene wear, aseptic loosening, instability, infection, arthrofibrosis, malalignment, component malposition, extensor mechanism deficiency, avascular necrosis of the patella, periprosthetic fracture, and isolated resurfacing of the patella. A comprehensive history and physical examination will often narrow the differential diagnosis. The surgeon must ask questions to include or exclude the presence of infection, instability, and loosening. Pain from an extrinsic source (hip, lumbar radiculopathy) must be excluded. An example of a patient-completed survey is found in Figure 22-1. The physical examination is useful to evaluate for instability, infection, arthrofibrosis, malalignment, and extensor mechanism deficiency. Furthermore, the soft tissues should be thoroughly evaluated, and if there is any question regarding the ability of the soft tissue envelope to heal, a plastic surgery consultation should be obtained. The overall constitution of the patient, including nutritional analysis, should be considered prior to offering TKR. In the absence of infection, conservative treatment appropriate to the patient's symptoms including physical therapy, bracing, and pain management should be exhausted prior to consideration of TKR. Revision within the first 6 months to 1 year after TKA is rarely indicated.

Standing AP, lateral, and sunrise radiographs are essential. Reviewing the preoperative radiographs, including those from prior to the index procedure, can give the surgeon an idea of the severity of the patient's degenerative disease, alignment, joint line, and AP femoral diameter. Serial radiographs are useful to demonstrate loosening, osteolysis, and wear. New radiographs are useful to demonstrate polyethylene wear, aseptic loosening, malalignment, component malposition, avascular necrosis of the patella, and periprosthetic fracture. Long-cassette (36") radiographs are often helpful for evaluation of alignment and for extra-articular deformities. Stress radiographs may be helpful in documenting instability. Computed tomography (CT) scans are occasionally indicated to evaluate osteolytic lesions. CT scan is also useful to assess component position and rotation.

Serologic markers such as the erythrocyte sedimentation rate (ESR) and C-reactive protein (CRP) are useful to exclude infection in the painful TKA.[3] Nuclear medicine modalities such as technetium 99-m bone scans are useful



Parvizi J, Klatt B.
*Essentials in Total Knee Arthroplasty* (pp 187-200).

In order to provide you with the best possible care, please try to complete the following questionnaire to the best of your ability.

Date: ____________________

NAME: ____________________

AGE: ____________________

OCCUPATION: ____________________

PRIMARY CARE PHYSICIAN: Name: ____________________
Address: ____________________
____________________
____________________
Telephone: ____________________

REFERRING ORTHOPEDIST: Name: ____________________
Address: ____________________
____________________
____________________
Telephone: ____________________

PLEASE CIRCLE THE AFFECTED JOINT(S):

| HIP | RIGHT | LEFT | BOTH |
|---|---|---|---|
| KNEE | RIGHT | LEFT | BOTH |

1. What is bothering you about the joint and when did the symptoms first appear?

____________________
____________________
____________________
____________________
____________________
____________________

2. DO THESE SYMPTOMS STOP YOU FROM DOING ACTIVITIES YOU ENJOY?

YES NO

Page 1 of 5

**Figure 22-1.** Survey to be completed by patient.

3. PREVIOUS HIP AND/OR KNEE SURGERY (if none please skip to question 8):
DATE ________________ WHAT WAS DONE ______________ SURGEON ______________________
WHY WAS IT DONE? ______________________________________________________________
______________________________________________________________________________
______________________________________________________________________________
______________________________________________________________________________
______________________________________________________________________________
______________________________________________________________________________

4. DID YOU HAVE ANY COMPLICATIONS SUCH AS (please circle):

| | |
|---|---|
| Wound Drainage | Blood Clots |
| Hematoma (Blood in the Joint) | Instability |
| Infection | Stiffness |
| Delayed wound healing | Trauma/Falls |

Other: ______________________________________

5. DO YOU CURRENTLY HAVE (please circle):

| | |
|---|---|
| Fevers | Instability |
| Chills | Stiffness |
| Wound drainage | Weakness |
| Night sweats | Pain at rest |

6. If you have had surgery, is the pain you have now the same or is it different than before surgery?
______________________________________________________________________________
______________________________________________________________________________
______________________________________________________________________________
______________________________________________________________________________
______________________________________________________________________________
______________________________________________________________________________

7. If you have had surgery, was there pain relief for a period of time before the pain returned?

YES NO



**Figure 22-1 (continued).** Survey to be completed by patient.

8. HOW FAR CAN YOU WALK?:

Wheelchair bound <1 Block 1 to 5 Blocks 5 to 10 Blocks >10 Blocks

9. DO YOU HAVE PROBLEMS WITH STAIRS? YES NO

10. DO YOU LIMP? YES NO

11. RATE YOUR PAIN:

No Pain 1 2 3 4 5 6 7 8 9 10 Severe Pain

12. TYPE OF PAIN:

SHARP DULL ACHING BURNING OTHER: ____________________

13. WHERE IS YOUR PAIN? (circle all that apply):

| LOW BACK | BUTTOCKS | GROIN | FRONT OF THIGH | SHIN |
|---|---|---|---|---|
| SIDE OF THIGH | BACK OF THIGH | FRONT OF KNEE | SIDE OF KNEE | |
| BACK OF KNEE | CALF | | | |

14. DOES THE PAIN GET BETTER AFTER A FEW STEPS? YES NO

15. What medications/natural supplements do you take for your pain? (please list):

______________________________________________

______________________________________________

______________________________________________

______________________________________________

______________________________________________

______________________________________________

16. HAVE YOU HAD PHYSICAL THERAPY? YES NO

17. HAVE YOU HAD CORTISONE INJECTIONS? YES NO

18. HAVE YOU HAD SYNVISC-TYPE INJECTIONS? YES NO

19. ASSISTIVE DEVICES: NONE CANE WALKER WHEELCHAIR

20. HAVE YOU USED BRACES? YES NO

Page 3 of 5

**Figure 22-1 (continued).** Survey to be completed by patient.

21. MEDICAL PROBLEMS (please list):

22. OTHER SURGERIES (please list):

23. MEDICATIONS/NATURAL SUPPLEMENTS/VITAMINS (please list):

24. ALLERGIES TO MEDICATIONS (please list):

25. DO YOU SMOKE? YES NO

26. REVIEW OF SYSTEMS:

| YES | NO | |
|---|---|---|
| ☐ | ☐ | 1. Have you ever had a problem with anesthesia other than nausea or vomiting? |
| ☐ | ☐ | 2. Has anyone in your family had a serious, life-threatening problem with anesthesia (not nausea)? |
| ☐ | ☐ | 3. Do you take drugs (over the counter or "street drugs") other than your regular prescription medications? |
| ☐ | ☐ | 4. Do you have high blood pressure requiring more than 2 drugs for control? |
| ☐ | ☐ | 5. Do you have heart trouble? |

Page 4 of 5

**Figure 22-1 (continued).** Survey to be completed by patient.

YES NO

- ☐ ☐ 6. Do you have angina or chest pain?
- ☐ ☐ 7. Do you have an irregular heartbeat?
- ☐ ☐ 8. Have you had a heart attack?
- ☐ ☐ 9. Have you ever had heart failure?
- ☐ ☐ 10. Do you have asthma that required oral steroid in the last 6 months?
- ☐ ☐ 11. Do you have a daily cough that produces fluid?
- ☐ ☐ 12. Do you have emphysema, bronchitis, or COPD?
- ☐ ☐ 13. Do you get short of breath after walking up a flight of stairs?
- ☐ ☐ 14. Do you use oxygen at home?
- ☐ ☐ 15. Do you have sleep apnea?
- ☐ ☐ 16. Do you have chronic kidney disease?
- ☐ ☐ 17. Do you receive dialysis?
- ☐ ☐ 18. Do you have diabetes?
- ☐ ☐ 19. Do you have a bleeding disorder?
- ☐ ☐ 20. Have you had problems with postoperative bleeding and needed a blood transfusion?
- ☐ ☐ 21. Do you take blood thinners?
- ☐ ☐ 22. Is there a family history of bleeding problems?
- ☐ ☐ 23. Have you had hepatitis, jaundice, or cirrhosis?
- ☐ ☐ 24. Do you have sickle cell anemia or thalassemia?
- ☐ ☐ 25. Do you weigh more than 250 pounds?
- ☐ ☐ 26. Could you be pregnant?
- ☐ ☐ 27. Have you had a stroke?
- ☐ ☐ 28. Do you have weakness or paralysis of an arm or leg?
- ☐ ☐ 29. Do you have a seizure disorder?

27. HEIGHT: __________ feet ________ inches

28. WEIGHT: _______ pounds

I have filled this form out as completely as possible and to the best of my ability.

Patient Signature: ______________________________________ Date: ____________________

Page 5 of 5

**Figure 22-1 (continued).** Survey to be completed by patient.

to exclude occult loosening, and when used in conjunction with Indium-111 white blood cell scans, are useful in inclusion or exclusion of the diagnosis of infection. If the index of suspicion for infection is clinically raised or if the ESR, CRP, or nuclear medicine tests are suspicious for infection, then an aspiration is warranted. The aspirate should be sent for a synovial white blood cell (WBC) count with visual differential, culture (aerobic, anaerobic, acid-fast bacilli, fungal) and sensitivity, and crystals. A synovial WBC count of more than 1700 with more than 65% neutrophils is suspicious for infection.[4] A positive culture is diagnostic of infection if the clinical picture supports this diagnosis, but a negative culture does not necessarily exclude infection. It is important to realize that there is no single test that is 100% sensitive and specific in the diagnosis of infection. The clinical presentation, serologic markers, aspiration, and nuclear medicine studies are used in combination to diagnose infection.

## Preoperative Planning

Preoperative planning is paramount to the success of TKR. The goal of preoperative planning is to allow the surgical procedure to flow in a smooth, well-organized, efficient manner. The surgeon must plan with a clear algorithm in mind, taking into account that his or her primary plan for the surgery may need to be altered due to unforeseen circumstances encountered during the case. For example, a typical error is to underestimate the degree of bone loss one will encounter as radiographs typically underestimate the actual degree of bone loss.[5] The surgeon must have a plan in place to manage larger defects than one would expect from the preoperative radiographs. The surgeon must first be aware of the reason or reasons for revision and plan accordingly. If the surgeon is planning on retaining one or more of the components, prior operative reports or so-called "parts stickers" will help to identify the current components and to determine if they are modular or if compatible components are available.

### Polyethylene Wear

Polyethylene wear can result in significant osteolysis and damage to the components such that simple exchange of a modular polyethylene insert is rarely indicated. The surgeon must be prepared to revise some or all of the components.

### Bone Loss

Bone loss can be classified according to several different systems. The authors prefer to use the classification system developed by Huff and Sculco.[6] This system is useful in that it allows for preoperative classification of the bone defect and for reconstructive planning. It subclassifies the defects into cystic, epiphyseal, cavitary, and segmental. There are multiple options for reconstructing each of these categories of bone loss, which will be addressed under the Surgical Technique section on p. 194. Classifying the bone defect via radiographs is a useful starting point for preoperative planning; however, one must plan for the intraoperative bone loss to be worse than that estimated by radiographs. Proper planning may require the availability of structural or cancellous allograft in varying quantities, which may need to be special ordered.

### Instability

There are 4 main types of instability after TKA: global, collateral ligament insufficiency, isolated flexion, and isolated extension. Global instability is manifested by laxity in extension and flexion. This problem may be solved by changing the polyethylene to a thicker insert. However, this approach must be used with caution as insert exchange will not solve inappropriate alignment, rotation, position, collateral ligament insufficiency, joint line, or flexion-extension mismatch. Collateral ligament insufficiency is treated with proper implant alignment, release of the tight side, and filling of the lax side with polyethylene. Ligament advancement should be considered. If there is no endpoint, then constrained implants may be necessary. Hinged implants should be reserved as a salvage procedure for instability that is not corrected by proper alignment, rotation, implant position, and joint line restoration. Isolated extension instability is treated by reducing the extension gap by moving the femoral component distally. One must be careful to exclude neurological conditions that may produce recurvatum. Flexion instability is treated by reducing the flexion gap by increasing the size of the femoral component or moving the femoral component posterior with the use of an offset stem. Subtle flexion instability can occur with some cruciate-retaining knees and may require revision to a posterior stabilized knee with reduction of the flexion gap.

### Infection

Infection that occurs acutely within the first 2 to 4 weeks after the arthroplasty or after an acute hematogenous infection can be treated with irrigation and débridement with exchange of the modular insert. The selection criteria include absence of sinus tract, loosening, radiographic evidence of infection, and the microorganism must be susceptible to antibiotics. The success of this approach has been variable with infection recurring in up to 77% of cases.[7] Two-stage exchange is the standard of care in subacute and chronic infections with success reported in 92% of cases as compared to 74% with one-stage exchange.[8] Antibiotic-impregnated spacers should be used in the interval between explantation and reimplantation to maintain ligament tension and to deliver a high local concentration of antibiotics.

### Arthrofibrosis

Stiffness after TKA can be a difficult problem to treat operatively. Prior to consideration of revision surgery, a correctable, intrinsic cause of stiffness should be identified. Extrinsic sources of stiffness such as hip osteoarthritis, muscle rigidity secondary to neurological conditions, and heterotopic ossification should be excluded. Patients with restricted preoperative range of motion are likely to have restricted postoperative range of motion and likely will not benefit from TKR. Correctable, intrinsic causes of stiffness include malrotation, malposition resulting in a reduced flexion and/or extension gap, so-called "overstuffing" of the patellofemoral joint by underresection of the patella or anterior translation of the femur, or a tight posterior cruciate ligament. The patient should be well motivated and alerted to the variability in results obtained after TKR for stiffness.

### Malalignment/Component Malposition

Malaligned or malpositioned components can lead to early wear and aseptic loosening, instability or stiffness, or patellofemoral maltracking, or can cause pain from asymmetric loading of the bone. Long-cassette standing radiographs can aid in assessing whether the malalignment is from the femoral side, the tibial side, or both. Rotational alignment is best assessed via CT. The surgeon should take into account any extra-articular deformity that may contribute to the overall alignment of the limb. Strict reliance on stems to guide alignment in the setting of extra-articular deformity will fail to restore the mechanical axis to neutral. Preoperative radiographs should be templated for sizing, position, joint line restoration, and alignment. Revision implants are typically available with a 5 or 7 degree valgus cut angle on the femur and varying degrees of offset for the femur and tibia that can help to restore the mechanical axis to neutral.

### Extensor Mechanism Deficiency

Extensor mechanism deficiency can occur from osteonecrosis of the patella with subsequent fragmentation, disruption of the patella ligament, or disruption of the quadriceps tendon. Although reconstruction of the deficient extensor mechanism is beyond the scope of this chapter, it is important to recognize that the TKA components must be evaluated for appropriate alignment, rotation, position, and sizing prior to reconstruction of the extensor mechanism. Failure to recognize implant malpositioning may doom the subsequent reconstruction to failure.

### Periprosthetic Fracture

The factors for determining how to treat periprosthetic (PP) fracture around a TKA involves determining the stability of the implant, quality of the remaining bone stock, age, and functional demands of the patient. PP fracture around the tibial component is usually due to osteolysis and the defect is bypassed with a stemmed component and the defect is bone grafted or replaced with metal augmentation. Fractures that are well distal to the tibial component are treated with standard fracture care. PP fracture of a loose femoral component is treated with revision of the component with stems and bone grafting or metal augmentation of the distal femur since the bone quality is often poor. PP fracture of a well-fixed femoral component is treated with either retrograde intramedullary nailing or plating of the fracture. PP fracture of the patella is fraught with a high complication rate. Treatment is based on the integrity of the extensor mechanism, the stability of the component, and the quality of the bone. Treatment options include patellectomy (partial or complete), revision of the component, or removal of the component and patelloplasty.

## Surgical Technique

TKR surgery should follow an algorithm of steps that will allow for consistent, reproducible, and efficient surgical results. The steps are as follows:

- Exposure and intraoperative evaluation
- Implant removal
- Bone defect reconstruction and implant selection
- Gap balancing and joint line restoration

Preoperative planning is essential so that the operation proceeds in a seamless manner. The appropriate personnel, instrumentation, implants, and allograft material should be readily available.

### Exposure and Intraoperative Evaluation

The primary approach for TKR is straight anterior. When feasible, the prior incision should be used to avoid compromise of the skin between the incisions. In the case

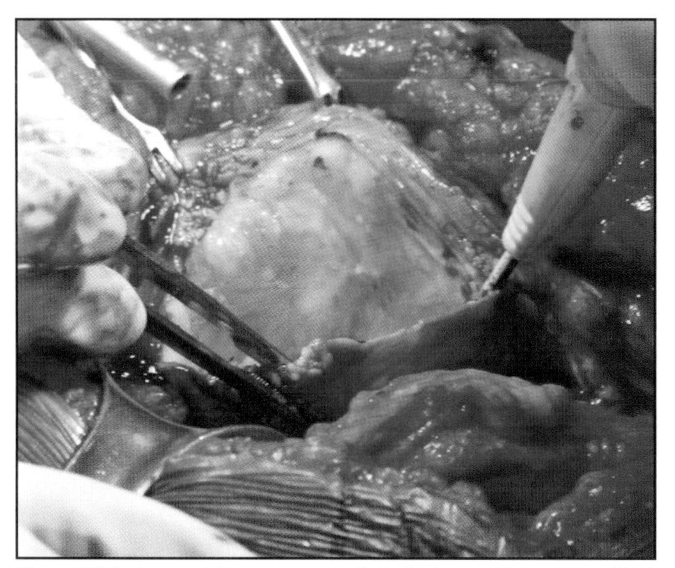

**Figure 22-2.** A thorough synovectomy allows for improved exposure of both bone and soft tissues.

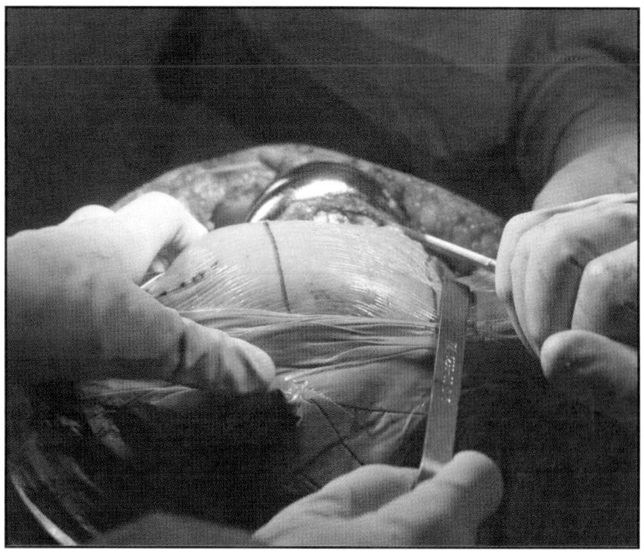

**Figure 22-3.** Thin osteotomes are used to disrupt implant-cement interface in removal of cemented TKA. This method may also be employed with cementless TKA.

of multiple incisions, one should choose the most lateral incision that can be used, as the blood supply to the skin in this area is based medially. Incisions that will cross old scars should be made perpendicular to the prior incision to avoid devascularization of the tissues.[9] Large subcutaneous flaps should be avoided. In more complex situations where there are multiple previous incisions or where the skins integrity is impaired (ie, prior irradiation or burn), one must consider plastic surgery consultation.[10]

The extensor mechanism is exposed and a medial parapatellar arthrotomy is performed. This arthrotomy allows for the necessary exposure for evaluation of the components and remaining bone stock. This is paramount in TKR surgery. The patella should not be everted to avoid disruption of the extensor mechanism. A thorough synovectomy should be performed to expose the remaining bone stock, components, and restore the medial and lateral gutters (Figure 22-2). Three separate synovial samples should be sent for culture. A frozen section can be helpful if infection has not been excluded prior to TKR. A medial retinacular release is performed. The patella is then subluxed laterally. If the patella cannot be subluxed laterally to allow for adequate visualization, then a quadriceps snip or tibial tubercle osteotomy should be performed.

Once adequate exposure is obtained, the knee is examined. The surgeon should note the range of motion; the presence of a flexion contracture; the condition of the extensor mechanism; the stability of the knee in full extension, midflexion, and flexion; patella tracking; alignment; and location of the joint line. The components should be evaluated for sizing, positioning, alignment, and condition of the implants. The preoperative diagnosis is confirmed and subsequent reconstruction begins.

## Implant Removal

Implant removal can often be challenging. Careful implant removal can facilitate subsequent reconstruction, while careless removal can complicate the reconstruction. It cannot be overemphasized that careful implant removal is essential. Several instruments and techniques are available to assist with removal of components and residual bone cement. The author prefers the use of a thin oscillating saw and osteotomes (Figure 22-3) to disrupt the implant-cement interface in cemented components and the implant-bone interface in uncemented implants. The implants should be carefully separated from the cement and/or bone to extent that they can be removed by hand. Forceful impaction of the implants may lead to fracture or catastrophic bone loss.

A fine tip burr can more clearly define the interface and ultimately allow for component removal with additional tools such as oscillating saws and osteotomes. Once the implant is removed, the remaining bone cement is removed with small osteotomes, curettes, and burrs. Any remaining osteophytes should be resected (Figure 22-4).

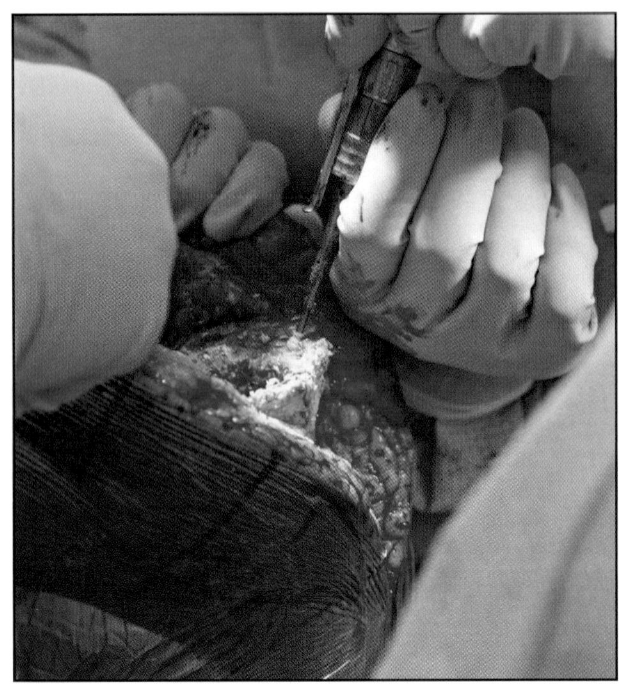

**Figure 22-4.** A fine-tip burr is used to more clearly define bony anatomy and remove residual bone cement.

## Bone Defect Reconstruction and Implant Selection

TKR has almost always some degree of bone loss, whether it is pre-existing or as a result of implant removal. Revision implants should be used in almost every revision case because primary implants have been shown to have poor results in the revision situation.[11] The classification system of Huff and Sculco (JOA) allows for the defect to be categorized into 1 of 4 types: cystic, epiphyseal, cavitary, and segmental. Each type has specific reconstructive options.

### Cystic

These defects are small, contained defects that do not compromise implant stability and are best treated with bone cement. Similar defects that are greater than 5 mm in diameter can be treated with bone graft.[12]

### Epiphyseal

Epiphyseal defects involve loss of cortical bone in the epiphyseal or metaphyseal bone. These defects can be reconstructed with metal augments and stemmed components. Long-term success of up to 92% has been reported when using metal augments in defects less than 2 cm in depth.[13]

### Cavitary

Cavitary defects are defined as massive metaphyseal defects. They require reconstruction with metal sleeves, cones, or structural allograft in conjunction with stemmed implants. Contained defects or defects that can be converted to contained defects can be treated with impaction grafting or bulk allograft. There is limited outcome data in the literature with regard to these reconstructive methods. Metal sleeves have had success of 100% reported in midterm follow-up.[14] Trabecular metal cones (Zimmer Trabecular Metal Technology, Inc, Allendale, NJ) have had short-term survivorship of 100% reported recently.[15] Clatworthy et al reported on the mid-term and long-term results of structural allografting in 52 cases.[16] The 5- and 10-year survivorship rates were 92% and 72%, respectively. The results of impaction grafting have been reasonable in the short-term but have had significant complications.[17,18] Bulk allograft has been demonstrated to have 77% to 87% good/excellent results at mid-term follow-up.[19,20]

### Segmental

Segmental defects are massive defects in which large portions of the femur or tibia have been lost. These are generally reconstructed with structural allograft or megaprosthesis. There is a dearth of outcome data for these types of reconstructions.

## Gap Balancing and Joint Line Restoration

This section will mainly focus on gap balancing and joint line restoration for the vast majority of revisions that do not present with massive bone, ligament, and extensor mechanism deficits. These types of revisions are beyond the scope of this chapter. The exact sequence of steps varies depending on the instrumentation system of the implant manufacturer. However, in general, the authors prefer to follow a step-wise method to TKR.

Gap balancing is crucial to the success of revision surgery. This task is often made complicated by the presence of bone loss, which can lead to detachment of the collateral ligaments. Restoration of the joint line is essential, as raising the joint line >8 mm has been shown to lower functional scores.[21] The joint line is 3.08 cm below the medial epicondyle and 2.53 cm below the lateral epicondyle.[22] This is used as a starting point and should be individualized to each patient's anatomy, the configuration of the prosthesis, and ligament tension. In general, the components should

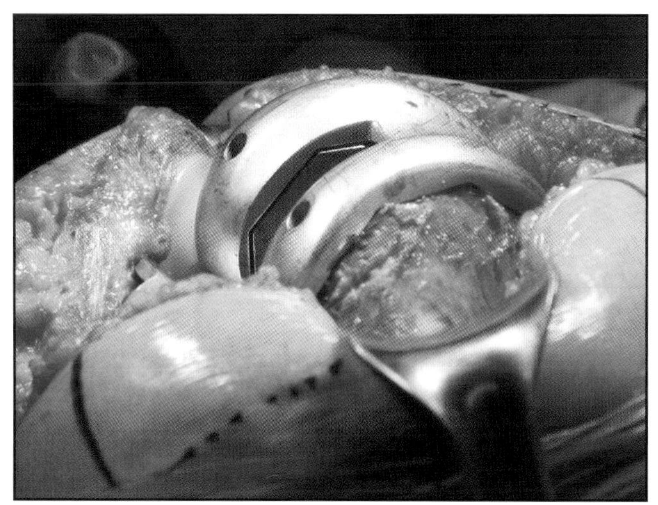

**Figure 22-5.** Femoral preparation demonstrating trialing of femoral component. Particular attention is paid to cortical contact and length of construct.

be stemmed. The choice of whether to cement or press-fit the stem remains an unanswered question and is left to the philosophy of the surgeon.

The authors prefer to start reconstruction on the femoral side. The femur is progressively reamed until good cortical contact is obtained at a depth that matches the overall length of the femoral construct from the distal aspect of the femoral component to the tip of the stem (Figure 22-5).

The joint line is recreated based on the distance from the transepicondylar axis (TEA) to the distal aspect of the femoral component (Figure 22-6). This may require augmentation of the distal femur (more common) or bone resection. Careful attention to the rotational alignment of femoral component parallel to the TEA is paramount. The AP diameter and offset of the femoral component will determine the flexion gap. The prior component can be used as a starting point for femoral sizing. The trial component can be upsized (requiring augmentation) or downsized (requiring bone resection) based on the flexion gap needs. One should not forget that posterior offset of the femoral stem can reduce the flexion gap and avoid overstuffing the patellofemoral joint by moving the anterior flange flush with the anterior femur. The box cut usually has to be enlarged or created if the authors choose to use a posterior stabilized TKR.

Attention is then turned to the tibial reconstruction. The previous tibial cut is assessed for alignment in the coronal and sagittal plane. The tibial cut should be freshened so that the tibial tray will be perpendicular to the mechanical axis of the tibia (Figure 22-7). The tibia is reamed progressively until good cortical contact is reached at a depth that matches the overall length of the tibial construct from the

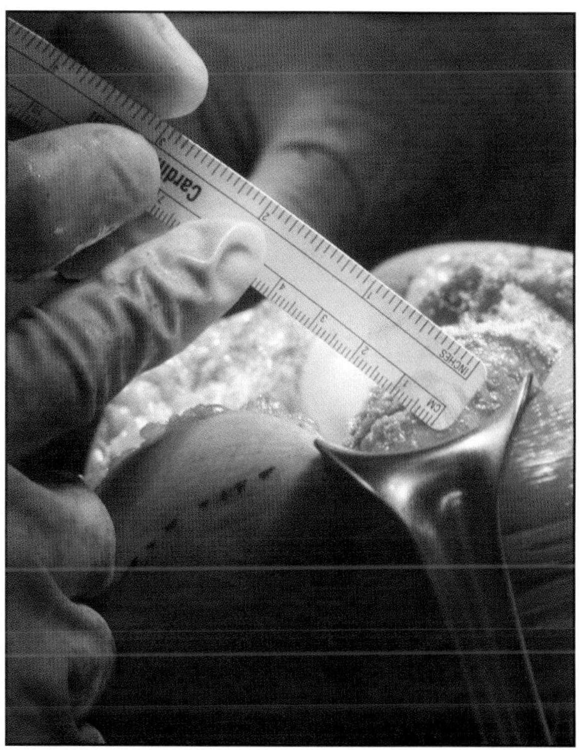

**Figure 22-6.** The joint line is recreated based on the distance from the transepicondylar axis (TEA) to the distal aspect of the femoral component.

inferior portion of the tray to the tip of the stem (Figure 22-8). The tibial trial is then inserted with careful attention paid to rotation. The center of the tibial tray should align with the medial third of the tibial tubercle. The size of the tray should be maximized to increase the surface area for force distribution without creating overhang. Pain in the area of overhang is a frequent problem. Augments and full block augments are tapered in some systems to prevent tibial overhang.

The patella is then assessed. Patella resurfacing is a controversial topic and if the patella has not been resurfaced, it may be left unresurfaced or resurfaced based on the philosophy of the surgeon. Patellae that were resurfaced during the index procedure should be evaluated for damage, fixation, and position. Lonner et al demonstrated that patellae may be retained at the time of TKR if the patella is undamaged, well-fixed, well positioned, and is not oxidized.[23] Patellae not meeting these criteria should be removed with care, provided that adequate bone stock remains. Reconstruction of the patella requires a thickness of 10 mm or more to obtain good fixation. If there is inadequate bone, there are several options for the patella. A patellectomy is probably the worst option, due to the loss in extension moment force. A patellar resection arthroplasty (also called a patelloplasty) involves

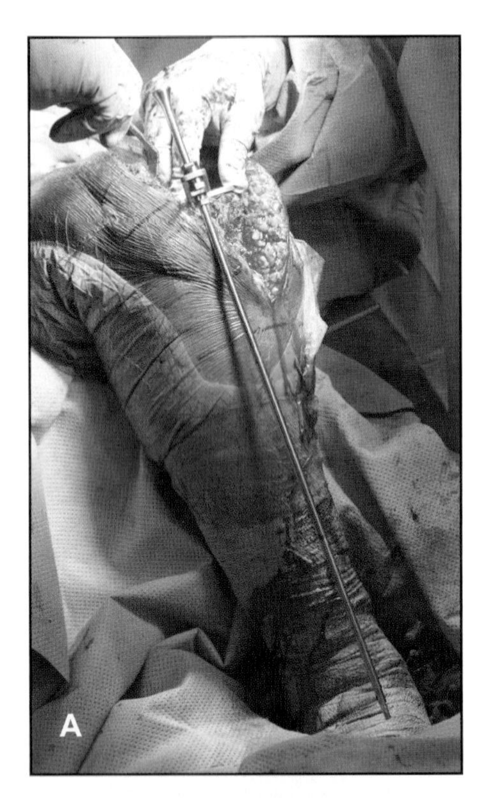


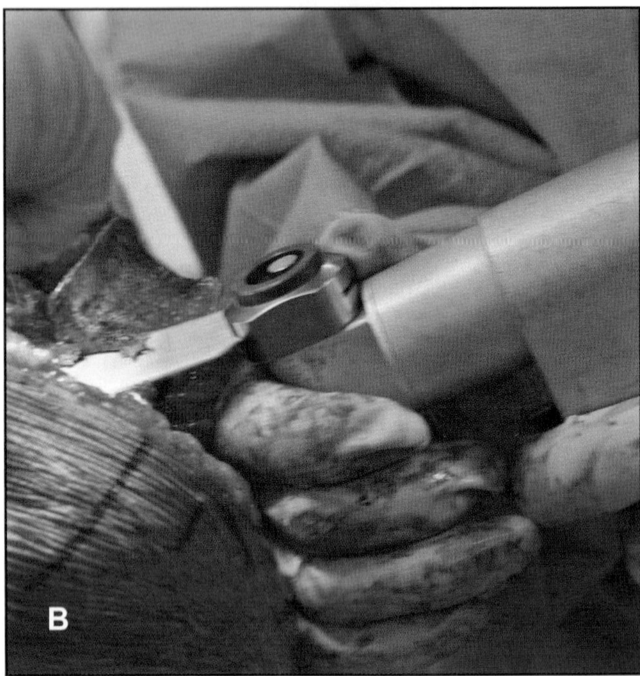


**Figure 22-7.** (A) The alignment of the tibial cut is checked intraoperatively. (B) The tibial cut is revised after assessment of alignment. The cut should be perpendicular to the tibias' mechanical axis.

removal of the patellar component. The residual bone is left intact to articulate with the femur. Some surgeons will split the residual patella longitudinally in a process called "gull winging." The patella will then form a V and this is

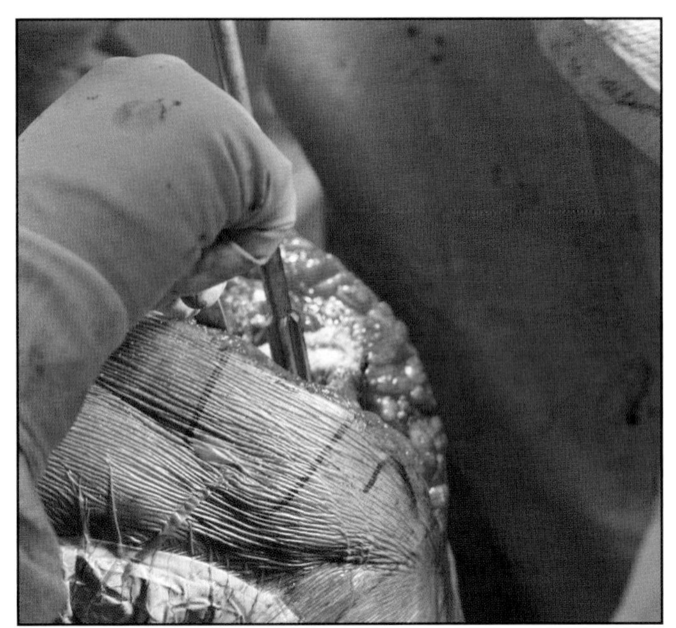

**Figure 22-8.** The tibia is reamed until good cortical contact is reached at a depth that matches the overall length of the tibial construct.

thought to improve tracking through the femoral trochlear groove. Another option is to restore bone stock to the patella. Allografting or autografting can be performed. This bone graft is held in place by suturing a flap of scar from the lining of the knee over the bone graft. A newer solution is reconstruction of the patella with a porous tantalum component (Zimmer Trabecular Metal Technology, Inc). The porous tantalum implant is sutured to the residual bone, and the patellar component is cemented to this implant.

The knee is then trialed to assess for alignment, stability, range of motion, restoration of the joint line, and patella tracking (Figure 22-9). If the knee is malaligned, an intraoperative radiograph may be helpful to determine if the intramedullary alignment of the stems is not ideal. Flexion-extension problems can be resolved with the algorithm shown in Table 22-1. The rotation, position, and sizing of the femoral, tibial, and patella components should be carefully assessed if the patella is not tracking well with the so-called "no thumbs" technique.

Once the TKR has achieved acceptable alignment, stability, range of motion, restoration of the joint line, and patella tracking, the final components are inserted with care taken to ensure that the trial components match the final implants prior to implantation. Closure then proceeds in meticulous fashion. Excessive tension encountered during skin closure should generate an intraoperative plastic surgery consultation. Postoperative radiographs are essential to evaluate the reconstruction and ensure that an intraoperative fracture does not go unrecognized (Figure 22-10).

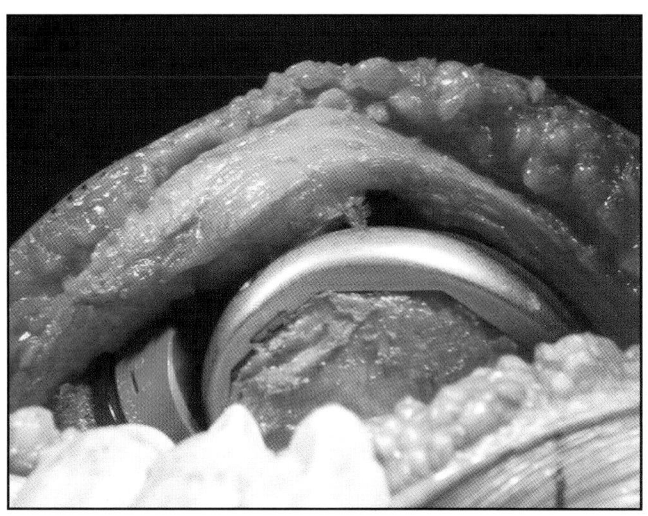

**Figure 22-9.** The knee is then trialed to assess for alignment, stability, range of motion, restoration of the joint line, and patella tracking.

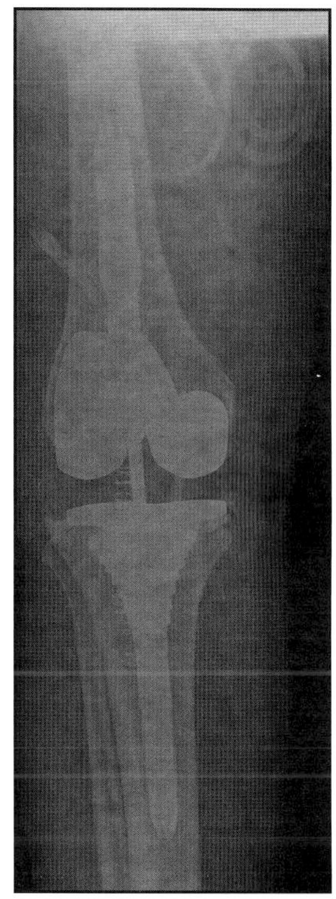

**Figure 22-10.** Postoperative radiographs are essential to evaluate the reconstruction and ensure that an intraoperative fracture does not go unrecognized.

Table 22-1

**OPTIONS FOR FLEXION-EXTENSION MISMATCH**

| | *Loose in Extension* | *Tight in Extension* | *Stable in Extension* |
|---|---|---|---|
| Loose in flexion | Increase tibial thickness | Upsize femoral component and resect distal femur<br>Resect more distal femur and increase tibial thickness | Upsize femoral component |
| Tight in flexion | Downsize femoral component and increase tibial thickness<br>Downsize femoral component with distal augments<br>Partial or full PCL release (CR only) | Thinner tibial component<br>Resect more tibia | Downsize femoral component<br>Increase tibial slope<br>Partial or full PCL release (CR only) |
| Stable in flexion | Augment distal femur<br>Downsize femoral component and increase tibial thickness | Resect more distal femur<br>Posterior capsular release | Finished |

## Summary

TKA has enjoyed immense success worldwide. Unfortunately, a certain percentage of these patients will require TKR. The success of TKR depends on appropriate patient selection; careful preoperative planning; meticulous surgical technique; and the availability of the appropriate personnel, instrumentation, implants, and allograft material. Strict adherence to these principles will maximize the patient's rehabilitation, function, and pain relief.

## References


1. Kurtz S, Ong K, Lau E, et al. Projections of primary and revision hip and knee arthroplasty in the United States from 2005 to 2030. *J Bone Joint Surg Am.* 2007;89:780-785.
2. Sharkey PF, Hozack WJ, Rothman RH, et al. Why are total knee arthroplasties failing today? *Clin Orthop Relat Res.* 2002;(404):7-13.
3. Austin MS, Ghanem E, Joshi A, Lindsay A, Parvizi J. A simple, cost-effective screening protocol to rule out periprosthetic infection. *J Arthroplasty.* 2008;23(1):65-68.
4. Trampuz A, Hanssen AD, Osmon DR, et al. Synovial fluid leukocyte count and differential for the diagnosis of prosthetic knee infection. *Am J Med.* 2004;117(8):556-562.
5. Rorabeck CH, Taylor J. Revision knee arthroplasty: how I do it? In: Insall JN, Scott WN, eds. *Surgery of the Knee.* Philadelphia, PA: Churchill Livingstone; 2001:1950.
6. Huff TW, Sculco TP. Management of bone loss in revision total knee arthroplasty. *J Arthroplasty.* 2007;22(7 Suppl 3):32-36.
7. Schoifet SD, Morrey BF. Treatment of infection after total knee arthroplasty by débridement with retention of the components. *J Bone Joint Surg Am.* 1990;72(9):1383-1390.
8. Leone JM, Hanssen AD. Management of infection at the site of a total knee arthroplasty. *Instr Course Lect.* 2006;55:449-461.
9. Insall JN, Scott WN, eds. *Surgery of the Knee.* Philadelphia, PA: Churchill Livingston; 135-148.
10. Dennis DA. A stepwise approach to revision total knee arthroplasty. *J Arthroplasty.* 2007;22(4 Suppl 1):32-38.
11. Bugbee WD, Ammeen DJ, Engh GA. Does implant selection affect outcome of revision knee arthroplasty? *J Arthroplasty.* 2001;16(5):5815.
12. Dorr LD, Ranawat CS, Sculco TA, et al. Bone graft for tibial defects in total knee arthroplasty. *Clin Orthop Relat Res.* 1986;(205):153-165.
13. Patel JV, Masonis JL, Guerin J, Bourne RB, Rorabeck CH. The fate of augments to treat type-2 bone defects in revision knee arthroplasty. *J Bone Joint Surg Br.* 2004;86-B:195-199.
14. Jones RE, Barrack RL, Skedros J. Modular, mobile-bearing hinge total knee arthroplasty. *Clin Orthop Relat Res.* 2001;(392):306-314.
15. Radnay CS, Scuderi GR. Management of bone loss: augments, cones, offset stems. *Clin Orthop Relat Res.* 2006;446:83-92.
16. Clatworthy MG, Ballance J, Brick GW, et al. The use of structural allograft for uncontained defects in revision total knee arthroplasty: a minimum five-year review. *J Bone Joint Surg Am.* 2001;83-A(3):404-411.
17. Whiteside LA. Cementless revision total knee arthroplasty. *Clin Orthop Relat Res.* 1993;(286):160-167.
18. Lotke PA, Carolan GF, Puri N. Impaction grafting for bone defects in revision total knee arthroplasty. *Clin Orthop Relat Res.* 2006;446:99-103.
19. Dennis DA. The structural allograft composite in revision total knee arthroplasty. *J Arthroplasty.* 2002;17(4 Suppl 1):90-93.
20. Ghazavi MT, Stockley I, Yee G, et al. Reconstruction of massive bone defects with allograft in revision total knee arthroplasty. *J Bone Joint Surg Am.* 1997;79:17-25.
21. Figgie HE, Goldberg VM, Heiple KG, et al. The influence of tibial-patellofemoral location on function of the knee in patients with the posterior stabilized condylar knee prosthesis. *J Bone Joint Surg Am.* 1986;68(7):1035-1040.
22. Stiehl JB, Abbott BD. Morphology of the transepicondylar axis and its application in primary and revision total knee arthroplasty. *J Arthroplasty.* 1995;10(6):785-789.
23. Lonner JH, Mont MA, Sharkey PF, et al. Fate of the unrevised all-polyethylene patellar component in revision total knee arthroplasty. *J Bone Joint Surg. Am.* 2003;85:56-59.

23

# Total Knee Arthroplasty Rehabilitation

*Catherine J. Fedorka, MD; Katie O'Shea, PT, DPT, MBA; Kristen Vogl, PT, DPT; and Kristen Huber, PT, MSPT*

Total knee arthroplasty (TKA) requires a well-designed rehabilitation program in order to achieve a rapid and complete recovery. A successful rehabilitation program requires cooperation of the orthopedic surgeon, the physical therapist, the occupational therapist, the case manager/social worker, the nurse, and the pain management team. The rehabilitation program begins with a preoperative evaluation and continues, on average, 6 months to 1 year postoperatively.

## Preoperative Care

Many rehabilitation programs today begin preoperatively as the surgeon and the therapists prepare the patient for surgery. Many physical therapists meet with the patient for at least one session preoperatively to teach him or her the exercises that will be preformed after the surgery and to instruct him or her on the proper use of assistive devices used for ambulation. Some physical therapists may also review transfers with the patient, such as from a bed to a chair, bathroom, and/or tub transfers. As a result of early instruction, some patients are able to achieve independence in activities of daily living (ADL) in a shorter amount of time than if they were to learn all of these activities postoperatively.[1]

## Postoperative Rehabilitation Program: Overview

The main goals of postoperative rehabilitation for patients undergoing a TKA are four-fold. The first focus of the program is to restore mobility, strength, and flexibility of the knee joint. Secondly, rehabilitation should focus on preventing complications such as infection, deep vein thrombosis (DVT), pulmonary embolism (PE), contractures, and to help reduce pain and swelling. Thirdly, therapy should also include restoration to independence in functional mobility and ADL such as getting in and out of a bed, up and down from chairs, transferring into or out of a car, and also climbing stairs. Finally, therapy should focus on teaching adherence to range of motion and also weight-bearing precautions. Although most rehab programs are designed to meet these goals, there have not been many clear randomized controlled trials on the most effective rehabilitation protocols. Therefore, the following chapter will focus on the most commonly used protocols and will incorporate those used at Thomas Jefferson University Hospital.

Rehabilitation programs are influenced by many variables. The therapist must take into account the patient's age, living situation, comorbid conditions, and level of function prior to TKA. Jones et al argued that patients who



Parvizi J, Klatt B.
*Essentials in Total Knee Arthroplasty* (pp 201-208).

demonstrated decreased levels of preoperative function will likely need further rehab than the acute care setting can provide.[2] Decreased preoperative function was defined as decreased joint function, decreased walking distance, and the use of an assistive device prior to TKA.[2] The techniques used by the surgeon in the operating room also affect the therapist's plan of care postoperatively. Type of fixation, type of bone cuts, and soft tissue balancing are all variables that will affect weight-bearing status. Patellar resurfacing may also increase anterior knee pain and joint effusion for several weeks following surgery, which may affect the patient's ability to participate in therapy sessions. In addition to the pain, which may limit progression, increased edema will decrease ROM and may impair recovery of gait. Finally, the extent of preoperative malalignment will influence which muscle groups will need to be focused on during rehab in order to achieve biomechanical balance and full function of the joint postoperatively.[3]

Many rehabilitation programs are broken down into 3 phases. Phase I extends from immediately postoperative until the patient is discharged from the acute care setting. Phase II is broken down into 2 subphases: IIa and IIb. Phase IIa includes patients who are unable to be discharged home secondary to medical and/or safety concerns and are therefore transferred to an inpatient rehab facility, extended care facility (ECF), or skilled nursing facility (SNF). Phase IIb refers to the time patients are homebound due to their decreased mobility and require home physical therapy. Phase III begins when the patient is no longer homebound and can attend outpatient physical therapy. This phase continues until the patient achieves his or her previous level of function or established therapy goals and/or his or her insurance no longer covers therapy.

## Phase I: Inpatient Acute Care

Goals of therapy during the acute care stay are directed at reducing medical complications, reducing pain and swelling, promoting range of motion, increasing quadriceps strength, and restoring safety and independence with functional mobility. In addition, therapists instruct on proper ambulation techniques as well as ADL to promote functional independence in the home environment. By the end of the acute care hospitalization, the patient will have achieved an independent level of function and will be able to safely return home alone or with family/friends.

### Medical Complications

The prevention and management of medical complications such as infection, DVT, PE, and joint contractures will be covered in Chapter 11. Rehabilitation contributes to the prevention of these complications. Early mobilization of the patient and many of the exercises performed during therapy reduce the risk of a DVT, PE, and also joint contractures.

### Pain Management

Anesthetic techniques and perioperative pain management play an integral role in recovery for patients undergoing a TKA. Uncontrolled pain can complicate the recovery. Management of pain has improved in recent times with the evolution of technology in analgesia. For example, regional anesthesia allows for less postoperative pain, nausea, and sedation, which enable the patient to begin participation in intense rehabilitation sooner. In addition, the advent of indwelling nerve sheath catheters with continuous nerve block analgesia, known as an epidural, have been particularly effective in reducing the early postoperative pain patients experience. This also allows the patient to participate in rehabilitation sessions earlier, which should help the patient achieve functional independence sooner.[3] However, therapists commonly will have to contend with altered cognitive status secondary to the side effects of strong-acting analgesics. Thorough cognitive screens and coordination of medication with the nurse can help to reduce these common side effects.

New anesthetic regimens being studied are aimed at decreasing anesthetic and narcotic side effects, allowing for accelerated short-term recoveries. Peters et al[4] studied a new multimodal regimen that involved the use of scheduled oral narcotics instead of IV narcotics, cyclooxygenase-2 inhibitors, femoral nerve catheters rather than intrathecal catheters, and local anesthetic wound infiltration. Early patient mobilization and physical therapy were started the same day as surgery as part of this protocol. Peters et al compared a group of 50 patients who underwent TKA using either the new multimodal protocol or the traditional anesthetic regimens that use general anesthesia, intrathecal nerve catheters, and IV narcotics.[4] They discovered that patients who underwent TKA using the newer multimodal regimen had improved rest pain postoperative days 1 and 2 and decreased total narcotic consumption. These patients also walked further on postoperative days 1 and 2 and had a shorter length of stay than the traditional regimen patients.[4]

### Weight-Bearing Status

The effect of weight-bearing status on the success of TKA rehabilitation has not been well documented in the literature. Therefore, the decision to limit weight bearing on the knee joint is ultimately the individual surgeon's decision. Most implants used today are cemented, and full weight bearing is usually well tolerated. However, there are a few indications for limited weight-bearing status on the knee joint such as concomitant osteotomies, structural bone grafting, and/or severe osteoporosis.[1] However, most rehabilitation programs promote weight bearing as tolerated in order to accelerate therapy. Therefore, it is of the utmost importance for the surgeon to indicate a specific weight-bearing status postoperatively to allow the therapist to plan the rehab program accordingly.

## Range of Motion

All TKA rehabilitation programs focus on achieving the degrees of knee range of motion required for daily activities. In general, one needs at least 65 degrees in flexion for the swing phase of gait, 90 degrees of flexion for daily activities (ie, transfers, lower body dressing, and stair negotiation), and 105 degrees of flexion to rise from a low chair/surface.[3] Multiple modalities are used to achieve adequate range of motion for TKA patients, including continuous passive motion (CPM) machines, neuromuscular electrical stimulation (NMES), and multiple exercises that focus on gaining quadriceps strength while also increasing knee range of motion.

Continuous passive motion machines have been a topic of controversy in the literature. Multiple studies have been performed on patients undergoing a TKA and the benefits of CPM machines, but the results are contradictory. Earlier studies demonstrated that the CPM machines help to achieve greater degrees of knee flexion earlier, may decrease the length of the inpatient stay, and may also decrease the need for manipulations.[3] However, more recent studies have demonstrated that CPM machines add no benefit to physical therapy in the short term.[5,6] Moreover, the literature has demonstrated that CPM does not add any long-term benefit and has been shown to help patients achieve the same functional ability at 6 months as patients who did not use CPM.[3]

The literature has demonstrated both benefits and disadvantages to CPM. Benefits include the ability to aid in wound healing and accelerate clearance of hemarthrosis. CPM also decreases adhesion formation and may help decrease the risk for DVT formation, although the literature is controversial on this issue.[4] There are multiple disadvantages to CPM. The patient must remain in bed while the machine is being used. This is in direct opposition to the early mobilization of the patient. More importantly, the studies that have demonstrated earlier gains in range of motion required up to 20 hours of use for the CPM machines, which is nearly impossible and definitely not realistic. Another disadvantage is that CPM requires additional staff to both teach the hospital staff how to use the machines and also to help with the machine's maintenance. CPM does not focus on knee extension, and those who rely only on the machine can get a flexion contracture. Finally, CPM machines are an expensive modality, therefore the cost:benefit ratio must be questioned.[7]

Current research indicates that CPM machines convey little benefit to TKA rehabilitation. Denis et al studied a group of 81 patients who underwent either conventional physical therapy alone, conventional physical therapy plus 35 minutes of CPM daily, or conventional physical therapy plus 2 hours of CPM daily.[5] No difference in AROM in knee flexion at discharge or length of stay was demonstrated between the 3 groups.[5] Leach et al did a similar study of 85 TKA patients and found that short-duration CPM does not influence range of motion or reported pain postoperatively.[6] These results do not support the use of CPM machines in addition to conventional physical therapy as it adds no benefit to the patient's recovery. Many institutions are discontinuing the use of CPM machines in postoperative TKA rehabilitation protocols.

Beaupre et al believed that a sliding board would produce the same results as a CPM machine at a much lower cost and hassle to patients.[8] A sliding board consists of a moveable heel cup that is fixed to a low friction sliding mechanism that allows the patient to actively flex and extend his or her leg with minimal active use of the quadriceps femoris and hamstring muscles. Beaupre et al proposed that the main benefit of using the sliding board is that patients can use it in either a supine or sitting position. In addition, the sliding board requires no maintenance and minimal, if any, nursing support. However, in their randomized control study of 120 patients, the research discovered there was no difference between using the sliding board in conjunction with standard exercises, using CPM machines with standard exercises, or using standard exercises alone. Beaupre et al therefore argued that neither CPM nor sliding board use is required in the standard rehabilitation programs of TKA patients, as patients will achieve the same functional status at 6 months regardless of their use.[8]

## Rehabilitation Exercises

The most important aspect of a rehabilitation program involves exercises designed to help patients regain the proper balance of range of motion and strength in the lower extremities. This will enable patients to participate in community and functional activities in addition to ADL. These exercises are either taught preoperatively or at the patient's bedside. If they are taught preoperatively, patients may begin some of the exercises, such as ankle range of motion, as soon as they are conscious postoperatively.[7] The ankle range of motion exercises, specifically pumping actions and circumduction, help engage the muscle, decrease edema, and avoid formation of a DVT.[7] Additional exercises that make up the core of the inpatient acute care physical therapy program include isometric gluteal sets, hamstring sets, quadriceps sets, heel slides, short-arc quads, long-arc quads, and straight leg raises. The patients should be instructed on how to properly perform quadriceps sets, gluteal sets, and ankle pumps on postoperative day 1. Patients should be encouraged to perform 10 repetitions of each exercise every hour and eventually progress to 20 repetitions 3 times a day.[7] The active assisted range of motion (AAROM) exercises (ie, heel slides, short-arc quads, long-arc quads) are therapist assisted during therapy sessions to help improve mobility and strength. The last stage of acute therapy should include straight leg raises and terminal knee extensions to further strengthen the dynamic stabilizing muscles of the knee.[8] At the time of discharge, the patient should be completing exercises independently.

## Gait Restoration

Acute care rehabilitation has one more very important goal before the patient can safely be discharged home, which is restoration of his or her gait. Postoperatively, many patients will ambulate with a shortened gait, half strides, or on tip toe. Antalgic gait patterns are not beneficial to healing and should be avoided by verbally cueing the patient to strike on the heel and roll over onto the ball of the foot with each step.[9] Walking in front of a full-length mirror may help the patient to develop a normal gait pattern. Asymmetrical joint loading forces may affect the fusion of the prosthesis. If the patient exhibits a stiff gait, the therapist may instruct the patient to exaggerate knee flexion and extension while walking. This may help the patient become more aware of the appropriate motions of the knee joint during the gait cycle.[3] Having the patient complete the previously described therapeutic exercises will allow the soft tissue to warm up and reach its elongated position with increased ease.

The physical therapist must also assist the patient in learning how to ambulate with an assistive device such as a walker, cane, or crutches. The physical therapist must evaluate the upper body strength and balance of the patient to identify which assistive device is best suited for each individual patient. Many patients will begin therapy with a walker and advance to crutches as they become more comfortable ambulating. Physical therapists instruct each patient on proper ambulation techniques over level surfaces, ramps, and stairs utilizing an assistive device.[7] Phase IIa and IIb will address progression of assistive devices.

## Occupational Therapy in Acute Care

Helping patients to safely and independently complete their ADL is an important aspect of therapy, as patients cannot safely return home until they are able to demonstrate independence in these activities. Activities such as dressing, bathing, reaching, and picking up items should be practiced during rehabilitation sessions. Usually, this falls under the instruction of the occupational therapist who has the responsibility of ensuring that the patient is able to safely move and function in his or her home environment.[7]

## Discharge Criteria

Discharge criteria from the acute care facility may vary slightly from hospital to hospital. The average length of stay in the acute care setting is 1 to 3 days with physical therapy sessions twice a day. First and foremost, the patient must be medically stable for discharge either to his or her home environment or to a rehabilitation facility. In order to be discharged home, the patient must be able to demonstrate 80 to 90 degrees AROM of knee flexion, ambulate 75 to 100 feet independently or with supervision from family members, and be able to independently or with supervision ascend and descend stairs. The patient must also be able to independently transfer from supine to sitting and sitting to standing positions. If the patient cannot perform these tasks or is not able to care for him- or herself at home for medical reasons, he or she must then be transferred to an extended care facility.[7] In cases in which the patient is medically stable, requires physical assistance, and has family members available, the family will be brought into the acute physical therapy/occupational therapy sessions to complete training. The goal is for the family member to be able to safely provide the patient with physical assistance with various functional activities. The rehabilitation protocol for the acute care stay including discharge criteria at our institution is included in Table 23-1.

# PHASE IIA: INPATIENT EXTENDED CARE OR SKILLED NURSING FACILITY

The goals of rehabilitation in the inpatient rehab, an ECF, or a SNF are similar to those for the acute care rehabilitation setting. The facilities allow for increased time for the patient to achieve these goals. The literature has demonstrated that the earlier the transfer from the acute care setting to the rehabilitation facility the better the outcome. Munin et al performed a randomized control trial of 86 high-risk TKA and total hip arthroplasty (THA)

Table 23-1

**THOMAS JEFFERSON UNIVERSITY TOTAL KNEE ARTHROPLASTY PROTOCOL**

*GENERAL INFORMATION*

- Physician must document
  - PT/OT orders
  - Activity orders
    - Activity as tolerated
    - OOB with assistance
  - Weight-bearing status
  - Brace orders if needed
  - CPM machines
    - Should not be used during sleep
- PT will evaluate patient POD 0 for exercise and ambulation
- OT will evaluate and treat patients targeted for home discharge
  - Will teach ADL
  - Patients going to rehab facilities will receive OT services at rehab facility
- PT/OT should document in medical record each time mobility or exercises are performed with the patient on any given POD
  - PT will document AROM and PROM
- A pillow or towel may be placed distal to the knee and proximal to calcaneus to promote complete knee extension and heel pressure relief for patients unable to actively reposition their lower extremities

*POD 0*

- PT evaluation at bedside
- Goals
  - Ambulation with walker
  - OOB to chair with PT or nursing staff
  - Initiation of knee ROM and exercises including:
    - Quad sets
    - Ankle pumps
    - Straight leg raises
    - Short arc quads
    - Heel slides
    - Sitting active knee flexion and extension
- If patient has an epidural, PT/OT must check thoroughly for adequate strength/sensation in both lower extremities prior to initiating transfer OOB
- Therapist should document BP and HR response to initial sitting, standing, and ambulation in the medical record

*POD 1 TO DISCHARGE*

- Patients seen 2 times per day for PT sessions
  - Patients start in gym PM of POD 1 after epidural removal
  - Patients who had Depodur may be able to attend gym AM of POD 1
  - Patients must be able to tolerate at least 1 hr of OOB and have appropriate vital sign responses to attend gym
  - If cannot travel to gym, patients will receive therapy at bedside twice a day
- Treatment focuses
  - Bed mobility
  - Transfer
  - Ambulation
  - ADL/home activities
  - ROM and HEP until
    - Independence achieved
    - Assistance is secured at home
    - Rehab transfer occurs

*POD 1 TO DISCHARGE*

- For D/C planning to home, anticipated date is POD 1
- If D/C plan is to rehab facility, anticipated date is POD 1
- D/C plan should be confirmed with team and patient on POD 1
  - If initial D/C plan is changed due to patient performance in therapy, the therapist will notify case management, social worker, and surgeon
  - If patients length of stay is increased due to medical issues, PT/OT will continue to asses patient for appropriate D/C plan
- All TKA patients receive home PT referral with eventual transition to outpatient PT once staples are removed
- PT will issue appropriate assistive device to patient
- OT will issue appropriate adaptive equipment
- Case management will order commodes as appropriate and set up home care referrals
- TKA patients can travel home via car provided they are able to perform car transfer, if not Case Management will make other arrangements.

POD = postoperative day; PT = physical therapy; OT = occupational therapy; OOB = out of bed; CPM = continuous passive motion; ADL = activities of daily living; AROM = active range of motion; PROM = passive range of motion; ROM = range of motion; BP = blood pressure; HR = heart rate; PM = post meridiem (afternoon); AM = ante meridiem (morning); HEP = home exercise program; D/C = discharge; TKA = total knee arthroplasty

patients at the University of Pittsburgh.[11] The researchers discovered that patients who entered the rehabilitation facility at postoperative day 3 compared to postoperative day 7 had a shorter overall length of stay, had faster attainment of short-term functional milestones, and had an equivalent functional outcome at the 4-month follow-up visit. Munin et al hypothesized that the increased number of therapy sessions attended per day for the group who entered the rehabilitation facility at postoperative day 3 was responsible for the earlier achievement of functional milestones.[11] The therapy sessions during a patient's stay in a rehab facility include the same exercises and modalities as the acute care sessions. The patient will be discharged home once he or she meets the same discharge criteria listed in the acute rehab section. However, sometimes it becomes necessary to begin to train family members and/or care takers to enable the patient to be safely discharged to home.[7] Elderly patients, patients with high anxiety, and patients with several comorbidities commonly fill the beds at these facilities.

## Phase IIb: Outpatient Home Therapy

Most patients are discharged home from the acute care setting by postoperative day 3 or postoperative days 7 to 14 if they require additional care in a rehabilitation facility. Regardless of the discharge disposition, once the patient is home, he or she should receive home therapy sessions 2 to 3 times per week for an average of 2 weeks. The goals of the home therapy sessions are to help the patient become safe in his or her home environment with transfers, gait, and ADL, and to begin community reintegration. The therapist is also responsible for assessing the patient's home for safety and making recommendations to improve conditions as necessary.

During this period of time, the physical therapist must also focus on further improvement of the patient's strength and range of motion. Patients are assisted on more progressive AAROM and functional strengthening exercises, specifically closed chain concentric exercises. These exercises are believed to limit anterior tibial displacement while strengthening the muscles in a more physiologic method.[3] These include bilateral toe raises, sit-to-stand exercises, one-quarter squats, and progressive step ups and step downs. All of these exercises have been shown to be effective in recruiting the vastus lateralis and vastus medialis oblique as compared with open chain exercises.[7] Recruitment of this musculature will enable the patient to ambulate in a more efficient pattern and provide increased control with dynamic activities.

Gait advancement, as indicated by patient progression, can also be done in the home setting. If a patient's balance is improving in cadence and symmetrical line weight bearing, he or she may be able to advance to crutches (bilateral to unilateral) or a cane. Also, the therapist should observe ambulation on uneven, ramped, and outdoor surfaces. Patients are discharged from home physical therapy when they are no longer home bound and can get to an outpatient rehabilitation center, usually after 2 weeks.[7]

## Phase III: Outpatient Care

Outpatient care can begin as early as postoperative week 1 for advanced patients or as late as postoperative week 3 or 4 for less advanced patients. Some advanced protocols call for outpatient therapy to begin on postoperative day 4 to 5. The goals of outpatient rehabilitation are to further increase range of motion of the knee joint; normalize the patient's gait; and to improve weight bearing, strength, endurance, and proprioception. The number of therapy sessions a patient will attend during this period will depend on the his or her progress, compliance, and insurance coverage.

Further improvement in the range of motion of the knee should be an important focus of outpatient therapy. According to Kendall and McCreary, full knee ROM is 0 degrees of extension and approximately 140 degrees of flexion.[12] Routine functional activities such as stair climbing, sitting on a toilet, and stationary bike riding require knee range of motion from 0 to 110 degrees.[7] Many patients will achieve this with the proper rehabilitation program. However, full range of motion may not be a realistic goal for all patients. For example, decreased postoperative range of motion may be evident in patients who had restricted range of motion preoperatively and/or intraoperatively. If motion is limited, manipulation under anesthesia (MUA) may be warranted. MUA is indicated if the patient has less than 70 degrees of flexion at postoperative week 4 or a progressive loss of flexion. Intensive physical therapy after MUA is essential to maintaining the increased motion. Contraindications to MUA include severe osteoporosis or markedly restricted intraoperative range of motion.[7] However, MUA may be avoided when patients are provided with a few extra therapy sessions with a special focus on range of motion exercises to achieve full functionality of the knee joint. Skilled outpatient physical therapists can use manual therapy and joint mobilizations in the clinic to decrease scar tissue and capsular restriction/adhesions to promote normal biomechanical movement.

As the patient regains his or her knee range of motion, the therapist can focus on further improving the patient's strength, weight-bearing capabilities, and endurance. A successful rehabilitation plan must include aerobic conditioning for weight reduction. Extra weight can cause increased forces that may lead to excessive wear on the joint surfaces. Low impact activities such as stationary bicycling, distance walking with proper footwear, and swimming should be encouraged. Some therapists may even include aquatic therapy as part of the outpatient rehabilitation program. The water is buoyant and warm, which can help with pain relief, may help to increase circulation, and decrease weight bearing for the patient. This also allows the patient to work on range of motion, strength, and gait without an assistive device. The patient is also able to increase his or her amount of weight bearing by progressing from shoulder deep water (~24% weight bearing) to waist deep water (~50% weight bearing) as he or she progressively becomes stronger and more independent.[7] All incisions must be fully closed before initiation of an aquatic therapy program, and the patient must be screened to ensure no other contraindications to aquatic therapy are present.

Outpatient rehabilitation should also focus on the patient's proprioception and correct any changes in equilibrium that may have occurred. Some patients may have postural changes as a result of decreased weight bearing on one side, altered gait, and/or pain. Single-leg exercises and mobilizing devices such as rocker boards and half form rollers can help the patient regain his or her balance and proprioception.[7]

The patient's discharge from rehabilitation depends on multiple factors. Some patients will achieve full range of motion and independence in a few months and will be discharged from therapy. However, many patients are discharged before full function of the knee joint is achieved due to insurance reasons. These patients should be instructed to continue the exercises on their own at home in order to achieve full range of motion and strength. They should also follow-up with their physicians who can monitor their progress. Finally, for some patients, full range of motion and strength may never be achieved, and therapy should be ended when further progression cannot be functionally achieved.

## Return to Sports and Activities

Return to low impact and noncontact sports is acceptable. Some of these activities are included in the rehab. Closed chain activities such as biking and elliptical are excellent activities for the patient with a total knee replacement. Implant survival may be negatively impacted by cutting sports and impact. Impact may weaken the bond between cement and bone and lead to early failure. Walking is a safe activity, but running should be discouraged. Doubles tennis is considered an acceptable activity also. Return to jobs and activities that require heavy, repetitive lifting should be discouraged for the same reasons.

## Summary

The ultimate goal of a successful rehabilitation program is to maintain a pain-free functional activity level for as long a period as possible. With a well-designed rehabilitation program, TKA patients should achieve an improvement in function and pain, allowing them to participate in low impact activities and achieve independence.

## References


1. Cameron HU, Brotzman SB, Boolos M. Rehabilitation after total joint arthroplasty. In: Brotzman SB, ed. *Clinical Orthopaedic Rehabilitation.* St. Louis, MO: Mosby, Inc; 1996:302-311.
2. Jones CA, Voklander DC, Suarez-Almazor, ME. Determinants of function after total knee arthroplasty. *Physical Therapy.* 2003;8(83):696-706.
3. Brander V, Stulberg SD. Rehabilitation after hip- and knee-joint replacement: an experience- and evidence-based approach to care. *Am J Phys Med Rehabil.* 2006;85(Suppl):S98-S118.
4. Peters CL, Shirley B, Erickson J. The effect of a new multimodal perioperative anesthetic regimen on postoperative pain, side effects, and length of hospital stay after total joint arthroplasty. *Journal of Arthroplasty.* 2006;21(6):132-138.
5. Denis M, Moffet H, Caron F, Quellet D, Paquet J, Nolet L. Effectiveness of CPM and conventional physical therapy after total knee arthroplasty: a randomized control trial. *Physical Therapy.* 2006;86(2):174-185.
6. Leach W, Reid J, Murphy F. Continuous passive motion following total knee replacement: a prospective randomized trial with one year followup. *Knee Surg Sports Traumatol Arthroscopy.* 2006;14:922-926.
7. Cacanian NP, Wong J, Ries MD. Total knee arthroplasty. In: Maxey L, Magnusson J, eds. *Rehabilitation for the Postsurgical Orthopedic Patient.* 2nd ed. St. Louis, MO: Mosby, Inc; 2007:400-414.
8. Beaupre LA, Davies DM, Jones CA, Cinats JG. Exercise combined with continuous passive motion or slider board therapy compared with exercise only: a randomized control trial of patients following total knee arthroplasty. *Physical Therapy.* 2001;81(4):1029-1037.
9. Petty W. Total knee arthroplasty: postoperative care and rehabilitation. In: Petty W, ed. *Total Joint Replacement.* Philadelphia, PA: WB Saunders Company; 1991:533-539.
10. Hozack W, Clark AD. *Total Knee Arthroplasty Protocol.* Philadelphia, PA: Thomas Jefferson University; 2008.
11. Munin MC, Rudy TE, Glynn NW, Crossett LS, Rubash HE. Early inpatient rehabilitation after elective hip and knee arthroplasty. *JAMA.* 1998;279(11):847-852.
12. Kendall F, McCreary E. *Muscles Testing and Function.* Philadelphia, PA: Lippincott, Williams and Wilkins; 1993.

# Financial Disclosures

Dr. Omar Abdul-Hadi has no financial or proprietary interest in the materials presented herein.

Dr. William V. Arnold is the principal investigator of a study sponsored by Stryker Orthopaedics.

Dr. Matthew S. Austin has a consulting agreement with Zimmer and research funding from DePuy.

Dr. Khalid A. Azzam has not disclosed any relevant financial relationships.

Dr. David Backstein is a consultant for Zimmer and Stryker. He receives no royalties or grants.

Dr. Hany Bedair has no financial or proprietary interest in the materials presented herein.

Dr. Benjamin Bender has not disclosed any relevant financial relationships.

Dr. Jennifer K. Bow has no financial or proprietary interest in the materials presented herein.

Dr. Carl A. Deirmengian is a consultant for Angiotech and Synthes.

Dr. Gregory K. Deirmengian has no financial or proprietary interest in the materials presented herein.

Dr. Craig J. Della Valle has not disclosed any relevant financial relationships.

Dr. Catherine J. Fedorka has no financial or proprietary interest in the materials presented herein.

Dr. Kishor Gandhi has no financial or proprietary interest in the materials presented herein.

Dr. Ashok L. Gowda has not disclosed any relevant financial relationships.

Dr. Nitin Goyal has no financial or proprietary interest in the materials presented herein.

Dr. Eric L. Grossman has no financial or proprietary interest in the materials presented herein.

Dr. Mark A. Hartzband has not disclosed any relevant financial relationships.

Dr. William J. Hozack is a consultant for Stryker Orthopaedics and receives royalties.

Dr. Bruce Hopper has not disclosed any relevant financial relationships.

Kristen Huber has no financial or proprietary interest in the materials presented herein.

Dr. Barry E. Kenneally has no financial or proprietary interest in the materials presented herein.

Dr. Brian Klatt has no financial or proprietary interest in the materials presented herein.



Parvizi J, Klatt B.
*Essentials in Total Knee Arthroplasty* (pp 209-210).

Dr. Gregg R. Klein has no financial or proprietary interest in the materials presented herein.

Dr. Sarah Lombardo has not disclosed any relevant financial relationships.

Dr. Alvin Ong is a consultant for Stryker Orthopedics.

Katie O'Shea has no financial or proprietary interest in the materials presented herein.

Dr. Michael R. Pagnotto has not disclosed any relevant financial relationships.

Dr. Javad Parvizi has no financial or proprietary interest in the materials presented herein.

Dr. Madhavi Pradhan has not disclosed any relevant financial relationships.

Dr. Manny Porat has no financial or proprietary interest in the materials presented herein.

Dr. Zachary Post has no financial or proprietary interest in the materials presented herein.

Dr. Luis Pulido has no financial or proprietary interest in the materials presented herein.

Dr. James J. Purtill has not disclosed any relevant financial relationships.

Dr. Arjun Saxena has not disclosed any relevant financial relationships.

Dr. Eric Schwenk has no financial or proprietary interest in the materials presented herein.

Dr. Peter F. Sharkey is a consultant for Stryker Orthopaedics and receives royalties from Stryker Orthopaedics and Stelkast, Inc.

Dr. Harvey E. Smith has no financial or proprietary interest in the materials presented herein.

Dr. Garen D. Steele has not disclosed any relevant financial relationships.

Dr. Eugene R. Viscusi is a consultant for Cadence, Merck, EKR, Pfizer, Adolor, GSK and receives research support from Merck.

Dr. Peter C. Vitanzo Jr has no financial or proprietary interest in the materials presented herein.

Kristen Vogl has no financial or proprietary interest in the materials presented herein.

Dr. Michael Williamson has not disclosed any relevant financial relationships.

# Index

accidental lateral parapatellar approach, 94–95
ACL (anterior cruciate ligament), 6, 10, 11, 36, 137, 176, 180
active, young patients, TKA in, 179
activities and sports, return to, 207
activity/exercise modification, as alternative to surgery, 24, 25
acupuncture, 26
acute care stay, rehabilitation for, 202–204
alignment instrumentation, 51, 81–85, 86, 111–112, 115–116, 123–124, 133, 152, 181
analgesia, 24, 25, 27, 28–29, 51, 101–107, 202
anatomic approach, 11, 44, 46–47, 81, 83, 85, 109
anatomy, 1–7, 9, 79–80, 81
anesthesia, manipulation under, 97, 133, 146, 149, 206
anesthesia for postoperative pain, 103–104
anesthesia for surgical procedure, 50, 51, 63, 73, 74, 101–102
anterior cruciate ligament (ACL), 6, 10, 11, 36, 137, 176, 180
anteroposterior (flexion instability), 136
antibiotic prophylaxis, 73–74, 96, 122, 131
antibiotic treatment of infection, 132, 163, 164, 194
anticoagulated patients, analgesia for, 102–103
anti-neuropathic analgesics, 105
arterial injuries, intraoperative, 91–92
arthritides
  complex primary TKA, 175, 176, 177, 179, 180, 181
  forms of, 19–22
  history of modern TKA, 51
  indications for TKA, 55, 56–58
  nonoperative treatments, 23–25, 28–29, 56
  patellar resurfacing, 114–115, 134
  patient evaluation, 56, 62, 63
  posterior cruciate ligament retention/substitution, 110, 111
  soft tissue considerations, 57, 137
  surgical alternatives to TKA, 33, 36, 37, 38
arthrofibrosis (knee stiffness), 96–97, 122, 125, 132–133, 168, 194
articular cartilage restoration, 34–35
aseptic loosening, 12, 15, 45, 93, 130–131, 137, 161, 163, 167–174
aspiration of knee joint, 57, 162, 193
assistive devices, 24, 26, 27, 56, 204
autologous chondrocyte transplantation, 34–35
avascular necrosis (AVN), 19, 22

backside wear, 15, 131, 169
bilateral knee arthroplasty, 74, 113–114
biomaterials, 13–15, 48–49
biomechanics, 9–13, 15, 79–80, 81, 96, 109, 111
blood supply, 3–4, 7, 65–66, 95, 141, 194–195
bone defect reconstruction, 50, 57, 143, 157–159, 176, 177, 178, 179, 193, 194, 196
bony architecture/landmarks, 2, 3, 9
buttress plating, 154

cartilage restoration, 34–35
cavitary bone defects, 196
cemented versus noncemented implants, 12, 13, 110, 124, 167–168, 179, 195

Charcot joint (neuropathic arthropathy), 57, 58, 182
chondroitin, 25–26
cobalt-chromium, 13, 15, 47, 48, 49
collateral ligaments, 5–6, 7, 9–10
computer navigation, 51, 83, 115–116, 124, 133
condylar prostheses, evolution of, 46–48
constrained implants, 11, 93, 94, 136, 137, 157, 171, 176, 177, 178, 181, 193
contact stress distribution, 12–13, 49, 137, 169, 170, 171
contraindications to TKA, 57, 58, 68, 114, 182
(COX-2) cyclooxygenase-2 inhibitors, 102, 104, 105
cross-linking polyethylene, 14, 49, 169, 170
cruciate ligaments, 3, 6, 7, 9–10
crystalline arthritis, 20–21
cystic bone defects, 196

débridement, 33, 94, 96, 132, 133, 163–164, 193–194
diabetes, 57, 182, 183
discharge criteria, 204, 205
distal femoral osteotomy, 39, 40, 41, 180, 181
distal femur, anatomy of, 2, 3, 9
dosing for oral opioids/nonopioid analgesics, 105, 106
draping, 75, 76–77
Duocondylar prostheses, 46, 47

epidural analgesia, 102–103
epiphyseal bone defects, 196
examination, physical, 1–2, 62
exercise/activity modification, as alternative to surgery, 24, 25
exercises, in rehabilitation, 203–204, 206, 207
extended care stay, rehabilitation for, 204–205
extensile approach, 69
extension balancing. *See* flexion/extension gap balancing
extensor mechanism deficiency, reconstruction of, 194
extensor mechanism preservation, 68, 71, 116
extensor mechanism rupture, 131
external fixation devices, 154
extra-articular deformity, 175–176, 177, 181, 194
extramedullary guides, 81, 82, 83, 111–112, 124, 181

fat pad, 4–5, 67, 94
female-specific implants, 50, 117, 152
femoral component, in patellofemoral mechanics, 85, 86, 125, 133–134, 136
femoral component, intercondylar opening by manufacturer/model, 156–157
femoral component loosening, 130–131, 136, 194
femoral component, sizing of, 83–85, 89, 96–97, 125, 136, 193, 197, 199
femoral deformity, extra-articular varus/valgus, 175
femoral fractures, periprosthetic, 135, 151, 152, 153, 194
femoral nerve block, 103–104
femoral "notching," 84–85, 135, 151, 152
femoral osteotomy, 39, 40, 41, 152, 176, 180, 181
femoral preparation, surgical principles of, 83–85, 111, 112, 115–116, 123–124, 136, 197, 199
fish oil, 26
fixation, as factor in loosening, 12, 13, 131
fixation, for periprosthetic fractures, 152, 153, 154–157, 158, 159, 194
fixation, in extra-articular varus/valgus deformity, 176
fixation, in osteotomy, 40, 41
fixation, in TKA for young active patients, 179
fixed angle devices, 154
fixed-bearing implants. *See* posterior stabilized implants
flexion instability (anteroposterior), 136, 193
flexion/extension gap balancing
  mechanisms of failure in TKA, 96, 123–124, 135, 136
  revision arthroplasty, 193, 196–197, 198, 199
  surgical principles of TKA, 83, 84, 86, 87, 88, 89, 176, 178
foot bump placement, 75
foot drop (peroneal nerve palsy), 95
fractures, 84, 131, 134–135, 141–149, 151–160, 168, 194
functional approach, 11–12, 44, 47–48

gabapentin, 105
gait restoration, rehabilitation for, 204, 206
gap balancing. *See* flexion/extension gap balancing
gender-specific implants, 50, 117, 152
Geometric prostheses, 48
global instability, 136, 193
glucosamine, 25–26
GUEPAR prostheses, 45, 46
"gull winging," 198

HA (hyaluronic acid), 24, 27–29, 56
hemophilic patients, 182–183
high tibial osteotomy (HTO), 39, 40–41, 179, 180–181
hinged knee prostheses, 44, 45–46, 47, 48, 86, 157, 159, 178, 182, 193
history of modern total knee arthroplasty, 43–53
home therapy, 206
hyaluronic acid (HA), 24, 27–29, 56

IM nails, 153, 155, 176
IM rods, 152, 155
imaging studies. *See* radiographic evaluation
implant removal in revision arthroplasty, 157, 195, 196
incisions. *See* skin incisions
indications for TKA, 51, 55–60
infection
  classification, 161
  complex primary TKA, 175, 178, 182, 183
  as contraindication to TKA, 57, 58
  diagnosis, 96, 131–132, 162, 163, 187, 193
  early failure in primary TKA, 121–123
  following revision arthroplasty, 121, 161, 162, 193–194
  history of modern TKA, 50
  operating room set-up, 74, 75–77, 122
  patient evaluation, 122–123, 129, 130, 131–132, 161–163, 172
  as percentage of failure in TKA, 122, 168
  postoperative wound complications, 95, 96
  revision arthroplasty for, 132, 163, 164, 193–194
  staged bilateral TKA, 113, 132, 163, 164, 194
  treatment, 96, 132, 163–164, 193–194
inpatient acute care, rehabilitation for, 202–204
inpatient extended care, rehabilitation for, 204–205
instability, partial knee replacement for, 36
instability, TKA for. *See* flexion/extension gap balancing
instability after TKA, 111, 122, 123, 135–137, 168, 181, 182, 193
instrumentation for TKA, 51, 81–85, 86, 111–112, 115–116, 123–124, 133, 152, 181
intercondylar opening of femoral component by manufacturer/model, 156–157
intra-articular (IA) steroid injections, 24, 27, 29
intramedullary guides, 81, 83, 111, 112, 124, 152, 181
intravenous patient-controlled analgesia, 105–106

joint fluid aspiration, 57, 162, 193
"joint fluid therapy" (viscosupplementation), 24, 27–29
joint injections, 24, 27, 29
joint line, anatomy of, 12–13, 79–80
joint line restoration, 12–13, 83, 87, 97, 134, 173, 193, 196–197, 198, 199
joint loading, mechanics/kinematics of, 10
joint stability, biomechanics of, 9–10, 11

ketamine, 102–103, 105
kinematics, 10–12, 109, 111, 112, 136
knee brace, 24, 26, 27, 56
knee capsule and surrounding soft tissue, anatomy of, 4–5

laboratory evaluations, 63, 130, 162, 187, 193
lateral closing wedge osteotomy, 39–40, 41
lateral collateral ligament (LCL), 2, 5, 6, 10, 177, 180
lateral parapatellar approach, 2, 68, 94–95
ligamentous laxity, severe, 36, 38, 86, 175, 178, 181
ligaments and tendons, anatomy of, 2, 3, 4, 5–6, 7
local anesthetics, 101–102, 103–104
locked plating, 154–155
loosening
  biomechanics, 12, 13, 15, 130–131
  complex primary TKA, 177, 179, 181, 182
  constrained implants, 93, 137
  contact stress distribution, 12, 49, 137, 169, 170, 171
  early mechanism of failure in TKA, 122, 124
  fixation, 12, 13, 131
  history of modern TKA, 45, 48, 49, 167–168
  infection, 132, 161, 163, 172
  MCL injuries, 93
  mechanical, 12, 112, 113
  patellar fractures, 135, 141, 143, 147–148
  patient evaluation, 130, 163, 172–173
  PCL sparing/substitution/sacrifice, 130, 131, 170–171
  periprosthetic fractures, 135, 153, 154, 159, 161, 194
  polyethylene, production and design of, 15, 131, 169–170
  recurvatum instability, 136
  revision arthroplasty for, 154, 157, 173, 194
  surgical technique, 130, 133, 171–172

lumbar plexus block, 103
lyme arthritis, 21

magnets, 26–27
malalignment following TKA, 81–82, 112, 116, 122, 123–124, 133, 134, 135, 136, 168, 171–172, 194
malpositioning, 116, 181, 194
manipulation under anesthesia, 97, 133, 146, 149, 206
manufacturers/models of intercondylar opening of femoral component, 156–157
medial collateral ligament (MCL), 1, 3, 5, 6, 7, 10, 92–94, 123, 177
medial opening wedge osteotomy, 40, 41
medial parapatellar approach, 2, 50–51, 65, 66–67, 68–69, 71, 116, 146, 147, 175, 195
medial-lateral instability, 136, 175
menisci, anatomy of, 6–7
menisci, radiographic evaluation of, 63
metal allergies, 14, 49
metals, types of, 13–14
metaphyseal sleeves, 50, 157, 158, 196
microfracture, in cartilage restoration, 34
midvastus approach, 67–68, 69, 71, 116
minimally invasive techniques, 2, 50–51, 94, 116
mobile-bearing implants (rotating platform), 36, 48, 50, 112–113
morphine, 101, 102, 103, 105 106
multimodal analgesia, 101–102, 104–105, 202
musculature about the knee
  anatomy of, 5, 80
  biomechanics of, 10

nerves, anatomy of, 2–3, 4
neuraxial analgesia, 101–103
neuropathic arthropathy, 57, 58, 182
neurovascular structures. *See* blood supply
nonopioid analgesics, 101–102, 103, 104–105
nonsurgical alternatives to knee replacement, 23–32, 56, 179
"notching," 84–85, 135, 151, 152
NSAIDs (nonsteroidal anti-inflammatory drugs), 24, 25, 27, 28–29, 104, 105

occupational therapy, 204
one-stage revision arthroplasty, 164, 194
operating room set-up, 73–77, 122
opioids, 101, 102–103, 104, 105–106
oral opioids, 103, 106
osteoarthritis/osteoarthrosis, 19, 23–25, 28–29, 55, 62, 114–115, 175, 176, 179, 181
osteochondral mosaicplasty, 35
osteotomy, 38–41, 69, 70, 152, 175, 176, 177, 179–181
Outerbridge classification, 34
outpatient care, 206–207
"overstuffing" of the patellofemoral joint, 84, 97, 125, 194, 197

pain management, 24, 25, 27, 28–29, 51, 101–107, 202
partial knee replacement, 35–38
patella, eversion of, 50, 67, 68, 94, 95, 116, 146–147, 180, 195
patella, resurfacing/nonresurfacing of, 114–115, 125, 134, 197–198
patella tendon rupture, 94, 95, 97
patella turndown, 69, 70
patellar clunk syndrome, 134
patellar component, in patellofemoral mechanics, 85, 125, 134
patellar component, in revision arthroplasty, 197–198, 199
patellar component loosening, 130, 135, 141, 143, 147–148
patellar fractures following TKA, 131, 134–135, 141–149, 168, 194
patellectomies, TKA following, 181–182
patellofemoral arthroplasty, 37–38
patellofemoral joint, "overstuffing" of, 84, 97, 125, 194, 197
patellofemoral mechanics, 11, 80, 81, 82, 84, 85–86, 94, 97
patellofemoral problems after TKA, 115, 122, 125, 133–135
patient education, 24–25, 63
patient history, 61–62
patient set-up on operating table, 74–75
patient-completed survey for revision surgery, 188–192
patient-controlled analgesia (PCA), 103, 105–106

PCL. *See* posterior cruciate ligament (PCL)
perioperative care, 63
peripheral nerve blocks, 103–104
periprosthetic fractures, 135, 151–160, 168, 194
peroneal nerve palsy (foot drop), 95
physical examination, 1–2, 62
physical therapy. *See* rehabilitation
pie-crusting technique, for valgus deformities, 2, 178
PMMA (polymethylmethacrylate) bone cement, 15, 46, 176
polyethylene
  contact stress distribution, 12, 169, 170, 171
  history of modern TKA, 46, 47, 48–49
  mobile-bearing implants, 112, 113
  production and design, 14, 15, 48–49, 131, 169–170
  revision arthroplasty, 193
  sterilization, 14, 131, 169–170
  varus deformity, 177
  wear/osteolysis, 12, 15, 130–131, 167–171, 179, 193
polymethylmethacrylate (PMMA) bone cement, 15, 46, 176
posterior aspect, anatomy of, 3, 7
posterior cruciate ligament (PCL)
  anatomy, 3, 6, 7
  arterial injuries, 92
  aseptic loosening, 130, 131, 170–171
  biomechanics, 10, 11–12, 109, 111
  complex primary TKA, 176–177, 180, 182
  history of modern TKA, 47
  mechanisms of failure in TKA, 133, 137, 182
  sparing/sacrificing/substituting controversy, 11–12, 109–112, 170–171, 182
posterior stabilized implants, 36, 44, 48, 93, 109, 110, 112–113, 134, 170–171, 172, 176, 177, 180, 197
postoperative analgesia options, 101–107
pregabalin, 105
preoperative care, rehabilitation for, 201
preoperative planning, 73, 122, 131, 181, 193–194
preoperative testing, 63, 130, 162, 187, 193
proprioception, 12, 110, 111, 207
psoriatic arthritis, 22

"Q" angle, 11, 50, 80, 85–86, 117
quadriceps snip, 69, 94, 95
quadriceps-sparing approach, 50, 68, 71, 116

radiographic evaluation for patient with failed TKA, 130
radiographic evaluation prior to TKA, 56, 62–63, 73
range of motion, rehabilitation for, 203, 206
recurvatum instability, 87, 111, 136, 193
rehabilitation
  as alternative to knee replacement, 24, 25
  arthrofibrosis (knee stiffness), 97, 125, 132–133
  history of modern TKA, 51
  indications for TKA, 57, 58
  minimally invasive techniques, 116
  overview, 201–202
  periprosthetic fractures, 151, 159
  phases of, 202–207
  postoperative pain, 101, 202
  staged bilateral TKA, 113
resurfacing versus nonresurfacing of patella, 114–115, 125, 134, 197–198
revision arthroplasty
  for arthrofibrosis (knee stiffness), 125, 133, 194
  extensile approach, 69
  fixed-bearing versus mobile-bearing knee replacements, 113
  history of modern TKA, 51
  infection, 121, 132, 161, 162, 163, 164, 193–194
  for instability, 111, 122, 135–137, 193
  for loosening, 154, 157, 173, 194
  for malalignment/malpositioning, 194
  patella tendon rupture, 94
  patellofemoral problems, 125
  PCL-sparing/substitution/sacrifice controversy, 110, 111, 130–131
  for periprosthetic fractures, 154, 157–159, 194
  preoperative evaluation/indications for, 130, 187–193
  preoperative planning, 193–194
  rates of, 121, 122, 187
  severe bone loss/ligamentous insufficiency, 178
  surgical technique, 194–199
  types of implants, 196
rheumatoid arthritis, 20, 111, 115, 179
rotating platform TKA design, 48, 112–113, 171
rotational instability following TKA, 136
rotational landmarks of the femur, 84

sciatic nerve block, 104
segmental bone defects, 196
selective patellar resurfacing, 115
septic arthritis, 21
serologic tests, 162, 187, 193
simultaneous bilateral versus staged bilateral TKA, 113–114
single-stage revision arthroplasty, 164, 194
sizing of components, 12, 82, 83–85, 89, 96–97, 117, 123, 125, 136, 193, 197, 198, 199
skin incisions
  accidental lateral parapatellar approach, 94–95
  anatomy, 2, 3
  complex primary TKA, 175, 180
  history of modern TKA, 50–51
  infections, 122
  minimally invasive techniques, 116
  patella fracture following TKA, 143
  patient set-up on operating table, 74, 76, 77
  revision arthroplasty, 194–195
  surgical approaches, 65–66, 67, 68
skin necrosis, 95–96
skin preparation for surgery, 75–76
SLE (systemic lupus erythematosus) arthritis, 20
slide approach/tibial tubercle osteotomy, 69, 70
soft tissue, anatomy of, 4–5, 80
soft tissue balancing
  as indicator for TKA, 57, 58
  in complex primary TKA, 86, 175, 176, 177, 178, 180
  PCL retention/sacrifice for, 111, 176–177
  surgical principles of, 83, 86–87, 88, 89, 123, 176, 177, 180
spinal analgesia, 101–102
sports and activities, return to, 207
stability, biomechanics of, 9–10, 11
staged bilateral versus simultaneous bilateral TKA, 113–114, 132, 163, 164, 194
stemmed components, fixation around, 157
Steri-Drape (U-drape), 75, 76
sterilization of polyethylene, 14, 131, 169–170
steroid injections, 24, 27, 29
stiffness (arthrofibrosis), 96–97, 122, 125, 132–133, 168, 194
subvastus approach, 50–51, 68, 69, 71
superficial infections, 96, 132
supplements, 24, 25–26, 159
supracondylar femoral fractures, 84, 135, 151, 153
surgical alternatives to TKA, 33–42
surgical approaches to TKA, 65–71
surgical instrumentation for TKA, 51, 81–85, 86, 111–112, 115–116, 123–124, 133, 152, 181
surgical management of periprosthetic fractures, 154, 194
surgical principles of TKA, 79–89
surgical techniques, evolution of, 50–51
surgical techniques for partial knee replacement, 36, 37
surgical techniques for patella fracture, 143–146, 147
surgical techniques, in aseptic loosening, 130, 133, 171–172
surgical techniques, in early failure of TKA, 121, 122, 123–124, 125
synovectomy, 195
systemic lupus erythematosus (SLE) arthritis, 20
systemic medications, as alternative to surgery, 24, 27

tantalum, 14, 49, 147, 148, 198
tendons and ligaments, anatomy of, 2, 3, 4, 5–6, 7
testing, laboratory, 63, 130, 162, 187, 193
Thomas Jefferson University total knee arthroplasty protocol, 205
tibial component, in patellofemoral mechanics, 85–86, 97, 125, 133–134, 136
tibial component loosening, 12, 130, 131, 170–171
tibial component, sizing of, 12, 82, 83, 89
tibial deformity, complex primary TKA for, 175
tibial fractures, in osteotomies, 41
tibial fractures, periprosthetic, 152, 159, 194
tibial osteotomy, 39–41, 69, 70, 152, 176, 177, 179, 180–181
tibial plateau, anatomy of, 6, 7
tibial preparation, surgical principles of, 81–82, 83, 89, 97, 111–112, 115–116, 123–124, 130, 136, 197, 198
tibial tubercle osteotomy/slide approach, 69, 70
tibiofemoral kinematics, 10–11
timeline for the development of modern total knee arthroplasty, 44
titanium, 13–14, 15
topical therapy, 24, 25

tourniquets, 74, 75, 76, 91, 92
two-stage revision arthroplasty, 132, 163, 164, 194

U-drape placement, 75
UHMWPE. *See* polyethylene
unicondylar knee arthroplasty (UKA), 35–37, 38, 62, 179
unicondylar prostheses, 46, 47
unloading knee brace, 26, 27, 56

varus/valgus deformities
- anatomy, 1–3, 5, 6
- history of modern TKA, 45
- nonsurgical alternatives, 26
- physical examination, 1–2, 62
- preoperative planning, 73
- surgical alternatives to TKA, 36, 38, 39–40
- surgical principles of TKA
  - complex primary TKA, 86–87, 175–178, 179–181
  - instability, 86–87, 123, 136, 175, 176, 177–178
  - intramedullary versus extramedullary guides, 81, 111–112
  - lateral parapatellar approach, 68
  - medial collateral ligament rupture, 93
  - mobile-bearing implants, 113
  - PCL-sparing/substitution/sacrifice controversy, 110, 111
  - postoperative foot drop, 95
  - tibial preparation, 81, 82

vastus-splitting approach, 67–68, 69, 71, 116
viral causes of joint pain, 21
viscosupplementation (or "joint fluid therapy"), 24, 27–29

wear/osteolysis, 12, 15, 122, 124, 130–131, 167–171, 172, 179, 193
weight loss, 23–25, 123, 206
weight-bearing status, in rehabilitation, 159, 202–203, 206, 207
wound complications after TKA, 95–96

young active patients, TKA for, 23, 51, 56–57, 58, 94, 96, 114, 179, 181

zirconium, 14, 49